Essentials of Long-Term Care Administration

Edited by

Seth B. Goldsmith, ScD, JD
University of Massachusetts
Amherst, Massachusetts

AN ASPEN PUBLICATION®
Aspen Publishers, Inc.
Gaithersburg, Maryland
1994

Library of Congress Cataloging-in-Publication Data

Essentials of long-term care administration/ (edited by) Seth B.
Goldsmith.
p. cm.
Includes bibliographical references and index.
ISBN: 0-8342-0567-X
1. Long-term care facilities—Administration.   2. Long-term care
facilities—Administration—Case studies.   3. Nursing homes—
Administration.   4. Nursing homes—Administration—Case studies.
I. Goldsmith, Seth B.
[DNLM: 1. Long-Term Care—in old age.   2. Long-Term Care—
organization & administration.   3. Nursing Homes—organization &
administration—United States.   4. Homes for the Aged—organization
& administration.   WT 30 E785 1994]
RA999.A35E87 1994
362.1'6'068—dc20
DNLM/DLC
for Library of Congress
94-13567
CIP

Editorial Resources: Jane Colilla
Library of Congress Catalog Card Number: 94-13567
ISBN: 0-8342-0567-X

Printed in the United States of America

1   2   3   4   5

Table of Contents

About the Editor/Contributor

Seth B. Goldsmith, Sc.D., J.D., editor of this book and author of a number of its chapters and cases, is presently Professor of Health Policy and Management at the School of Public Health of the University of Massachusetts at Amherst. Additionally, Dr. Goldsmith is editor of *The Journal of Ambulatory Care Management* and Counsel to the law firm of Bowditch and Dewey in Worcester, Massachusetts. Professor Goldsmith's involvement in long-term care has included teaching both graduate and continuing education courses in long-term care, membership on the New York State Board of Examiners for Nursing Home Administrators, consulting to nursing homes as well as board level appointments to various organizations including membership in the House of Delegates of the American Association of Homes for the Aging, The Association of Massachusetts Homes for the Aging, and the Jewish Nursing Home of Western Massachusetts. In 1990, Dr. Goldsmith's book, *Choosing a Nursing Home,* published by Prentice Hall, was selected as a Book of the Year by *Library Journal.* Additionally, in 1991, the American Association of Homes for the Aging honored Dr. Goldsmith with its Chairman's Citation.

About the Contributors

Roberta A. Bergman is a teacher who lives in Longmeadow, Massachusetts.

Howard L. Braverman, M.H.A., L.N.H.A., is president and CEO of Jewish Nursing Home of Western Massachusetts and its parent holding company, Jewish Geriatric Services, Inc., both in Longmeadow, Massachusetts. He has 18 years experience in senior management positions in the acute and long-term care industries and is active in professional and community organizations.

James N. Broder is an attorney with the Portland, Maine, law firm of Curtis Thaxter Stevens Broder & Micoleau. A former two-term member of the Federal Council on Aging, his national law practice focuses on the representation of nonprofit and proprietary developers and providers of a wide range of residential and long-term care services.

Marian C. Broder, J.D., an attorney, is a consultant to nursing homes on federal and state regulations regarding long-term care. She serves on the adjunct faculty of Western New England College School of Law. She is currently chairperson of the board of the Jewish Nursing Home of Western Massachusetts and has chaired its ethics committee for four years.

Janet Courtney, R.N., M.S.N., is a professor of nursing at Holyoke Community in Holyoke, Massachusetts. In this position, she plans and supervises classroom and clinical learning experiences in care of elderly nursing home residents for nursing students who are preparing for registered nurse practice. She has presented lectures at local and national conferences related to the teaching of geriatric nursing theory and skills as part of an integrated nursing curriculum.

Joan Marie Culley, R.N, M.S., M.P.H., is an associate professor of nursing and coordinator of the Nursing Career Pathway Program at Holyoke Community College in Holyoke, Massachusetts. She is a consultant to hospitals and other health care organizations regarding the teaching of "critical thinking" skills in nursing, and the development of programs for nontraditional learners, and has presented papers on these topics at local and national conferences. She has over 23 years of experience in nursing both as a nursing instructor and practicing clinician. Her specialties include medical/surgical nursing, nursing administration, and public health.

Marvin A. Goldberg, M.S.W., is executive director of the Jewish Home for the Aged in Worcester, Massachusetts.

Solomon Goldner, M.B.A., M.P.H., is vice president and chief financial officer of Golden State Health Centers, Inc., a multi-facility chain of skilled nursing facilities in Sherman Oaks, California. He was formerly with Coopers and Lybrand and National Medical Enterprises', Hillhaven Division. His degrees in accounting and public health are both from Columbia University.

Anne K. Harrington, Ph.D., is an independent consultant, writer, and gerontologist working in the Boston area. She writes, edits, and produces two publications on aging (one of which she co-founded in 1989) and consults on industry trends, strategic planning, public policy, and communications.

H. Ralph Hawkins, A.I.A., M.P.H., is executive vice president of HKS, Inc., an architectural, planning, and engineering firm specializing in the design of health care facilities. In this position, Mr. Hawkins has worked for more than 17 years in over 35 states designing and planning health care facilities from tertiary medical centers to long-term facilities.

Lorrie A. Higgins, B.A., is director of human resources for the Jewish Nursing Home of Western Massachusetts in Longmeadow, Massachusetts.

Richard S. Lamden, B.B.A., is executive vice president of Handmaker Jewish Services for the Aging, Inc., in Tucson, Arizona, a nonprofit, nonsectarian long-term care organization. He is also the president/CEO of Handmaker Management Enterprises, Inc., a for-profit subsidiary specializing in consultation and management services to long-term care facilities and housing. He is a former officer of the American Association of Homes for the Aging.

Steven A. Levenson, M.D., is the medical director of Asbury Methodist Village in Gaithersburg, Maryland. He has been a long-term care physician full time since 1978, and medical director since 1982. He has written over 30 articles, book chapters, and monographs in the areas of geriatrics, medical ethics, medical computing, quality assurance, and medical direction. He is also the editor and principal author of *Medical Direction in Long-Term Care* and *Medical Policies and Procedures for Long-Term Care,* two widely used comprehensive reference sources for the nursing home medical director.

Robert R. Merry, B.S., is director of finance for the Jewish Nursing Home of Western Massachusetts in Longmeadow, Massachusetts.

Donna G. Michaels, Ph.D., is president and executive director of Kids Voting Florida, Inc., based in Miami. Her experience includes service as a senior development officer in a university and as a program developer and administrator in state and local level human services organizations. She has also held senior management and marketing positions in the media and communications industry.

Marianne Raimondo, M.S., Ph.D., is a vice president of Applied Management Systems, a consulting firm for health care organizations. Her expertise is in the area of total quality management. She has been involved in quality management in health care for 10 years.

Stephen R. Roizen, M.H.A., is executive director of the Willows at Westborough, a continuing care retirement community in Massachusetts. Previous positions include being director of cost settlement and audit for the Medicaid Program of the Commonwealth of Virginia and associate director of the Jewish Home for the Aged in Detroit, Michigan.

Linda J. Shea, Ph.D., is an associate professor of marketing in the Department of Hotel, Restaurant, and Travel Administration at the University of Massachusetts at Amherst. Her research and teaching emphases are in marketing management, marketing research, and consumer behavior—particularly the elderly consumer. She specializes in marketing applications to the service sector, including health care, education, and hospitality organizations.

Charles D. Schewe, Ph.D., M.B.A., is a full professor at the University of Massachusetts at Amherst and president of University Research Associates, a management and marketing consulting firm offering a broad range of marketing and strategic consultation to health care providers and other organizations. Dr. Schewe has developed a particular expertise in understanding the marketing implications of our 50+ population. He is presently the president of the American Association for Advances in Health Care Research.

Herbert H. Shore, Ed.D., is the executive vice president of North American Association of Jewish Homes and Housing for the Aging in Dallas, Texas. He is also the director of field instruction in the Center for Studies in Aging at the University of North Texas in Denton, Texas.

Ronald L. Skaggs, F.A.I.A., is chairman and CEO of HKS, Inc., an architectural, planning, and engineering firm specializing in the design of health care facilities. During the past 25 years, Mr. Skaggs has been responsible for the planning and design of more than 250 health care projects including many long-term care facilities.

Mark E. Toso, M.S.B.A., C.P.A., is president of TriNet Healthcare Consultants, Inc. Mr. Toso has worked in the health care industry for over 18 years. His broad range of experience includes strategic, financial, and organizational analysis for hospitals, nursing homes, and physicians. Before starting TriNet, he was the eastern regional vice president of Amherst Associates Inc. from 1976 to 1985.

Concetta M. Tynan, R.N.N.P., serves as vice president of senior services with Handmaker Jewish Services for the Aging, Inc., a nonprofit, nonsectarian health care facility. She also is the vice president of Handmaker Management Enterprises, Inc., a for-profit subsidiary specializing in consultation and management services to long-term care facilities and housing. Mrs. Tynan has 13 years of expertise in the long-term care field.

James E. Wallace, Jr., J.D., L.L.M., is a senior partner and co-chair of the Labor/Employment Practice Group with Bowditch & Dewey in Worcester, Massachusetts.

Janice Warnke, M.S.W., serves as the director of adult day care services with Handmaker Jewish Services for the Aging, Inc., a nonprofit, nonsectarian long-term care agency in Tucson, Arizona. Ms. Warnke administers three distinct programs that serve disabled, demented, and elderly persons. Ms. Warnke is a licensed nursing home administrator who has held administrative positions in California and Arizona.

Susan Krauss Whitbourne, Ph.D., is a professor of psychology at the University of Massachusetts at Amherst and has extensive experience in gerontological research, teaching, and practice. Her areas of research interest include psychological adaptation to the aging process, personality development in adulthood, and the provision of clinical services to older adults.

Karen-Jo Wills, M.S., is a Ph.D. candidate in clinical psychology at the University of Massachusetts at Amherst. She has experience in direct care to the elderly and in providing psychotherapy to adults of various ages. In addition, she is an active researcher who recently co-authored a major longitudinal investigation of adult personality development.

Charles S. Wolfe, M.A., Ed.S., is a consultant and lecturer in Adventura, Florida. He formerly served as executive director of the Jewish Home of Detroit for 16 years prior to becoming the executive director of the Mt. Sinai Medical Center Foundation.

Acknowledgments

This book evolved from a related project that produced the 38-chapter book, *Long-Term Care Administration Handbook.* In thinking about the applicability of that volume to teaching students of long-term care administration, it became clear that the handbook was too long, too expensive, and not primarily organized as a teaching-oriented textbook. After discussions with various colleagues and reviewing my own experiences as an administrator, consultant, and educator, I decided to develop this textbook, which utilizes some of the original chapters of the handbook, along with 23 new case studies designed to provide students with an opportunity to develop a range of skills by working on "real" problems.

I want to thank a number of people for their contributions to this effort. First, I am grateful to my fellow chapter authors whose work is proving so invaluable. Next, I thank Roberta Bergman, Howard Braverman, James Broder, Marian Broder, Marvin Goldberg, Lorrie Higgins, Bob Merry, Stephen Roizen, Janice Warnke, and Chuck Wolfe for their efforts at developing cases for this book. A special thanks to John Kress and the Association of University Programs in Health Administration for permission to republish the case I authored, "A Dietary Dilemma," which originally appeared in their book, *Cases in Long Term Care Management* (AUPHA Press, 1989).

I would also like to thank the "crew" at Aspen for their encouragement and help: Mike Brown, Jack Bruggeman, Cynthia Smith, Lenda Hill, Trudy Graham, Sandy Cannon, Barbara Hoffmann, and Jane Colilla.

Additionally, thanks to my students at the University of Massachusetts, who have had to test and be tested by many of these cases and whose feedback has been most appreciated.

Finally, thanks to my wife Sandra and sons Ben and Jonas who have supported me all the while I have been in the cellar working on this project.

xv

A Note about the Cases

The cases appearing in this text present a range of different problems for students and administrators to analyze. Each case is designed to highlight issues developed and discussed in the base chapter. However, it should be noted that not every case covers every issue, and in some instances the case itself may introduce entirely new material to the chapter.

Further, the cases do not follow a uniform format or length. Some cases are short and provide discussion questions; others develop a protracted scenario with a clear assignment; and some merely present a problem, leaving the student and instructor to decide on the next steps.

All of the cases are real. As is evident from the case authorship, several were developed by distinguished practitioners, but most are based on my own experience in the long-term care field and others on several reported legal cases.

It is my hope that these cases will prove to be both interesting and provocative.

Introduction

The field of long-term care administration offers students an extraordinary personal and professional challenge. The problems administrators face touch the heart and spirit of our nation's elderly and their families and the purses of these same people as well as those of state and federal governments. To deal effectively with the myriad problems of managing long-term care organizations and programs, administrators must understand a number of essential issues and be able to operate effectively in the dynamic milieu of long-term care. This book is designed to meet that need by providing students with a substantive understanding of the theoretical issues through the various chapters and the practical aspects of managing in long-term care through the 23 related case studies that follow all but the first chapter.

The first chapter of this book is by Dr. Herbert Shore, one of America's most distinguished leaders in long-term care. In this historic overview of the history of long-term care, Dr. Shore establishes the context for understanding the field. In the next chapter, Dr. Susan Krauss Whitbourne, a psychologist and gerontologist, and Karen-Jo Wills present an important and thoughtful analysis of the psychological issues that arise in institutional care for the aged. The chapter provides a conceptual and theoretical framework for understanding aging and also describes how the infantilizing behavior of caregivers can adversely affect residents.

In Chapter 3, Marian Broder, an attorney with extensive experience in long-term care, discusses ethical issues that providers must confront, including health care proxies, living wills, advance directives, and durable powers of attorney.

Chapter 4, which I authored, analyzes the functions of management, the special challenges in long-term care, and expectations from managers and makes some practical suggestions on the subject of entering management. In the next chapter, I examine another classical issue, that is, the care and feeding of boards of directors.

In Chapter 6, Steven Levenson, MD, a leading authority on long-term care medical departments, analyzes the role of the medical director in nursing homes. Next, professors of nursing Joan Culley and Janet Courtney focus on the delivery of nursing services.

Chapter 8, by Jim Wallace, a lawyer specializing in employment law, presents a comprehensive discussion of the critical issue of employment law.

The next chapter, by professors Linda Shea and Charles Schewe, provides a conceptual overview of the marketing basics that long-term care administrators need to understand in order to develop effective marketing plans.

Chapter 10, by Marianne Raimondo, focuses on one of the most interesting and, in some ways, controversial innovations in health care, total quality management.

My co-author for Chapter 11 is Sol Goldner, an experienced nursing home executive and former consultant. This chapter covers the financial organization, the elements of financing, and the budgetary process. Then Chapter 12, by Donna Michaels and Charles Wolfe, examines the issues of capital fund raising in long-term care.

In Chapter 13, architects Ron Skaggs and H. Ralph Hawkins provide a comprehensive analysis of architectural issues of importance to long-term care administrators, including the likely impact on design of the Americans with Disabilities Act. Chapter 14, by Dick Lamden, Concetta Tynan, and Janice Warnke, provides an excellent introduction to planning day care services. Following this chapter is a case prepared by Janice Warnke that focuses on empowerment of day care center clients. Then Chapter 15, by Anne Harrington, provides an important overview and analysis of assisted living for the elderly. Following this chapter, Steve Roizen has developed several cases from his own experience as a director of a continuing care retirement community. Finally, Chapter 16, by Mark Toso, concludes the book with an overview of strategic planning in long-term care.

In sum, this book includes 16 chapters as well as 23 case studies, which taken together will provide students of long-term care administration an important introduction to what may become a lifetime commitment.

Chapter 1

History of Long-Term Care

Herbert H. Shore

HISTORICAL SURVEY

The Patriarch Abraham (Gen. 12:6) is credited with originating institutions such as hostels, hospitals, and homes by legends that tell of his tent in the plain of Moreh at the junction of important trade routes. It had openings on four sides and was accessible from every direction. Strangers were welcomed, given food and drink, and made comfortable for the night, and in the morning they were set upon the road headed in the right direction.[1]

"God loves the stranger" (Deut. 10:18) served as inspiration to those who made an effort to accommodate journeyers to Judea. It was the aspiration to holiness that resulted in a whole range of amenities and comforts for those in the community who were deprived. The furnishing of food, clothing, education for children, dowries for maidens, subsidies for orphans, visitors to the sick, support for pregnant women, money for free burials, ransom for captives, aid to the ailing, and shelter for the aged was placed among the highest ideals of mankind (Talmud, B.B. 8b). Maimonides, a physician and Judaic philosopher, supported the position that helping others in need should be a goal not only of the Jewish constituency but of all people alike.

In Ecclesiastes and the Psalms, there are references to the infirmities of the declining years, the failing powers of the aged. Old age was pointed to as a state of inactivity. As a balance, upon the young was placed an obligation to provide for the support and comfort of the old (Ruth 4:5), and without question the Fifth Commandment (Exod. 20:12), asserting that honor should be given to one's father and mother, is in a similar vein.

Accurate information about the origins and early history of institutions for the aged is scanty. Garrison attributes "the credit of ministering to human suffering on an extended scale" to the teachings of Christianity and traces the development of institutions for the sick in the Byzantine Empire following the conversion of Constantine.[2]

Among the specialized hospitals that gradually developed during the fourth century, he mentions *Gerontochia,* for the aged; *Nosocomia,* for the care of the sick alone; *Brephotrophia,* for foundlings; *Orphanotrophia,* for orphans; *Ptochia,* for the helpless poor; and *Xenodochia,* for poor and infirm pilgrims. These functions undoubtedly overlapped in many of the local foundations that grew up in the Middle Ages, especially during the Crusades, under the inspiration of priests and with the support of nobility. In many cases, these foundations were managed and staffed by Catholic orders devoted to the care of the sick.

Medieval and Renaissance hospitals were in actuality only places of refuge for sick strangers and infirm aged individuals without family or friends. There was no organized supervision by physicians. In the poem "The Hye Way to the Spytell Hous" (c. 1536), the author, Robert Copland, inquires from the porter of a London hospital what sort of people obtain help there and receives this reply:

> Forsooth they that be at such myschefe,
> That for they'r lyvying can do no labour
> And have no frendes to do them socour
> As old people seke and impotent...

R.M. Clay, in *The Medieval Hospitals of England,* points out that these homes were called indiscriminately "hospital," "Maison Dieu," "almhouse," or "bedehouse."[3] The oldest in England are St. John's in Canterbury, founded by Archbishop Lanfranc in 1084, and St. Cross' in Winchester, founded in 1132 by Henry de Blois, Bishop of Winchester and brother to King Stephen.[4] Both these institutions are still in existence. Ewelme, in Oxfordshire, founded in 1437 by William de la Pole and completed by his wife Alice, a granddaughter of Geoffrey Chaucer, is of particular interest because the mastership of the almshouse is an obligation and also a source of revenue for the Regius Professor of Medicine at Oxford. Sir William Osler's interest in the pensioners and his discovery of priceless old documents in a locked chest are described in Cushing's biography.[5]

W.J. Marx traced the development of charity in medieval Louvain and mentions, among others, the hospice of St. Barbara, which was begun in the last half of the 13th century.[6] Belgium is the chief site of activity of the Béguines, members of lay sisterhoods founded in 1170 by Lambert le Bégue, a priest of Liege. The Béguinage of St. Elizabeth of Ghent, famous for its architecture, has about a thousand sisters, nearly all elderly women, who devote themselves to a life of service without taking monastic vows. The Béguines wear the old Flemish headdress and a dark costume.[7] They support themselves by the manufacture of fine laces and are noted for their kindness to the poor and the sick.

The deterioration and breakdown of the monastic charities all over Europe as well as in England and their gradual supplementation by the action of municipal authorities has been well covered by the Webbs in their classic study of the Old

English Poor Law.[8] The English were stimulated into action by the Spanish scholar Juan Juis Vives (1492–1540), who became friendly with Henry VIII at Bruges and frequently visited England. In his *De subventione pauperum sive de humanis necessitatibus* (1526), he told the authorities of Bruges that they must help the destitute in order to prevent rebellion and because slums are centers of infection and moral contamination. He divided the indigent into three classes: those sheltered in hospitals and almshouses, homeless beggars, and the honest and shamefaced poor living in their own homes. He insisted on an accurate census and recommended medical aid for the sick and segregation of the insane.

The earliest English law for relief of the poor, the statute of Henry VIII (1531), empowered justices to issue licenses to beggars. The parliamentary statue of 1597–1598 authorized the appointment in each parish of overseers of the poor and imposed on them, and on the churchwardens, the duty of providing for all of the destitute, whether able-bodied or impotent, young or old, lame or blind, and gave them the right to raise funds by taxing parish residents. The courts were empowered to jail anyone refusing to work or anyone refusing to pay the poor rate. This poor law, enacted in the reign of Queen Elizabeth, became part of the English common law that was brought to America by the colonists and has formed the basis of our local government activities on behalf of the poor.

With the growth of modern medicine, the hospital became gradually the center for active treatment of the sick, but in France and Germany homes for the aged also took on important functions as centers of medical study and research, often furnishing to distinguished investigators material on which to base valuable contributions to our knowledge, not only of old age and its associated diseases but also knowledge in other areas of medicine. This rich medical tradition is nowhere better exemplified than in Paris, where the Salpétrière (for women) and the Bicêtre (for men) provided refuge for the aged, the chronically ill, and the insane and were even used at various times for the incarceration of criminals. Guillain and Mathieu have written a vivid history of the achievements of the Salpétrière.

> Refuge of thousands of aged, great center of neurology, great center of psychiatry, the Salpétrière has only become adapted to its actual role by stages. It has seen within its walls the men of the 17th, 18th, 19th and 20th centuries according to their successive conceptions, attempt to solve the great problems of public and private charity, of aid to the poor and the aged, of the protection of society against the insane and the defective, of the protection of the defective and insane against society; it has seen. . . the creation of scientific psychiatry."[9]

Charcot left us an unforgettable picture of this great institution, where he himself worked and taught so brilliantly for many years.[10]

At the Bicêtre, Pinel in 1798 first struck the chains from the insane, as we learn from the often told story of the earliest efforts toward humane care of the mentally affected. Magendie, Cruveilhier, Rostan, Prus, Durand-Fardel, Landré-Beauvais, and Dechambre were only a few of the great French physicians who made important studies of the aged in these Parisian institutions. In the provinces, Emil Demange made excellent clinical and pathological observations during 500 postmortem examinations of the old residents of the St. Julien Hospice at Nancy.[11] Jules Boy-Teissier of Marseille, physician to the Hôpital St. Marguerite, a home for the aged, published in 1895 *Lectures on the Diseases of the Aged,* based on lectures given at the Marseille Medical School.[12] In recent times, Adrien Pic utilized the clinical material of the Hospice of Perron, near Lyon, for his textbook on the diseases of old age.[13]

In the first monograph on the anatomy of the aged by Burkhard Wilhelm Seiler, *Anatomia Corporis Humani Senilis Specimen,* which appeared at Erlangen in 1800, we find the author admonishing physicians connected with homes for the aged to take advantage of the material at their disposal and stressing the necessity for repeated observations before ascribing any manifestation to old age itself.[14] Lorenz Geist based his 1860 monograph *Klinik der Greisenkrankheiten* on his studies of the residents of the Pfrundner Anstalt zum Heiligen Geist in Nürnberg.[15] Carl Mettenheimer (1824–1898) worked at the Frankfurt Home for the Aged for many years.[16] In Austria, the Vienna municipal hospital for the aged was a source of inspiration for Mueller-Deham's *Innere Krankheiten des Greisernalters,*[17] which owes much of its value to some 2,000 autopsies of old people supervised by the distinguished pathologist Jakob Erdheim.

In England, the Royal Hospital in Chelsea, a medical establishment for old soldiers, gave MacLachlan, in 1863, and Lipscomb, in 1932, the motivation to write texts on the medical aspects of old age, and it later stimulated the efforts of Dr. Trevor Howell, who has written so interestingly of its history as well as of its pensioners' maladies.[18]

THE AMERICAN EXPERIENCE

The colonists came to the New World seeking religious and political freedoms and economic opportunity. In addition to their meager possessions, they brought hope, faith, determination, and dreams. They also brought, consciously and unconsciously, the systems of law and the communal structures that had evolved over many centuries in their native lands.

They continued a Calvinistic approach exemplified by Elizabethan poor laws, which attempted to limit and control mendancy by requiring able-bodied individuals to work. They agreed that the lame, sick, blind, orphaned, and elderly could be cared for in communal facilities, which became known as almshouses. (Almshouses were built in Boston in 1622, in Philadelphia in 1713, and in New York in 1736.)

Early in the history of our country, there were no government agencies or programs. Relief was a local responsibility and was dispensed either by the local community or church or by organizations formed to meet the social, cultural, and religious needs of the immigrant groups. Thus there were associations, clubs, and societies to ensure that the poor would be clothed, housed, and fed, the sick visited, the prisoners ransomed, and the deceased buried. These early organizations, some known as the "Ladies Sheltering Aid Society" and similar names, were established so that those without families and in need of help would be cared for.

These "societies" often purchased private houses and converted them into "homes." Whatever was provided for the wards, referred to as inmates, was expected to be appreciated. The facilities, based on the poor farm or asylum model, were created primarily by nonprofit communal groups, but county-run homes were instituted for individuals who were unaffiliated with any such group.

There were several streams of experience. Immigrants who came from Eastern Europe brought with them the communal "collection pot." This "home" served the aged and orphaned, the handicapped and disabled, the mentally deficient and the mentally ill. It was a feared and dreaded fate and was accepted only when there was no other alternative or recourse.

Immigrants from Germany and Scandinavia brought a different model—the Altenheim, a kind of a club-residence for those who had saved and planned for a respectable retirement. These two distinctly different types of facilities coexisted until virtually the end of World War II.

The voluntary, philanthropic, fraternal, ethnic, church-related home was the primary type of facility providing services throughout the 19th century and up to the early 1920s.

The federal government pursued a philosophy of studied avoidance of intrusion into the lives of citizens. It was not until the late 1890s that the Public Health Service was established, not until 1909 that a president used his good offices to call for a White House Conference (on children), and not until 1916 that Congress authorized a study of the problems of housing and the nation's slums.

There were several factors that maintained the status quo. First, the average life expectancy was low, and therefore the need to develop institutions for the elderly was relatively small. Second, every winter fully one-fourth of the population of existing homes (and those on the waiting lists) would die of pneumonia. Pneumonia was popularly called the "old man's friend" because it was most often accompanied by death, resulting in an end to the burdens of old age.

The major economic upheaval of 1929, the Great Depression, proved to be the undoing of the system of welfare on the county and state level. Unemployment and need was so great that the local church and community groups did not have the resources to cope.

Fearful of the "Army of the Aged," the movement begun by Dr. Francis Townsend, which had grown into a significant political force, President Franklin Roosevelt instructed Frances Perkins (the first woman cabinet member and Secretary of Labor) to propose legislation that would deal with the demands for pensions and welfare reform.

In August 1935, the Congress of the United States passed, and the president signed, the Social Security Act. This legislation was designed to accomplish several things and was indirectly responsible for the growth of the nursing home industry.

The Social Security Act provided for a national, unified welfare system through "categorical assistance" programs. In effect, it said that those already aged (over an arbitrary age of 65), those who were blind, and families with dependent children would receive assistance from a federal and state program. The second part of the act established a form of old age and survivors insurance. The idea was that workers, in conjunction with their employers, would contribute to a fund that in their retirement years would provide income security. If a contributing worker died before age 65, his survivors (wife and children to age 18) would be assured a monthly income.

The Social Security Act has been amended a great many times to provide coverage for the "permanently and totally disabled," coverage for certain special refugee groups, and universal coverage.

In the language of the original act were two provisions for the exclusion of beneficiaries. One of these indicated that if an individual had contracted for life care, he or she would be ineligible for old age assistance. The second provision stated that if an individual was in a government or "county" facility, he or she would be ineligible for old age assistance. Consequently, many local (county) homes recognized that if they continued to operate, the residents would not receive Social Security income. If the residents were discharged or transferred, however, they could become eligible, and thus many county homes moved toward closing.

Another result of the Great Depression was that many people were close to losing their homes (due to severe unemployment). Some of these individuals, seeking income to help them make their mortgage payments, were happy to welcome relatives and those being discharged from county homes into their own homes. This gave rise to a new cottage industry consisting of private homes converted into rest homes. In that era of meager regulation, there were no standards of care and no licensing requirements. And finally, once older people had some income and were no longer totally indigent, there was a dramatic shift from thinking of them as inmates to recognizing them as individuals. They became "residents" rather than "wards" or "patients."

THE DEMOGRAPHIC CHANGES

The increased sophistication of medicine, the discovery of new drugs, various technological breakthroughs, changes in rehabilitation, and the shift from acute to chronic care altered forever the demographic landscape and led to the "graying of America."

In the late 1930s and 1940s, the discovery of broad spectrum antibiotics virtually eliminated infectious diseases (the use of sulfa, penicillin, and the myecins reduced the risk of death from surgical interventions).

World War II made drastic changes imperative in the treatment and repair of orthopedic injuries and gave birth to the field of physical medicine and rehabilitation. Previously, older people who had broken a hip were subjected to long periods of traction and often died from other complications. Now age was no longer a factor in treatment. With replacement hardware, antibiotic medication, and transfusable blood, people could recover from or live for long periods with chronic disabilities.

The next major breakthrough was the discovery of the psychotropic drugs. The psychopharmacological revolution made the treatment of depression and aggressive behaviors possible. Individuals who previously could only be cared for in state hospitals could be maintained at home, in the community, or in a nursing home.

The progress of medicine thus altered the demand for services, and the demographic revolution led to the need for a modified health benefits insurance program for the aged.

COLLATERAL DEVELOPMENTS

Licensing of Facilities

In the amendments to the 1950 Social Security Act, Congress mandated that, by 1953, if a facility housed and cared for four or more unrelated individuals receiving Social Security income, the facility would require a license from the state in which it was located. Thus for the first time on a national scale, physical and service standards were established, and nomenclature began to define care facilities.

Introduction of Specially Designed Facilities

The nature of the population in care facilities was changing. Familyless immigrant residents were being replaced by nativeborns. The residents were older (average age on admission increased from around 60 in the 1940s to around 86 in the early 1990s), sicker (they had four or more chronic disabilities and more than half suffered from some form of dementia), and poorer (they had exhausted their funds or divested them prior to institutionalization).

Because of the increased age and enfeeblement of the residents, the federal government, in 1958, convened the first national Conference on Homes for the Aged and Nursing Homes, and the thrust of that effort was to focus on unsafe, unsanitary conditions and to eliminate the possibility of nursing home fires. A steady stream of regulations came forth, calling for fire-resistant structures, sprinkler systems, smoke and heat detectors, and alarm systems. Several federal loan programs made loan guarantees available to replace the fire-hazardous facilities, and a new era of facilities designed for use as nursing homes was ushered in. Some of these new and efficient designs became the foundation for the growth of nursing home chains.

National Organizations

Although there were some sectarian nursing home organizations (Protestant, Catholic, and Jewish), there was no unified national organization representing all nonprofit homes. In 1960, the American Association of Homes for Aging was organized to represent those facilities. There already was an association representing for-profit homes, the American Nursing Home Association, which later changed its name to the American Health Care Association. This group also accepts nonprofits into its membership.

These organizations primarily serve institutions. The American College of Nursing Home Administrators (name changed to the American College of Healthcare Administrators) serves the professionals who manage nursing homes.

The American Association of Homes for Aging became the force for recognition of the "social components of care," which introduced the psychosocial model to long-term care.

With the virtual elimination of infectious diseases and pneumonia, homes began to have large waiting lists, the elderly were increasing in number, as were organizations serving the elderly, and their political clout was felt at the First White House Conference on Aging, authorized by Congress in 1960.[*] At that conference, delegates urged that some form of national health insurance be enacted.

Though originally introduced in the Congress in 1942 by Murray, Wagner, and Dingill, it was not until 1965 that Congress passed the Health Insurance Benefits

---

[*]President Harry Truman called for a National Conference on Aging, which was held in 1950, but the first White House Conference on Aging was officially held in 1960.

for the Aged Act, which established Medicare (an insurance program primarily for physician benefits and hospital and home care payments) and Medicaid (an assistance program for extended care, etc.).

The belief that the government was going to underwrite posthospital extended care was the impetus for an enormous growth in nursing homes and also for the linking of many free-standing facilities to form chains. The emergence of nursing homes as major players in the health delivery system permitted them to create corporate entities and, by going public, to get their stocks traded on the big board. Some of these corporations were bought and sold and traded and were as much economic entities as care-providing entities.

With reimbursement comes regulation, and during President Nixon's adminis- ✶✶
tration a major nursing home reform initiative was established that placed new emphasis on the provision of services as well as on the physical plant of nursing homes. Nixon also appointed a special Commissioner for Nursing Homes.

The U.S. Senate Subcommittee on Aging has been interested for many years in the conditions in America's nursing homes. In 1967, Congress passed legislation ✶ mandating that every administrator of a nursing home be licensed by 1970, and each state has now established a board of licensure.   Higher reqs. than any other

The Congress called upon the National Academy of Science's Institute of Medicine to conduct a study to improve the quality of care in the nation's nursing homes. After several years of work and in an effort to identify quality indicators, the report was issued and served as the basis of the Nursing Home Reform Act of 1988, part of the Omnibus Budget Reconciliation Act. The reforms were the most sweeping in ten years and will contribute to the empowering of residents, the creation of restraint-free environments, and the upgrading of nurse aide training.

✶ The modern nursing home is the result of centuries of evolution and refinement. Only a very small portion of the elderly are cared for in institutions (approximately 5 to 6 percent at any given moment), yet those who are in homes tend to be especially frail, fragile, vulnerable, and cognitively impaired.

Free-standing and single-function nursing homes are disappearing. In their place are campuses for serving the elderly in housing and nursing homes and in continuing care retirement communities, which offer a vast array of services.

The modern nursing home offers inpatient, outpatient, and outreach services. In addition to direct services, it can provide education (to its own staff and to college students or others) and can engage in research and demonstration projects.

The nursing home today is the foundation for a comprehensive, community-based continuum of care. With its range of services, it can utilize care management to provide the right service at the right time and at the right cost.

The nursing home is no longer the point of no return. It is the "aging person's destination" and the "thinking person's choice" when the need for long-term care arises.

NOTES

1. J.G. Gold and S.M. Kaufman, Development of Care of Elderly: Tracing the History of Institutional Facilities, *The Gerontologist* 10 (1970):262–274.

2. F.H. Garrison, *An Introduction to the History of Medicine,* 4th ed. (Philadelphia: W.B. Saunders, 1929).

3. R.M. Clay, *The Medieval Hospitals of England* (London: Methuen, 1909).

4. H. Moody, *A History and Description of the Hospital of St. Cross* (Winchester: G. & H. Gilmour, 1844).

5. H. Cushing, *The Life of Sir William Osler* (Oxford: Clarendon Press, 1925).

6. W.J. Marx, The Development of Charity in Medieval Louvain (Thesis, Columbia University, 1936).

7. G. Van Bever, *Les Béguinages* (Brussels: Editions due Cercle d'Art, 1944). See also the *Catholic Encyclopedia* and the *Encyclopedia Britannica.*

8. S. Webb and B. Webb, The Old Poor Law, in *English Poor Law History* (London: Longmans Greedn & Co., 1927).

9. G. Guillain and P. Mathieu, *La Salpétrière* (Paris: Masson & Cie, 1925).

10. J.M.A. Charcot, *Clinical Lectures on the Diseases of Old Age,* trans. by L.H. Hunt (New York: William Wood & Co., 1881).

11. E. Demange, *Étude Clinique et Anatomo-Pathologique Sur la Vieillesse* (Paris: F. Olean, 1886).

12. J. Boy-Teissier, *Leçons sur les Maladies des Vieillards, Faites a l'école de Médecine de Marseille* (Paris: O. Doin, 1895).

13. A. Pic and S. Bonnamour, *Précis des Maladies des Vieillards* (Paris: O. Doin & Fils, 1912).

14. B.W. Seiler, *Anatomia Corporis Humani Senilis Specimen* (Erlangen, Germany: J.J. Palm, 1800).

15. L. Geist, *Klinik der Greisenkrankheiten* (Erlangen, Germany: F. Enke, 1860).

16. C.F.M. Mettenheimer, *Sectiones Longaevorum* (Frankfurt, Germany: Sauerlander, 1863).

17. A. Mueller-Deham, *Innere Krankheiten des Greisenalters* (Vienna: Julius Springer, 1937).

18. D. MacLachlan, *A Practical Treatise on the Diseases and Infirmities of Advanced Life* (London: J. Churchill's Sons, 1863); F.M. Lipscomb, *Diseases of Old Age* (London: Bailliere, Tindall & Cox, 1932); T. Howell, *Old Age: Some Practical Points in Geriatrics* (London: H.K. Lewis & Co., 1944). For further information, see T. Faulkner, *A Historical and Descriptive Account of the Royal Hospital and the Royal Military Asylum at Chelsea* (London: T. Faulkner, 1805); G.R. Gleig, *Chelsea Hospital and Its Traditions* (London: Richard Bentley, 1839).

SUGGESTED READINGS

Abel, N.E. A short history of long term care. *Modern Healthcare,* July 1976, 13–16.

McArthur, R.F. The historical evolution from almshouse to ECF. *Nursing Homes,* April–August 1970.

Rogers, W.W. Historical institutions of long term care. *The Southwestern Journal of Aging* (Southwest Society on Aging) 7, no. 1 (1991).

Tobriner, A. Almshouses in sixteenth-century England: Housing for the poor elderly. *Journal of Religion and Aging* 1, no. 4 (1985):13–41.

U.S. Department of Labor. Bureau of Labor Statistics. *Care of aged persons in the United States.* Pub. No. 489, Oct. 1929.

U.S. Department of Labor. Bureau of Labor Statistics. *Homes for the Aged in the U.S.* Pub. No. 677, 1941.

Zeman, F.D. The institutional care of the aged: Scope and function of the modern home. Unpublished, 1952.

Chapter 2

Psychological Issues in Institutional Care of the Aged

Susan Krauss Whitbourne and Karen-Jo Wills

The psychological concerns of aging individuals have been the focus of four decades of research, beginning with the publication in 1959 of the first *Handbook of Aging and the Individual.*[1] At that time, it was generally believed that aging brought with it a diminution of happiness, level of activity, and self-esteem and an increase in anxiety, susceptibility to stress, and rigidity. However, even in this first edition, Kuhlen[2] pointed out that age alone is not a sufficient basis for predicting adjustment and that personality and life circumstances interact in important ways to influence the individual's level of happiness and adaptability. The theme of personal variability and the influence of situational determinants remained an important concept throughout the subsequent 40 years, serving as the basis for hundreds of investigations into factors affecting adjustment in later life.

PERSON-ENVIRONMENT CONGRUENCE MODELS OF ADAPTATION

Among the variables studied as predictors of adjustment in old age, one of the most important has been the individual's living situation. With the growth of institutions designed to care for the infirm elderly, psychological gerontologists have maintained a commitment to understanding the effect of institutional life on the individual's adjustment, a commitment that began with the early publications in this area by Carp, Coe, Lawton, and Lieberman.[3] Implicit in this research is the understanding that most elderly persons in need of supervised medical care would prefer to live independently in their own homes and fear the institutionalization process,[4] yet health problems and the unavailability of caregivers prevent them from living at home.[5] When institutional care becomes a necessity, the question is to determine how to reduce the negative impact of forced dependence on the psychological health of older people.

Over the past 25 years, the search for ways to minimize the negative effects of institutionalization has led to the development of a model focusing on the concept of congruence, or a matching of the needs of the individual with the characteristics of the institutional environment.[6] According to this model, individuals vary in their needs and perceptions of the environment and are best adapted when they are in a state of congruence (i.e., the environment both meets their needs and is positively perceived). The central assumption is that there are large individual differences in the person-environment congruence equation. Elaborating on the congruence model, the competence model adds the notion that the demands of the environment must be considered in relation to the capacities of the resident.[7] Severely impaired residents are unable to function in environments that are too challenging; conversely, highly competent residents have difficulty adapting to environments that are insufficiently demanding of their abilities. Thus, not only must needs and interests be taken into account when considering the person-environment match, but so must the resources and demands of the person and the environment.

As helpful as the congruence and competence models have proven in stimulating further theory building and research, they have obvious limitations as models for practice when they are implemented in the real world. Institutions, by their very nature, must provide for the "average" person; they are not easily molded to meet the idiosyncratic needs of the varieties of people who live in them. To take a simple example, some individuals prefer rooms that are warm and others prefer rooms that are cool. Yet the heating system of the institution must be set at some average temperature, and by definition this average will fail to satisfy people who prefer or require environments that are warmer or cooler.

Consideration of the emotional climate of the institution leads to more puzzling dilemmas. The emotional needs of institutional residents can be regarded as revolving around the important theme of autonomy-security,[8] a dimension regarded as contributing to personal growth as well as physical and emotional well-being in institutional residents.[9] Apart from their physical needs, some older adults may desire a nurturant environment that fosters dependence; others value their emotional autonomy and wish to preserve it as long as possible. Yet, as with the setting of temperature, the institution adjusts the level of independence to an "average" amount and in the process creates tension between the needs of individuals and the ability of the institution to meet those needs. The natural tendency of caregivers is to err on the side of dependence, as the institution runs more smoothly if staff rather than residents organize daily schedules, decide on activities, plan meals, and structure activities of daily living such as bathing, dressing, and feeding.[10] In the area of toileting, for example, it is more efficient for staff to change a patient than to rely on the patient's schedule of voiding.[11] This tendency to encourage dependence is also fostered by the medical model, in which the resident is regarded as a patient who passively receives treatment.[12] Ironically, although institutions may pride themselves on providing as much support as possible for residents by meeting their daily needs for care, activity, and stimulation, too much support can actually be detrimental, because it will tend to reduce the individual's efforts at self-direction and mastery, leading to greater psychological dependence on the institution.[13]

Even if it were not more efficient to run an institution by having the staff in control, the roles of resident and caregiver almost naturally foster the development of dependence in residents. The resident, whose responsibilities for taking care of home, family, and finances have been removed in the institutionalization process, is placed in a dependent or childlike relationship to the staff, who have taken over the management of the resident's affairs. A self-fulfilling prophecy is set in motion when the caregiver views the resident as too infirm to take independent action, which causes the resident, in turn, to lose self-maintenance skills.

THE INFANTILIZATION PROCESS

Underlying the issue of dependence versus independence is a process that is discussed less frequently in the gerontological literature but seems to play a fundamental role in the lives of the institutionalized elderly. This is the process of infantilization, which involves treating an elderly individual like a child.[14] The infantilization of older adults is reflected in the characterization of later life as a "second childhood."[15] Older adults are seen as unproductive, undisciplined, disruptive, cranky, irrational, silly, and impulsive. Their need for help with the activities of daily living that small children need help with—eating, dressing, and toileting—further supports this characterization of older adults as infantile. Activities that are planned for older adults typically include arts and crafts, birthday parties, and play with toys, all of which are activities that adults make available to children.

Infantilization can also be seen in the way an older person is dressed by caregivers. A woman may have bows, ponytails, or pigtails put in her hair. The clothes she is given to wear are pastel colored, like those used to dress small infants, and on holidays she may be outfitted using colors or pins that are symbolic of the season. Elderly men are often subjected to a similar kind of treatment. For example, a male resident wearing a necktie or a suitcoat might be responded to by flirtatious remarks on the part of female caregivers, who might declare how "handsome" he looks. At the opposite extreme, caregivers may pay little attention to dressing the residents in proper attire, leaving them in pajamas and bathrobes, much as infants are left in their sleepers during the day. Finally, infantilization may take the form of lack of respect for a resident's need for privacy—by dressing or undressing the resident in a public location or without proper safeguards to prevent intrusion.

The language directed at residents is another area in which infantilization manifests itself.[16] Referring to an elderly man as "handsome" is not in and of itself an instance of infantilization; it is when the term is used as synonymous with "cute" that the compliment becomes condescension. Similarly, referring to a resident as "sweetie," "grannie," and "dearie," or using first names only, is patronizing and violates the resident's dignity.[17] Baby talk—speaking with intonations and words that would be used to address a small child—is another manifestation of infantilization.[18] Although it may be argued that such verbalizations can be reassuring and consistent with the role of nurse as caregiver,[19] it is just as likely that the use of baby talk results from a lack of knowledge of alternate methods of communication.[20]

Caregivers may also decorate the environment so that it resembles a kindergarten or preschool rather than a residence for adults. For weeks before the next major holiday, the institution may be decorated with hearts, pumpkins, turkeys, or Santa Clauses (or Hanukkah decorations in a Jewish institution), just like a classroom in an elementary school. At other times, mobiles, stickers, or the artwork of residents may be placed in the hallways and common spaces as a way to add color, contributing further to the school-like appearance of the institution.

It is, perhaps, in the attitudes and general behaviors directed toward residents that infantilization occurs in its most extreme form. These attitudes and behaviors include rewarding residents by patting, touching, or kissing them, which is like cuddling or hugging babies when they are good. Similarly, a caregiver may reinforce childlike fantasies in a resident by giving the resident a doll, for example, and calling it "baby" when the resident starts to treat it as a child. Residents are also given little freedom of choice in the areas of food, dress, and activities, just like children, who typically lack the authority to control the decisions made by parents. If a resident balks or objects to a particular choice, the caregiver is likely to respond in ways similar to those adopted by a parent handling a difficult child. The resident may be publicly scolded or punished by having certain benefits withheld, whereas compliant behavior is rewarded.

WHAT CAUSES INFANTILIZATION?

The most straightforward explanation of infantilization is that it occurs as a function of the elderly adult's being placed in a dependent position with regard to the caregiver. As a result of being placed in this dependent position, the elderly person acquires by association the status of a child, who is also dependent relative to caregivers.[21]

Although both resident and caregiver are likely to make this association between dependence and childlike attributes, it is more probable that the caregiver will act on this association. The resident has an identity as an adult and a sense of continuity of the self over time. The caregiver, who has only seen the resident in the dependent position within the institution, lacks this reference point and sees the resident only as a frail elderly person no longer capable of self-care. In many ways, this situation is comparable to the fundamental attribution error described by social psychologists[22] in which observers discount the importance of situational variables when making judgments about the causes of a person's behavior. The caregiver attributes childlike qualities to the resident despite the obvious fact that the resident's physical frailty or illness has contributed to his or her need for institutional care.

The forming of an association between dependency and childlike status may begin the process of infantilization. Once set in motion, though, infantilization becomes a vicious cycle. The resident, feeling increasingly helpless and dependent, begins to regress behaviorally to the level of a child, and the more helpless the resident feels, the more this regression occurs. Regressive behaviors on the part of the resident trigger complementary behaviors in the staff as their view of the elderly person as a child is borne out. There is a tendency for staff to encourage dependent, compliant behavior and to ignore and even punish more competent, self-reliant behavior.[23] Furthermore, the control that caregivers have over the consequences of residents' behaviors makes residents highly dependent on how caregivers evaluate them. Scolding by caregivers or encouragement to be "good" only aggravates this regressive pattern.[24]

Adding to the regression shown by each resident individually may be interactive behaviors among residents that further confirm the caregiver's view that they are like children. The lack of privacy and space, combined with loss of control over their environment, may lead residents to become competitive and territorial about their claims to occupy certain areas of the institution or to receive certain rewards, such as food and materials. Residents may be drawn into fights and bickering among themselves as they struggle to maintain possession of what they perceive as limited resources to which they have no independent access. Such disputes may be likened by staff to the way that children fight in the playground for desirable toys or access to equipment. Similarly, if a resident complains about having a valued item taken away, this behavior can be used to justify the assertion that residents are like children who cry or become angry when they must give up or share a desired possession.

Not only are residents dependent on caregivers for material rewards, but they are also dependent on them for much of the affection and approval they experience in their lives. Seeing that childlike behaviors are given attention and rewarded may lead residents to enact these behaviors as a route to affection.[25] Furthermore, residents may be willing to put up with the patronizing behaviors of kissing, hugging, and touching for the sole purpose of maintaining human contact, even if it is degrading. In this regard, it is important to point out that caregivers who infantilize in this manner may be doing so out of the best of intentions, because they believe that the elderly residents appreciate this treatment, and, perhaps, because they have no other model of positively relating to residents. Indeed, when interviewed about their feelings toward their work, one sample of nursing assistants described themselves as nurturing, caring, and compassionate individuals who help the infirm elderly.[26]

Finally, infantilization may be furthered by sensory losses, disorientation, and confusion, which make the resident feel more helpless and lead to even greater dependence on caregivers for help in negotiating the environment. Caregivers also take on heightened importance for residents who feel isolated, abandoned, and lonely and cannot bring themselves to interact with other residents. The clearest way to receive attention from caregivers is to comply with the infantilization process by taking on childlike personal qualities.[27]

Professional caregivers are not the only individuals likely to infantilize the elderly. Family members may also become caught up in the process of seeing their elders as children. In part, this attitude is encouraged by popular characterizations of aging families, in which role reversal between adult children and their parents is regarded as almost an inevitable concomitant of the parents' aging process. Adult children may come to anticipate the moment when they will begin to parent their parents, and elderly parents, exposed to similar social attitudes, may unquestioningly follow through with complementary behavioral changes. An unfortunate consequence of the infantilization process when it occurs in the home is that the older adult's grandchildren are likely to take on similar infantilizing attitudes through modeling their own parents. In addition to developing this unfortunate way of behaving toward older adults, young people are more likely to develop negative attitudes toward old age because they associate it with childhood, a period of life they have just left behind. Similarly, adults are more likely to become "gerontophobic," because they are facing the prospect of an old age in which they will be treated like a child.[28]

WHO BECOMES INFANTILIZED?

The infantilization process may be expected to vary according to the individual characteristics of the resident and the standards or norms of the particular institution. The person-environment congruence model predicts that there are individual variations in the way that older adults adapt to the institutional environment. These variations are based on differences in physical status, functional competencies in the physical and cognitive domains, personal needs and motivations, and prior socialization. Two psychological constructs particularly relevant to institutional adaptation are expectancy of personal control[29] and coping strategy.[30]

By expectancy of personal control is meant the individual's sense of whether the outcomes of events in his or her life are determined by factors internal to the individual, such as quality of judgment or appropriateness of decision making, or by external factors, such as fate, chance, luck, or religious or political forces. Although having a sense of internal control over one's life is generally regarded as more adaptive and as enhancing feelings of well-being,[31] there are potential drawbacks, especially when, as in an institution, control is shifted to an external agency (i.e., the institutional staff and administration). In such cases, the individual might maintain adaptability by relinquishing personal control rather than fighting against a system which now, in fact, has control over his or her life.[32] The exception is if the individual is residing in a malleable environment in which autonomy and personal responsibility are fostered.[33]

The coping strategies an individual uses to manage stress are a separate but related dimension influencing quality of adjustment to the institution. Stress, in the context of the institution, may be seen as involved in the initial phases of relocation and as further involved in the day-to-day adaptation to the demands of institutional life, which are different from the demands of living in the community. Rather than being a direct function of events in the environment, stress is regarded as dependent on the individual's perception of a situation as overwhelming. The two types of coping strategies identified within the stress and coping literature are emotion-focused coping and problem-focused coping.[34] In emotion-focused coping, the individual attempts to reduce stress by changing the way the event is perceived so that it is no longer regarded as threatening. Emotion-focused coping strategies include avoidance, escape, and wishful thinking. None of these strategies causes the stressor to disappear, but the individual may feel less stressed and therefore better adapted. In problem-focused coping, the individual attempts to lower stress by changing something in the situation. There are also coping strategies that involve a combination of emotion- and problem-focused coping, such as seeking social support. When people reduce stress through social support, the situation may or may not be changed, but the actions involved in finding others to confide in can lower the perception of stress.

As with locus of control, coping strategies may be seen as more or less adaptive for certain situations. In a situation that cannot be changed, such as bereavement, emotion-focused coping is more adaptive in that the individual can at least eventually come to feel better about the loss. Conversely, problem-focused coping will be more successful if the threat represented by a situation can be reduced by taking some sort of action. In the institutional setting, emotion-focused coping would appear to foster adaptation to the environment. Assuming that the institutional environment is relatively unmalleable, the individual will adapt better by finding ways to feel better rather than by engaging in futile attempts to bring about change.

For the average institutional resident living in the average institutional environment, having an external locus of control and relying on emotion-focused coping would seem to result in the most positive adaptation, at least in terms of the individual's ability to fit into the surroundings.[35] Institutions run more smoothly when residents do not question or challenge the authority of staff, and those residents who manifest a compliant pattern of behavior are likely to be given more positive regard by staff and administrators. Some variation around this normative pattern may be satisfactory, though, particularly in institutions that allow greater autonomy for residents, have active resident governments, or have a resident population that is functioning at high levels of physical and cognitive ability.

In summary, to answer the question of who becomes infantilized, it seems reasonable to predict that this process will develop more rapidly in individuals who live in an environment that fosters compliance and who use modes of adapting to the environment that combine an external locus of control and emotion-focused coping. Less likely to become infantilized are those individuals who have an internal locus of control and rely on problem-focused coping. Whether these individuals continue to resist pressure to become infantilized may depend on the response of the environment to their behaviors and on their ability to resist the pressure to conform.

OUTCOME OF INFANTILIZATION

As the above discussion implies, individuals who have an external locus of control and use emotion-focused coping may be "happier" in the institutional setting because they see no reason to complain about what they are being offered. They may feel comforted by the knowledge that the institution is taking care of them and that the burden of decision making has been lifted from their shoulders. At a deeper level, the infantilization to which they become subject may provide them with feelings of being nurtured, of returning to an earlier state of dependence on parents. If these individuals have been socially isolated before their entry into an institution, the care and concern shown by staff may provide reassurance that they are valued for their personal qualities.

By contrast, individuals who maintain a sense of personal control, try to force change in a rigidly controlling institutional environment, and in the process take offense at being infantilized face a more difficult process of adjustment. It is likely that they will be labelled "troublemakers" and have even more of the autonomy they seek withheld from them. A vicious cycle is set into motion, in which the more these individuals protest, the more they stand to lose and the more likely it is that their resolve will give way to compliance at best or isolation at worst.[36] Unlike their counterparts who entered the institution with a more compliant attitude, these defiant individuals will find great difficulty in accepting institutional control and do so only at a great emotional cost.

Although it is important to identify both the favorable and unfavorable outcomes of infantilization, it is also crucial to identify the potential dangers of infantilization. As was just described, the autonomous individual is likely to become demoralized in an environment that stresses infantilization. The more compliant individual, though perhaps happier, nevertheless loses important adaptational skills. Just because it is more comforting to be infantilized does not mean that the individual is better served when treated like a child. Researchers have consistently demonstrated that the loss of autonomy and control has negative effects on the emotional, physical, and behavioral well-being of nursing home residents.[37] The encouragement of a more adultlike status and set of behaviors would seem to be advantageous for all institutional residents, since it would maximize their functional capacities for as long as possible. Unlike children, these older individuals have developed a set of adult coping skills and behaviors. Divesting them of these through infantilization leaves them as helpless as children at a time in their lives when they should be able to benefit from their wisdom, maturity, and life experiences.

HOW INFANTILIZATION CAN BE AVOIDED

If it is assumed that the outcome of infantilization is more negative than positive, then it would seem that this process should be averted in any way possible. Given the many factors that make it likely to occur in any given institution, administrators and staff must be vigilant in their efforts to eradicate infantilization and maintain an environment in which residents receive more adultlike treatment.

Perhaps the first step in avoiding infantilization is to change the perception by staff that the residents are dependent, and to do this, the residents need to be encouraged to act in more independent, adultlike ways. To facilitate this process, ingrained patterns in which staff take over the daily maintenance functions for residents must be broken by having staff make a conscious decision to encourage residents to do more for themselves without help. To implement this decision, staff can be trained in methods of reinforcing residents to become more independent, such as self-shaving, self-dressing, and self-eating.[38] With residents behaving more independently, staff will be less likely to regard them as childlike and helpless. Even when residents need assistance, they can be encouraged to make their own decisions.[39] To the extent that the institution can foster autonomy by giving residents a voice in the administrative policies, the sense among residents of personal independence can also be enhanced.[40]

A second method of combatting infantilization is to encourage staff to become more empathic to the feelings of residents when they are treated as children. One technique helpful in sensitizing students enrolled in courses on the psychology of aging is to use an infantilization exercise. In this exercise, an activities program is simulated in the classroom, and the students are put in the role of residents and are required to make "decorations" for the "dining room."[41] The decorations consist of simple drawings that the students color using crayons that are passed around. The students are infantilized by the instructor, who behaves toward them in an exaggeratedly patronizing manner, calling them "sweetie" and "dearie," insisting that they "color between the lines," and making a number of intrusive or embarrassing remarks about their personal appearance and demeanor ("Doesn't your hair look pretty today?"). Students resent this treatment, and although they soon gather that the exercise involves role-playing, they nevertheless demonstrate some of the key signs of infantilization, such as regression and compliance. Some students become enraged within the context of the role-playing, however, and refuse to follow the rules set by the instructor. After approximately 15 minutes, the instructor stops the exercise and opens the floor for discussion. Students express their feelings of powerlessness and irritation and recognize that if they were in such a situation in real life, they would feel humiliated and angry. Students who work in institutional settings claim that the experience alters their way of relating to the residents and that they will be on guard against infantilizing them in the future. Such an exercise, if redesigned to be more appropriate for institutional staff, could provide a valuable lesson in the dangers of infantilization.

A third way of focusing the attention of caregivers on the elderly resident as an adult is to emphasize the resident's life history and past accomplishments.[42] The assumption is that the more the resident is presented as an individual rather than as one of many people being cared for, the more likely it is that the resident will receive treatment that respects the resident's rights and adult status. Further, by emphasizing the resident's past achievements, in whatever arena these might be, caregivers can come to appreciate the talents and skills that the individual possesses and will thus be less likely to reduce the individual to the status of a helpless child.

Changes in the physical environment can serve to reduce infantilization by enhancing the resident's ability to negotiate that environment independently. In an environment in which the markings and directions are clear, residents will be able to find their way around without staff assistance. The more the environment encourages orientation, the less confused residents will be, decreasing their reliance on staff for assistance and contributing to the perception by staff that the residents are self-reliant. An environment that is decorated to reflect the personal interests of residents rather than the interests of staff can add to the focus on residents as adults with diverse and mature interests. Caregivers may be less likely to treat residents as children if the environment is not school-like in its appearance. With their personal possessions available in their surroundings, residents can gain greater satisfaction[43] and a sense of connectedness to their preinstitutional existence.

Providing an environment that allows for high levels of personal comfort, as perceived by residents, can also serve to enhance independence. In a more comfortable setting, residents are more likely to initiate activities themselves, to inter-act with each other socially, and to use their time more productively.[44] When residents are in surroundings they perceive as pleasant, they may feel more sup-portive of each other and are also more likely to find activities that they find per-sonally involving. Such changes not only build the self-esteem of residents but also lead to their behaving in ways that reinforce the staff's perception that resi-dents are self-directed and mature adults rather than children in need of guidance.

The last suggested intervention involves a more general approach—respecting the dignity of each resident as well as his or her feelings, type-of-care prefer-ences, and expressions of emotion. This intervention may require a two-way process, since residents, as a result of becoming infantilized, sometimes develop ways of relating to caregivers that are insulting, abusive, retaliatory, and deper-sonalizing. Staff also wish to be treated politely and with respect.[45] Helping resi-dents to recognize their own responsibility to treat staff courteously and considerately may break the destructive cycle that lowers the quality of interac-tions for both groups of participants.

IMPLICATIONS

This focus on infantilization as a central psychological issue in institutionaliza-tion has led to a set of recommendations that have broader implications for the long-term care of older adults. Infantilization is assumed to be a pervasive but relatively unrecognized problem of institutional life, and it is proposed that by reducing its prevalence some of the other difficulties involved in caring for the elderly can be ameliorated as well. If residents could live up to their functional capacity potential, the person-environment congruence model predicts that the institutional environment could be made more challenging. Caregivers would therefore find their workload reduced, if not made less burdensome, as more resi-dents become capable of self-care. For those residents who cannot achieve higher levels of self-care, staff would have more time available to provide support and structure.[46] Unfortunately, changes that promote independence may meet with resistance or with unresponsiveness on the part of caregivers unless caregivers have continuous in-service training.[47]

Improvements in the environment, such as increasing the level of stimulation, can indirectly enhance the morale of residents through the positive effects such stimulation has on caregivers.[48] Interventions designed to increase the quality and quantity of interactions between residents and caregivers can also be of value to residents,[49] since staff nurses can serve as an important source of social sup-port for residents.[50] Heightened contact of a social nature in a context in which residents and staff respond appropriately to one another can further break down the stereotypes that each group has of the other.[51]

By recognizing variations in the ways that people respond to the institutional environment, caregivers can become more attuned to the variations in people's needs for nurturance, on the one hand, and autonomy, on the other. Although attention to the psychological needs of residents cannot eliminate the physical diseases that require institutional care, such efforts can reduce the emotional discomfort of these diseases, both for the elderly residents and the caregivers.

NOTES

1. J.E. Birren, *Handbook of Aging and the Individual* (Chicago: University of Chicago Press, 1959.)

2. R.G. Kuhlen, Aging and Life-Adjustment, in *Handbook of Aging and the Individual,* ed. J.E. Birren (Chicago: University of Chicago Press, 1959).

3. F.M. Carp, The Impact of Environment on Old People, *The Gerontologist* 7 (1967):106–108; R.M. Coe, Self-Conceptions and Institutionalization, in *Older People and Their Social World,* ed. A.M. Rose and W.A. Peterson (Philadelphia: Davis, 1965); M.P. Lawton, How the Elderly Live, in *Housing and Environment for the Elderly,* ed. T.O. Byerts (Washington, D.C.: Gerontological Society, 1971); M.A. Lieberman, Institutionalization of the Aged: Effects on Behavior, *Journal of Gerontology* 24 (1969):330–340.

4. P.J. Biedenharn and J.B. Normoyle, Elderly Community Residents' Reactions to the Nursing Home: An Analysis of Nursing Home-related Beliefs, *The Gerontologist* 31 (1991):107–115.

5. S.J. Newman et al., Overwhelming Odds: Caregiving and the Risk of Institutionalization, *Journal of Gerontology: Social Sciences* 45 (1990):S172–183.

6. E. Kahana, A Congruence Model of Person-Environment Interaction, in *Aging and the Environment: Directions and Perspectives,* ed. M.P. Lawton, P.G. Windley, and T.O. Byers (New York: Garland STPM Press, 1980); M.F. Nehrke et al., Toward a Model of Person-Environment Congruence: Development of the EPPIS, *Experimental Aging Research* 7 (1981):363–379.

7. M.P. Lawton, Activities and Leisure, *Annual Review of Gerontology and Geriatrics* 5 (1985): 127–164.

8. J. Grimley-Evans, Prevention of Age-associated Loss of Autonomy: Epidemiological Approaches, *Journal of Chronic Disease* 37 (1984):353–363; P.A. Parmelee and M.P. Lawton, The Design of Special Environments for the Aged, in *Handbook of the Psychology of Aging,* ed. J.E. Birren and K.W. Schaie, 3d ed. (San Diego: Academic Press, 1990).

9. B.F. Hofland, Autonomy in Long Term Care: Background Issues and a Programmatic Response, *The Gerontologist* 28, suppl. (1988):3–9; S. Lemke and R.H. Moos, Measuring the Social Climate of Congregate Residences for Older People: Sheltered Care Environment Scale, *Psychology and Aging* 2 (1987):20–29.

10. R.A. Kane et al., Everyday Autonomy in Nursing Homes, *Generations* 14, suppl. (1990):67–71; S. Stein et al., Patients and Staff Assess Social Climate of Different Quality Nursing Homes, *Comprehensive Gerontology* 1 (1987):41–46.

11. J.F. Schnelle et al., Reduction of Urinary Incontinence in Nursing Homes: Does It Reduce or Increase Costs? *Journal of the American Geriatrics Society* 36 (1988):34–39.

12. C.W. Lidz and R.M. Arnold, Institutional Constraints on Autonomy, *Generations* 14, suppl. (1990):65–68; J. Wack and J. Rodin, Nursing Homes for the Aged: The Human Consequences of Legislation-shaped Environments, *Journal of Social Issues* 34 (1978):6–21.

13. J. Avorn and E.J. Langer, Induced Disability in Nursing Home Patients, *Journal of the American Geriatrics Society* 30 (1982):397–400; M.P. Lawton, Community Supports for the Aged, *Journal*

of Social Issues 37 (1981):102–115; P.A. Parmelee and M.P. Lawton, The Design of Special Environments for the Aged, in *Handbook of the Psychology of Aging,* ed. J.E. Birren and K.W. Schaie, 3d ed. (San Diego: Academic Press, 1990).

14. I. Milton and J. MacPhail, Dolls and Toy Animals for Hospitalized Elders—Infantilizing or Comforting? *Geriatric Nursing* 6 (1985):204–206; A.R. Tarbox, The Elderly in Nursing Homes: Psychological Aspects of Neglect, *Clinical Gerontologist* 1 (1983):39–52.

15. A. Arluke and J. Levin, Another Stereotype: Old Age as a Second Childhood, *Aging,* August 1984, 7–11.

16. E.H. Dolinsky, Infantilization of the Elderly, *Journal of Gerontological Nursing* 10 (1984):12–19.

17. D.C. Kimmel and H.R. Moody, Ethical Issues in Gerontological Research and Services, in *Handbook of the Psychology of Aging,* ed. J.E. Birren and K.W. Schaie, 3d ed. (San Diego: Academic Press, 1990).

18. L.R. Caporael, The Paralanguage of Caregiving: Baby Talk to the Institutionalized Aged, *Journal of Personality and Social Psychology* 40 (1981):867–884.

19. L.K. Wright, A Reconceptualization of the "Negative Staff Attitudes and Poor Care in Nursing Homes" Assumption, *The Gerontologist* 28 (1988):813–820.

20. M.D. Shulman and E. Mandel, Communication Training of Relatives and Friends of Institutionalized Elderly Persons, *The Gerontologist* 28 (1988):797–799.

21. A.R. Tarbox, The Elderly in Nursing Homes: Psychological Aspects of Neglect, *Clinical Gerontologist* 1 (1983):39–52.

22. L. Ross, The Intuitive Psychologist and His Shortcomings: Distortions in the Attribution Process, in *Advances in Experimental Social Psychology,* vol. 10, ed. L. Berkowitz (New York: Academic Press, 1977); see also S.T. Fiske and S.E. Taylor, *Social Cognition* (Reading, Mass.: Addison-Wesley, 1991).

23. M.M. Baltes et al., Further Observational Data on the Behavioral and Social World of Institutions for the Aged, *Psychology and Aging* 2 (1987):390–403.

24. A.R. Tarbox, The Elderly in Nursing Homes: Psychological Aspects of Neglect, *Clinical Gerontologist* 1 (1983):39–52.

25. L. Herst and P. Moulton, Psychiatry in the Nursing Home, *Psychiatric Clinics of North America* 8 (1985):551–561.

26. T. Heiselman and L.S. Noelker, Enhancing Mutual Respect among Nursing Assistants, Residents, and Residents' Families, *The Gerontologist* 31 (1991):552–555.

27. A.R. Tarbox, The Elderly in Nursing Homes: Psychological Aspects of Neglect, *Clinical Gerontologist* 1 (1983):39–52.

28. A. Arluke and J. Levin, Another Stereotype: Old Age as a Second Childhood, *Aging,* August 1984, 7–11.

29. J.B. Rotter, Generalized Expectancies for Internal versus External Control of Reinforcement, *Psychological Monographs* 80, no. 1, whole no. 609 (1966).

30. R.S. Lazarus and S. Folkman, *Stress, Appraisal, and Coping* (New York: Springer, 1984).

31. J. Rodin, Aging and Health: Effects of the Sense of Control, *Science* 233 (1986):1271–1276.

32. A. Antonovsky, *Health, Stress, and Coping* (San Francisco: Jossey-Bass, 1979); N. Krause, Stress and Coping: Reconceptualizing the Role of Locus of Control Beliefs, *Journal of Gerontology* 41 (1986):617–622.

33. E.J. Langer and J. Rodin, The Effects of Choice and Enhanced Personal Responsibility for the Aged: A Field Experiment in an Institutional Setting, *Journal of Personality and Social Psychol-*

ogy 34 (1976):191–198; J. Rodin and E.J. Langer, Longer Term Effects of Control-Relevant Intervention within the Institutionalized Aged, *Journal of Personality and Social Psychology* 35 (1977):897–903.

34. R.S. Lazarus and S. Folkman, *Stress, Appraisal, and Coping* (New York: Springer, 1984).

35. H.A. Davidson and B.P. O'Connor, Perceived Control and Acceptance of the Decision To Enter a Nursing Home as Predictors of Adjustment, *International Journal of Aging and Human Development* 31 (1990):307–318.

36. A. Arluke and J. Levin, Another Stereotype: Old Age as a Second Childhood, *Aging,* August 1984, 7–11.

37. M.M. Baltes and P.B. Baltes, *Aging and the Psychology of Control* (Hillsdale, N.J.: Lawrence Erlbaum, 1986).

38. D.J. Sperbeck and S.K. Whitbourne, Dependence in the Institutional Setting: A Behavioral Training Program for Geriatric Staff, *The Gerontologist* 21 (1981):268–275.

39. B.J. Collopy, Autonomy in Long Term Care: Some Crucial Distinctions, *The Gerontologist* 28 (1988):10–17.

40. J. Rodin et al., The Construct of Control: Biological and Psychosocial Correlates, *Annual Review of Gerontology and Geriatrics* 5 (1985):3–55.

41. S.K. Whitbourne, The Infantilization Exercise as a Teaching Tool in Courses on the Psychology of Aging, in preparation.

42. M.E. Pietrukowicz and M.S. Johnson, Using Life Histories To Individualize Nursing Home Staff Attitudes toward Residents, *The Gerontologist* 31 (1991):102–106.

43. G.C. Smith and S.K. Whitbourne, Validity of the Sheltered Care Environment Scale, *Psychology and Aging* 5 (1990):228–235.

44. C. Timko and R.H. Moos, Determinants of Interpersonal Support and Self-Direction in Group Residential Facilities, *Journal of Gerontology: Social Sciences* 45 (1990):S184–192.

45. T. Heiselman and L.S. Noelker, Enhancing Mutual Respect among Nursing Assistants, Residents, and Residents' Families, *The Gerontologist* 31 (1991):552–555.

46. S. Lemke and R.H. Moos, Personal and Environmental Determinants of Activity Involvement among Elderly Residents of Congregate Facilities, *Journal of Gerontology: Social Sciences* 44 (1989):S139–148.

47. J.F. Schnelle et al., Management of Patient Continence in Long-Term Care Nursing Facilities, *The Gerontologist* 30 (1990):373–376.

48. E. Kahana et al., Alternative Models of Person Environment Fit: Prediction of Morale in Three Homes for the Aged, *Journal of Gerontology* 35 (1980):584–595.

49. D.J. Sperbeck et al., Determinants of Person-Environment Congruence in Institutionalized Elderly Men and Women, *Experimental Aging Research* 7 (1981):381–392.

50. J.E. Bitzan and J.M. Kruzich, Interpersonal Relationships of Nursing Home Residents, *The Gerontologist* 30 (1990):385–390.

51. F.J. Vaccaro, Application of Social Skills Training in a Group of Institutionalized Aggressive Elderly Subjects, *Psychology and Aging* 5 (1990):369–378.

The Residents Speak Out

Seth B. Goldsmith and Roberta A. Bergman

An increasing number of complaints from the families of residents as well as an informal meeting with the ombudsman from the state department of elder affairs led the administrator of the Green Meadow Home to hire Gary Newman as an outside consultant to clarify the problems residents and their families were having with the home. Newman met with a number of residents and their families and felt the following four situations exemplified the state of affairs at the home.

1. Miss Fish, a 74-year-old woman who was never married, was admitted to the home six months before the meeting with Newman. Prior to her admission, which was precipitated by two massive strokes, she had lived independently and for 35 years had been an active volunteer at the Green Meadow Home. Her two sisters attended the meeting with Newman and told him that their formerly vivacious sister was now very withdrawn. After some probing by Newman, it came out that the sisters were quite frustrated because none of the staff seemed to have the time to deal with Miss Fish. In their opinion, this appeared to be because Miss Fish had lost her ability to communicate verbally. One sister said she was particularly disappointed because it seemed that everyone in the home was just interested in forcing Miss Fish to "become part of the system, you know what I mean: getting up when the nurses or aides want you up, eating when they want you to eat, going to the bathroom when it is convenient for the aides, sitting around the nurses' station ten hours a day, and going to sleep like a baby at 6:30 P.M. even in the summer when the sun is still shining!" The sister added that Miss Fish "deserves much better treatment, particularly in light of her years of contributions to the home."

2. Mr. Lester Mead is an 88-year-old man who has been a resident of the home for two years. In his meeting with Newman he stated, "Forty years ago I was a pretty well-off businessman in this town, and in fact I was one of the guys who raised the money to build this home. I frankly never thought I would ever live here. And when my wife and I moved to Sun City in Arizona, I never thought I would ever move back here to Metropolis. But here I am, my wife is dead, and my

only son lives 100 miles away. I look around and see many people who I used to associate with and see what they have become, and it is a scary sight! The thing I hate about this place is that there are many staff who don't respect old people. This is our home and we should be treated accordingly and we are not. And particularly me—I'm private pay, not one of those Medicaid patients."

3. Mrs. Meg Douglas also had some things that she wanted to share with Gary Newman: "I have been a resident of the home for four years. As you can see, I have had one leg amputated because of my diabetes. A few weeks ago I cut my index finger and told the aide that it looked like it was getting infected and asked her to tell the nurse. The nurse told her to tell me not to worry—so I didn't, until a few days later when my son came to visit and saw it and made a whole big stink on the floor about my care. He also called the administrator, and finally I was taken care of. But what could have been a small problem now took weeks to clear up, and because of my diabetes it might have had to be cut off. When the nurse was asked about it, she said she was never informed.... So she sided with the aide. I wish I could get out of this place!"

4. Mr. Max Stein is an 81-year-old man who has been a resident of the home for five years. He is one of ten Jewish residents in the home. Still ambulatory, Mr. Stein is one of the most physically active residents in the home. He met with Gary Newman to express his anger and outrage at the antisemitism displayed by some of the other residents, who he said have called him a range of offensive names. Mr. Stein said he handles these slurs by occasionally "smacking the bastard," but he added that he only does this if no one is looking. He also stated that he does not like to take the law into his own hands, "but nobody is doing anything about this problem here because we are such a small minority." Mr. Stein would not provide Newman with the names of the residents who had slurred him. In checking with the director of nursing and the administrator, Newman found no recollection of any resident complaining of being hit by another resident.

* * *

Discussion Questions

1. What problems are likely to be identified by Newman at the nursing home?
2. To what extent do the problems learned about by the consultant relate to the issues discussed in this chapter?
3. What steps can administration take to correct or minimize the problems presented in these situations?

Ethical Decision Making in Long-Term Care

Marian C. Broder

INTRODUCTION

Ethical issues have always been an integral part of health care delivery. Historically, discussion about these issues occurred primarily in hospitals. However, recently ethical issues are being examined in the long-term care setting.[1]

Nursing homes, having to cope with instituting ethical decision making, are attempting to redefine ethical principles to fit the long-term care environment. They are concerned with establishing policies, guidelines, procedures, and educational programs to guide residents, families, and staff in making ethical determinations. With the availability of technology and more skilled staff, higher levels of care are now being provided in nursing homes. Important decisions on how long technological support should continue and when appropriate circumstances exist for termination of care are being made with increasing frequency.

DIFFERENCES BETWEEN HOSPITALS AND LONG-TERM CARE FACILITIES

Consideration of ethical issues in hospitals is different than in long-term care institutions. In hospitals the patient is admitted, treated, and discharged. The length of stay is short. Medical treatment focuses on acute illness and recovery and, in many instances, uses technology. "Do not resuscitate" orders are for brief periods or for the duration of the hospitalization. Physicians dominate the decision-making process. Autonomy issues are dealt with according to a traditional model. If the patient has decision-making capacity, the patient makes the medical decisions. If the patient lacks the necessary capacity, a surrogate makes decisions on behalf of the patient using either the substituted judgment or the best interest standard.

The situation is totally different in long-term care facilities. In a nursing home, the stay is generally prolonged. The term *resident* instead of *patient* and the term *placement* instead of *admission* correctly suggest that a long-term care facility is primarily a home rather than a health care institution. The care is more often based on medical treatment or rehabilitative or palliative care rather than equipment and procedures. Treatment issues and decisions are made over a longer period of time rather than in response to an acute illness. The care team is interdisciplinary. The nursing staff is primarily responsible for providing care, and physicians play a smaller role than in the hospital. Physicians join with nursing staff; social workers; physical, occupational, and recreational therapists; and others in developing care plans. Because many residents have varying degrees of diminished mental capacity, decisions involving autonomy and other issues must respect individual variations and not be based on simple categorizations of residents as having or not having capacity. Finally, because of the length of the residents' stays, orders and directives for care must be periodically reviewed and kept current.

ADVANTAGES OF THE NURSING HOME ENVIRONMENT FOR ETHICAL DECISION MAKING

The nursing home has a responsibility to provide opportunities for ethical decision making. Education and communication must take place between the resident, the family, and the staff. Planning can be done in advance; the resident's values can be documented prior to a crisis. Conflicts can be anticipated and attempts made to avoid them. The interdisciplinary team of daily caregivers can be involved in decision making. As the resident's values or medical condition change, decisions can be reviewed, updated, and documented. Rather than merely mirror the hospital situation, the nursing home can proactively assist its residents and staff.

BASIC PRINCIPLES OF BIOMEDICAL ETHICS

Among the most basic principles of biomedical ethics are the principles of autonomy and beneficence.[2]

The term *autonomy* is derived from the Greek *autos* (self) and *nomos* (rule) and means self-rule. The principle of autonomy is that each individual should be in control of his or her own person, both body and mind. In the health care environment, the principle entails that each individual has a right to be free from nonconsensual interference with his or her body. Justice Cardoza, in 1914, stated that "every human being of adult years and sound mind has a right to determine what shall be done with his own body."[3] The doctrine of informed consent grew out of this. A competent individual has the right to accept or refuse medical treatment.

The principle of beneficence is that what is best for each person's welfare should be accomplished. It incorporates two obligations: the first is to do that which is for the good of the individual; the second is to do no harm to the individual (nonmaleficence). In some instances the two obligations must be balanced against one another, that is, the amount of good to be done balanced against the amount of harm. For instance, a resident with advanced terminal cancer may be offered chemotherapy, but the adverse side effects of the drug might increase the pain and suffering. Or in the case of a resident undergoing cardiopulmonary arrest, resuscitation may be offered. Although the procedure is frequently successful when administered to healthy individuals whose attack is witnessed by someone else, the procedure, when performed on nursing home residents, often results in fractured ribs, punctured lungs, and increased pain and suffering and has little chance of success.[4]

The principles of autonomy and beneficence come into conflict when an individual wishes to refuse a treatment that others believe would be beneficial. Generally the principle of autonomy has been accepted as primary in medical ethics and the principle of beneficence as secondary. However, in the nursing home setting, where state and federal regulatory policies to provide care must be complied with, the principle of beneficence may override the principle of autonomy.

Residents who are admitted to nursing homes with their full capacities can consent to admission and to medical treatment. However, residents who are suffering from substantial physical and mental difficulties are not able to exercise autonomy.

Autonomy in a nursing home environment must be defined and measured differently than autonomy in an independent living situation. In the latter, autonomy is characterized as freedom, self-choice, privacy, and control of decision making. Placement occurs when the individual, because of age, illness, dependent behavior, or dementia, requires personal and medical support. The nursing home, to meet both state regulatory standards and provide care in a cost-effective manner, has routines and schedules for eating, bathing, dressing, medications, activities, and bedtime that deprive residents of choices they would have had in independent living. Privacy in both living space and public space is limited. Some autonomy is sacrificed for the benefits of the care offered.

A report based on the Hastings Center Project on Responsible Caring: New Directions in Nursing Home Ethics urges that the concept of autonomy be rethought in the nursing home setting.[5] "Because of the limitations most residents face...and the social functioning of nursing homes,...autonomy and dependency cannot be seen as opposites. Instead, they must be seen as intertwined facets of one's life and one's state of being." Furthermore, the difficult problem of "justifiable limitations on individual freedom of choice and the institutional management of behavior" must be reconsidered.[6]

Some elderly residents prefer to delegate the primary responsibility for making their medical decisions to others (e.g., their physicians, family members, or friends). Although health care institutions and physicians should do all that is possible to encourage residents to make their own decisions, they should also recognize that autonomy includes the freedom of the individual to waive decision-making rights. However, before accepting and acting on the waiver of these rights, the physician should be certain that the person's preferences have been expressed unambiguously, that they are documented in the medical record, and that guidance has been given to the surrogate decision maker by the resident.[7]

MAXIMIZING AUTONOMY

An ethical goal of a long-term facility should be to maximize the autonomy of all residents within the facility. Historically, elderly patients have been treated in a paternalistic manner by physicians, staff, and family. Misconceptions exist about the degree of dementia in the elderly. Residents must be viewed individually and given the greatest possible opportunity to make their own decisions.

Initially the decision has to be made about whether the resident is competent or has decision-making capacity. Competency is a legal concept, and only through a formal legal proceeding can the determination be made that a person cannot make legally effective decisions regarding his or her own affairs. If the person is judged incompetent, a guardian is appointed by the court to make personal, financial, and medical decisions on the person's behalf.

Medical decision-making capacity is not strictly a legal issue. It must be determined by the physician in relation to the specific medical decision that must be made. Individuals with capacity are able to make their own decisions about medical care whereas those without capacity must have decisions made by a surrogate. The Massachusetts Health Care Proxy Law defines "capacity to make health care decisions as the ability to understand and appreciate the nature and consequences of health care decisions, including the benefits and risks of and alternatives to any proposed health care and to reach an informed decision."[8]

Residents should be given an opportunity to demonstrate their highest level of functioning. To protect the rights of the residents, facilities should develop guidelines to assist the medical staff in assessing a resident's capacity to give informed consent. Many different types of tests of capacity exist, and physicians should be able to provide the staff with examples of available tests.[9] Four standards that have been suggested are (1) the ability to communicate choices, (2) the ability to understand information about treatment decisions, (3) the ability to appreciate the situation and grasp the relevant consequences, and (4) the ability to manipulate the information provided in order to compare the benefits and risks of the various treatment options.[10]

Decisional incapacity is not always clear-cut. A medical determination should be made about the underlying cause of the loss of capacity. Capacity can fluctuate or waver. Incapacity can be a temporary condition resulting from a reversible physiological abnormality such as an illness, a physical or emotional trauma, overmedication, or another treatable condition. Efforts should be made to change the underlying situation. It is critical to identify and evaluate depression when determining competency to make medical decisions.[11]

To enhance the resident's autonomy, the assessment of capacity should provide specificity about particular decision-making responsibilities and not be global. Simple mental status tests can be used for an initial screening of mental function but do not provide details. Health care team members who observe the resident daily often can provide the necessary details better than a psychiatric or neurologic evaluation. For instance, a resident who cannot manage financial decisions may be able to decide about a roommate or surgery. Residents should be able to make the decisions that they are capable of making (e.g., residents who can no longer dress themselves should be encouraged to select the clothes that they wish to wear). Recognition should be given to lifetime patterns[12] (e.g., the resident who never ate breakfast should not be forced to eat in order to comply with state regulations). Expanded autonomy within the community improves the institutional environment and enhances the quality of the resident's life.[13]

The principle of autonomy must be balanced against the principle of beneficence when health care staff believe that the resident is making an incorrect treatment choice. The risks and benefits must be weighed. The resident's values, history, personal goals, motivation, immediate care goals, and long-term goals must all be built into the equation.

AUTONOMY IN MEDICAL DECISION MAKING

The Patient Self-Determination Act

Long-term care facilities can foster autonomy in medical decision making for their residents through policies and guidelines, an environment that fosters full disclosure, and a commitment to gaining truly informed consent regarding medical treatment. Residents must be informed of diagnosis, treatments, risks and benefits of treatments, prognosis with and without treatment, and alternatives. Paternalistic patterns of behavior by physicians and families, who tend to shelter the elderly from information in the belief that they do not want to or are unable to make decisions, must be changed.

The Patient Self-Determination Act requires facilities participating in Medicare and Medicaid to provide at time of admission written information about the rights of a patient under state law to make health care decisions.[14] Providers are required to provide state-specific information and documents. Included is the right to accept or refuse treatment and the right to execute advance directives. Facilities must inform residents of their policy on implementing advance directives. Documentation of whether or not an individual has executed an advance directive is to be placed in the medical record. The law does not require execution of an advance directive, nor can the provision of care be conditioned on whether or not an individual has executed an advance directive.

The Use of Agents and Directives

Autonomy for the resident can be furthered by encouraging the competent resident to appoint an agent to make future medical decisions for the resident when the resident can no longer do so and by encouraging the resident to express and document his or her values and opinions on treatment issues to that person. The resident is able to choose a person whom the resident trusts and who he or she believes will express his or her preferences.

The appropriate timing for this undertaking is difficult to determine. Each facility must establish a policy or set guidelines that reflect state regulations. Some facilities ask for this information at the time of placement. State regulations for nursing homes may require advance directive data to complete the medical record. Facilities subject to such regulations sometimes find it convenient to have new residents and their families complete the paper work at the time of admission. Family members, who are not always available, may be gathered together for this process.

Some argue, however, that admission is not a good time to complete advance directive documents. The process is stressful to a new resident and his or her family, and the resident should be given the opportunity to adjust to the facility prior to making advance directive decisions.

Many documents and planning tools are available: health care proxies, durable powers of attorney, advance or medical directives, living wills, and values statements. These documents vary according to state, and any documents completed by residents must conform to state law. Through a combination of one or more of these documents, the resident will be able to designate a surrogate and provide the information necessary to make the surrogate's decision reflective of the resident's viewpoint.

Health Care Proxy

A health care proxy is a legal document that allows a resident ("the principal") to appoint a person (the "proxy" or "agent") to make health care decisions for the resident if the resident no longer has the capacity to make or communicate those decisions. The proxy has the same access to medical information and the same authority to make decisions that the resident would have had if she or he could make decisions.

Durable Power of Attorney

A power of attorney is a legal document that allows a competent person to appoint an agent to act on his or her behalf for purposes that are described and limited in the document. Traditionally, the power of attorney has been used for financial and real estate purposes. A problem with the document was that its authority expired upon the "incapacity" of the principal and it could not be used for managing the affairs of elderly individuals who lost their capacity. To solve this problem, a durable power of attorney was developed. The authority of this document is not affected by the incapacity of the principal.

Durable powers of attorney for health care list specific powers to make health care decisions regarding, for example, the admission, discharge, or transfer of an individual to or from a health care facility; the selection of health care professionals to treat the individual; access to medical records; and consent to the provision of medical treatment, including the withholding or withdrawal of medical care.

Responsible Party

Responsible parties are required to cosign admissions agreements with the residents in many nursing homes. Generally they agree to fulfill certain obligations related to financial matters. The designation of someone as a responsible party does not give that person any power to make medical decisions; thus, a health care proxy or durable power of attorney must also be completed.

Advance Directive

An advance directive is a written statement that is prepared in advance of any serious illness and indicates how the person completing it wants medical decisions to be made if he or she no longer has the capacity to make or communicate the decisions. Included are instructions about medical treatments that the person wants or does not want and circumstances in which these instructions are to apply.

Advance directives take a number of different forms. Where state laws exist, the directives need to comply with the regulations or the form adopted in the state. Sometimes the health care proxy or durable power of attorney for health care document includes instructions about medical treatments that the person wants or wishes to avoid. Instructions may be included in a private letter using the person's own language or in a printed form. Forms are titled "Advance Directive" or "Medical Directive" or "Living Will" and include choices about specific treatments in specific situations.[15] For example, the form may list a treatment such as cardiopulmonary resuscitation or mechanical breathing and then list various situations in which a person may wish to have or not to have the treatment.[16]

Living Will

A living will is a type of advance directive or medical directive. It is a document in which a competent person provides directions regarding medical treatment in the event that the person can no longer communicate or make medical decisions. It is called a *will* because it expresses a person's will regarding medical treatment. It is called a *living* will because it takes effect before a person dies. Over 40 states have passed living will statutes. These statutes specify the types of decisions that a person can make and provide immunity to physicians and health care professionals for following the directives. Many living wills are limited to medical decisions regarding the withholding or withdrawal of medical treatment when an individual is terminally ill, is in an irreversible coma, or has "an incurable or irreversible mental or physical condition with no hope of recovery."[17]

Values History

A values history is a questionnaire that can assist a surrogate decision maker in predicting the preferences of the principal. Rather than asking a person about specific types of medical treatment, the questionnaire focuses on the "premises and processes" a person uses. It contains questions about "preferences in specific medical circumstances, general values, medical values, relationships with family, friends, and health care providers, religious views, financial preferences and other issues."[18] A values history can be used to motivate conversation between the resident and the surrogate. Through such conversations, the surrogate's ability to exercise accurate substituted judgment will be strengthened.

Periodic reviews of the directives and values history are necessary. Unlike hospitals, where the medical orders are of short duration, nursing homes may have residents with medical orders that are in effect for longer periods of time. It is necessary to have residents periodically review the documents to be certain that they still reflect their views. Some nursing homes look at these documents during regular review of residents' care plans. In addition, they request that, when there is a significant change in the resident's condition, the resident or his or her family review and update them.

Some ethicists and physicians advocate the use of the health care proxy or durable power of attorney for health care decisions. The advantage of these documents is that the physician can discuss the medical treatment with a person who has the legal authority to make a health care decision. Unlike a living will or medical directive, which specifies consent to or rejection of specific medical treatments and may be limited to certain medical conditions (such as terminal illness), a health care proxy or durable power of attorney gives the agent the flexibility to make all types of medical decisions in all circumstances. To safeguard this flexibility, it is advised that specific limitations not be written into the health care proxy or durable power of attorney document.[19] Principals are encouraged to inform their agents either orally or in a private letter of their preferences.

Selection of the Surrogate Decision Makers

Generally, when a nursing home resident no longer has the capacity to make health care decisions, an agent or a surrogate makes the decision on behalf of the resident. Deciding who is to be the surrogate decision maker is critical for ensuring the autonomy of the resident, whose own desires and preferences are intended to be reflected in the surrogate's decisions.

A clear-cut choice is made when the surrogate is appointed by a court through a guardianship proceeding or is designated by the resident through advance planning in the form of a health care proxy or a durable power of attorney. In some states, when there is no specific surrogate, statutes, regulations, or judicial precedents provide guidance. Without such guidance, it is customary for the decisions to be made by family members. This policy is based upon the belief that the family knows best what the resident would have wanted and has the resident's best interests in mind.

Although the process is time consuming and difficult, a nursing home, in order to protect the residents and itself, must develop policies and guidelines for informal substitute decision making. Copies of these policies and guidelines should be provided to residents and families at the time of admission. Consideration should be given to requiring a consensus among family members for any substitute decision. When there is disagreement among family members or the decision appears to contradict the implied preferences of the resident or contradict the position of the physician or staff, then the facility, for its own sake as well as for the sake of the resident, should encourage the family to initiate a formal legal intervention or should initiate a legal intervention itself to resolve the disagreement.[20]

Surrogate Decision Making

The surrogate, in making a decision, employs the substituted judgment standard, which requires the surrogate to try to determine what decision the principal would make if confronted with the situation at that time. In making the decision, the surrogate should have the same medical information that the principal would have had available, such as descriptions of diagnosis, prognosis, treatment, and risks and benefits. In addition, the surrogate must search for information that indicates how the principal would have decided. The surrogate may consider the resident's past preferences (expressed in writing or orally) and religious beliefs, the impact on the family, the extent of suffering, present and future incompetency, and other relevant factors. If the surrogate lacks such information, then the surrogate can make the decision based on the best interests standard, which requires the surrogate to choose what he or she believes would be in the best interests of the patient.

WITHHOLDING OR WITHDRAWING MEDICAL TREATMENT

One of the most critical ethical decisions in nursing home care is whether to administer or to withhold treatment that is within the scope of usual medical care. Withholding treatment is considered only when an individual is suffering, beyond hope of recovery, unable to respond to therapy, or living a life that the individual would not want to live. Withholding a necessary treatment might allow death to occur naturally and with dignity. Deciding whether to withhold treatment might involve subsidiary decisions regarding transfer to the hospital, surgery, cardiopulmonary resuscitation, the use of antibiotics, and nutrition and hydration. These decisions are made more difficult when the resident lacks the capacity to make them and had expressed no preferences prior to incapacity.

The objectives of the care for the resident must be set by the resident, the physician, and the family prior to making any decision regarding the withholding or withdrawal of medical treatment. Is the objective to restore the resident to a previous state? Is it to provide rehabilitation? Is it to prolong life? Is it to provide comfort? Is it to provide relief of pain and suffering?

Care planning requires adequate data. In the nursing home environment, there is generally adequate time for the compilation of the necessary information. Included should be an assessment of the resident's physical and emotional status; the prognosis with and without treatment; the risks and burdens of treatment; the resident's level of intellectual functioning; an assessment of the resident's quality of life; the previously expressed wishes of the resident and family; and the recommendations of caregivers, the family, and the physician. Ordinarily there should be consensus among the resident's family, the physician, and other health care workers. Data and decisions should be documented in the resident's medical record.[21]

Following is a suggested list of 11 questions that might provide a framework for making a morally and legally sound decision:[22]

1. Does the resident have a severe, progressive, imminently fatal disease?
2. Is the resident in an irreversible coma or a chronic vegetative state?
3. What steps have been taken to substantiate the diagnosis?
4. Is the therapy beneficial or is it burdensome or futile?
5. Does the patient want the therapy under consideration continued or stopped?
6. If the patient cannot communicate, what evidence is there of his or her wishes?
7. What does the family want?
8. Is the family united in their wishes for the resident?
9. Are all concerned parties communicating?
10. Has any concerned party been omitted from the decision-making process?
11. What is the law in the state regarding withholding or withdrawing therapy?

Facilities should have policies or guidelines on the process available as well as required information before making withdrawal or withholding decisions.

"DO NOT TRANSFER" AND "DO NOT HOSPITALIZE" DECISIONS

Decisions about where to undertake treatment occur frequently in nursing homes. Determining whether to issue a "do not transfer" or "do not hospitalize" order is among the most important ethical decisions made in long-term care. Hospitalization is required for evaluation and treatment, including surgery. Hospitalization decisions should be made in accordance with the treatment objectives for the individual. The benefits of hospital treatment must be measured against the risks of hospitalization. Frequently nursing home residents transferred to hospitals suffer confusion, falls, adverse drug reactions, bed sores, and infections.

Decisions not to hospitalize should not be absolute. In some instances, hospitalization may be required to alleviate pain and maintain comfort. For example, surgery may be necessary for broken bones or a laparotomy for a mechanical intestinal obstruction. Pneumonia or respiratory distress may require oxygen or parenteral antibiotics.

ALLEVIATION OF SUFFERING

The alleviation of suffering and pain and the provision of care and comfort should be part of every nursing home's medical treatment program. No resident should suffer from physical pain. Analgesic or psychoactive drugs used appropriately can provide comfort. Care plans that include skin care, turning, bowel and bladder management, and oral and eye hygiene can provide comfort to both residents and their families.

DEVELOPING AN INSTITUTIONAL FRAMEWORK FOR ETHICAL DECISION MAKING

Institutional policies and guidelines for ethical decision making have been devised by committees or departments, depending on the organization of the facility. Administrative, medical, and nursing staff adopt policies in response to government regulations. The Omnibus Budget Reconciliation Act of 1987 set the standards for patient rights. In some states, the Department of Public Health requires policies about cardiopulmonary resuscitation. Treatment, care, and competence decisions are made by the physician in consultation with the family and the resident. Issues of patient autonomy and self-determination are concerns of interdisciplinary committees developing individual care plans. Social workers deal with the issues of identifying surrogates for residents who are unable to speak for themselves.

Although nursing homes already have mechanisms for considering ethical issues, a centralized ethics committee can foster an institutional environment that is especially sensitive to such issues. The ethics committee can also bring medical, legal, social, and religious issues into consideration as well, and it can develop policies (mandatory) and guidelines (advisory) to handle ethical issues; educate residents, staff, family members, and the community about ethical issues and ethical analysis; perform case reviews; and provide consultation to residents, staff, and families.

Prior to developing guidelines and policies on specific issues, the ethics committee must define the value system or orientation of the institution. This is particularly true in a nonprofit religious institution, where religious views may establish the parameters for decision-making guidelines. When policies reflect these views, residents should be informed of them prior to admission.

Among the topics that the ethics committees consider are those related to end-of-life decisions (e.g., "do not resuscitate" and "do not transfer" orders and decisions to withhold or withdraw medical treatment or technology). When many residents have some form of cognitive impairment, the topics of competency, autonomy, valid informed consent, decision-making capacity, surrogates, and the role of the family in decision making become prominent. Legal and legislative changes as well as policies for advance directives, living wills, and durable powers of attorney for health care are also addressed. In addition, the ethics committees will probably be involved in case consultation regarding these very issues.

THE ETHICS COMMITTEE

There are guides published on how to start an ethics committee.[23] Defining the mission and purpose of the ethics committee will help determine its size and composition. Membership on a typical committee includes nurses, social workers, an administrator, a physician, an attorney, a clergy representative, and a resident or resident representative. Ombudsmen, family members, community members, and representatives from the board of trustees can also be included. If education is an important role of the committee, participation of the education director is essential. All participants must be aware of resident privacy and the duty of confidentiality in the discussion of cases.[24]

Educational Role

The educational role of the ethics committee is an important one. Through educational programs, the ethics committees can help to create an environment that supports ethical decision making by residents, family members, the clinical team, and the physician.

Initially, ethics committee members themselves need to be educated and oriented. Committee members must be given a common background understanding of the field of biomedical ethics and health care decision making. The concepts of autonomy, beneficence, and nonmaleficence must be defined and discussed. At each meeting, a case study or an article related to ethical issues can be reviewed. New members should be briefed on past committee decisions.

Educational programs should be planned for staff and families as well as residents. Movies, videos, discussion of articles, speakers, brochures, and visual displays can be used for educational purposes, as can ethics conferences or ethics rounds.[25]

Case Review Function

An ethics committee does both retrospective and concurrent case reviews. Retrospective case reviews assist the committee to identify clinical situations that require policies, guidelines, or educational programs. They assist committee members in evaluating their own ability to provide guidance on a particular issue and to interact with other nursing home committees.

In concurrent or advisory case review, the committee acts in a consultative capacity, providing assistance to residents, families, and staff. The committee must act skillfully and cautiously in order not to intrude on the physician-resident relationship or assume direct responsibility for resident care decisions. The advisory function should be assumed by the ethics committee only after it has completed its education and has developed policies and guidelines.

Each institution should have its own process for determining how cases are to be brought before its ethics committee and how the committee is to transmit its opinion to the parties. The process should identify who can contact the committee and how the contact should be made. Information gathering may be done by the whole committee or selected members. The committee generally meets in private and communicates its recommendations, either orally or in writing, to the person or persons referring the case and to the physician. Typically the recommendations of the committee are advisory and not binding.

CONCLUSION

There are many ethical issues that need to be resolved in the long-term care setting. As the resident population becomes more acutely ill and more cognitively impaired, residents, families, and staff will need to confront these issues. Facilities should develop and implement policies and guidelines. There should be an initial focus on methods to increase the autonomy of each resident. Equally important are policies related to termination of medical treatment, resident competence, resident autonomy, and choosing surrogates. Staff particularly need educational programs and case review to assist them in understanding and carrying out clinical decisions based on bioethical principles.

NOTES

1. P. Boyle and B. Jennings, eds., *Responsible Caring: Ethics Resources for Nursing Homes* (Briarcliff Manor, N.Y.: The Hastings Center, 1991); R.A. Kane and A. Caplan, eds., *Everyday Ethics: Resolving Dilemmas in Nursing Home Life* (New York: Springer, 1990); M. Waymack and G. Taler, *Medical Ethics and the Elderly* (Chicago: Pluribus Press, 1988).

2. T. Beauchamp and J. Childress, *Principles of Biomedical Ethics* (New York: Oxford University Press, 1989).

3. Schloendorf v. Society of New York Hospital, 211 N.Y. 125, 105 N.E. 92 (1914).

4. D.J. Murphy, Do-Not-Resuscitate Orders: Time for Reappraisal in Long-Term-Care Institutions, *JAMA* 260:2098–2101.

5. B. Collopy et al., New Directions in Nursing Home Ethics, *Hastings Center Report* 21, suppl. (March-April 1991):1–16.

6. Ibid., 3.

7. M. Knapp, Medical Empowerment of the Elderly, *Hastings Center Report* 19 (July-August 1989):5–7.

8. *Massachusetts General Laws,* Chapter 201D.

9. J. Janofsky et al., The Hopkins Competency Assessment Test: A Brief Method for Evaluating Patients' Capacity To Give Informed Consent, *Hospital and Community Psychiatry* 43 (February 1992):132–136.

10. P. Appelman and T. Grisso, Assessing Patients' Capacities To Consent to Treatment, *New England Journal of Medicine* 319 (1988):1635–1638.

11. E. Howe et al., Medical Determination (and Preservation) of Decision-Making Capacity, *Law, Medicine, and Health Care* 19 (Spring-Summer 1991):27–33.

12. B. Collopy, Autonomy in Long Term Care: Some Crucial Distinctions, *The Gerontologist* 28, suppl. (June 1988):10–17.

13. B. Collopy et al., New Directions.

14. The Patient Self-Determination Act, passed as Sections 4206 and 4751 of the Omnibus Budget Reconciliation Act of 1990.

15. L. Emanuel et al., Advance Directives for Medical Care: A Case for Greater Use, *New England Journal of Medicine* 324 (1991):889-895; L. Emanuel and E. Emanuel, The Medical Directive: A New Comprehensive Advance Care Document, *JAMA* 261 (1989):3288–3293.

16. Ibid.

17. Living Will Declaration, Society for the Right to Die, 250 West 57th Street, New York, NY 10107.

18. P. Lambert et al., The Values History: An Innovation in Surrogate Decision-making, *Law, Medicine, and Health Care* 18 (Fall 1990):202–212.

19. G. Annas, The Health Care Proxy and the Living Will, *New England Journal of Medicine* 324 (1991):1210–1213.

20. M. Knapp, Family Decisionmaking for Nursing Home Residents: Legal Mechanisms and Ethical Underpinnings, *Theoretical Medicine* 8 (1987):259–273.

21. R. Besdine, Decisions To Withhold Treatment from Nursing Home Residents, *Journal of the American Geriatric Society* 31 (1983):62–66; J. Lynn, Ethical Issues in Caring for Elderly Residents of Nursing Homes, *Primary Care* 13 (June 1986):295–306.

22. R. Carlton, Defining the Limits of Treatment: When May It Be Withheld or Withdrawn? *Journal of Critical Illness* 6 (February 1991):138–147.

23. J.W. Ross, *Handbook for Hospital Ethics Committees* (Chicago: American Hospital Publishing, 1986); R.E. Cranford and A.E. Doudera, eds., *Institutional Ethics Committees and Health Care Decision Making* (Ann Arbor, Mich.: Health Administration Press, 1984).

24. B. Brown et al., The Prevalence and Design of Ethics Committees in Nursing Homes, *Journal of the American Geriatrics Society* 35 (1987):1028–1033.

25. L. Libow et al., Ethics Rounds at the Nursing Home: An Alternative to an Ethics Committee, *Journal of American Geriatrics Society* 40 (1992):95–97.

Ethics in Long-Term Care: Withholding or Withdrawing Artificial Nutrition and Hydration

Marian C. Broder

Mr. M. is an 85-year-old nursing home resident with Alzheimer's disease, intermittent confusion, and memory loss. Two years ago, following the death of his wife, he entered the nursing home. Although he needed assistance with most activities of daily living, Mr. M. could walk without help and was oriented to place and time. He was sociable and engaged in conversation. His daughter visited daily, and his son, who lived out of town, telephoned his father monthly but had not visited his father in the two years since his mother's funeral.

Recently, Mr. M. began to refuse food and lost a great deal of weight, then had pneumonia and congestive heart failure. His physician recommended transfer to the hospital for treatment with intravenous antibiotics and the possible insertion of a nasogastric tube to help maintain adequate nutrition. These medical treatments would treat his illness and maintain him at his previous level of function.

The physician did not think that Mr. M. had sufficient decision-making capacity to make medical decisions regarding hospitalization, antibiotics, or the insertion of a feeding tube. He had no advance directives, health care proxy, or durable power of attorney for health care. His daughter was away on a vacation and could not be reached. The physician therefore telephoned the son to discuss the recommendations. The son agreed with transfer to the hospital and treatment.

After admission, Mr. M. was started on antibiotic therapy and a nasogastric tube was inserted. During his hospitalization, Mr. M. suffered a stroke that left him totally disoriented, confused, and unable to speak or move his right side. He made minor movements of his head and neck. He did not apparently recognize anyone, but he could follow people with his eyes although he generally kept them closed. He moaned a lot. The hospital discharged Mr. M. back to the nursing home with the nasogastric tube still in place as he was totally dependent on the tube for nutrition and fluids.

The physician and the nursing home staff developed a care plan to introduce food to Mr. M. and to remove the tube. He refused to eat, turned away his head, and kept his lips closed. He tried to pull out the tube. The nursing home staff had to restrain his left hand so that he could not remove the tube. The hand restraint made him very agitated. Mr. M.'s health continued to deteriorate and he developed decubitus ulcers and a recurrent urinary tract infection.

Upon her return, the daughter told the physician that her father never would have wanted to live like this. She said he used to say that he had lived long enough. She felt that when his death was imminent, nothing extraordinary should be done for him. Although he could not talk, she was certain that by refusing food and trying to pull out the tube he was trying to say that he had had enough. She said that had she not been on vacation she would never have approved having the tube inserted in the first place since that is not what her father would have wanted. The daughter asked the physician to remove the nasogastric tube.

The physician said that she did not believe that the resident's condition would change or that medical intervention would produce any improvement or promote the restoration of health and function. The tube feedings merely maintained the status quo and if the feeding tube were removed, death would probably result within a few days or weeks. She believed that its removal would not cause him discomfort and that he could be provided with supportive care and comfort measures such as skin care, ice chips, lip lubricant, turning, and eye and mouth hygiene.

The physician discussed the removal of the tube with Mr. M.'s son as well and learned that the son still wanted everything done. He told the doctor that his sister might not be thinking clearly about the tube removal since she frequently expressed to him how burdened she felt by the responsibility of always having to visit the father.

Members of the health care team were divided on the issue of removing the nasogastric tube. Some of the nurses who had cared for him prior to his stroke believed that he would not have wanted to live this way. Other nurses said that removal of the tube would be killing him and that they would have no part of it.

The physician asked that the case be referred to the ethics committee for guidance. The ethics committee members asked the social worker to compile information from each of the parties to present to the committee. The following is a summary of the social worker's report.

Daughter. The daughter lived in the same city as her father and had been involved with the medical care of both her parents. Her mother had died two years ago. After her mother's death, she did everything possible to keep her father at home because his independence was important to him. She hired private duty companions for him. However, when he became a physical danger to himself, leaving the gas stove burners on or wandering out at night, she had to admit him to the nursing home. He always said when he watched his wife suffer and lie in a coma before her death that he never wanted to live that way and never wanted anyone to keep him alive with tubes and machines if he did not know who or where he was.

The daughter said that her brother had not been home during the two years since their mother's funeral. She believed that her brother was remembering their father as he last saw him and that he might not insist on continuing life support measures if he could see their father as he was today. She also felt that her father and brother had a difficult relationship and speculated that some of those feelings might be influencing her brother in his recommendations.

Individual nurses had spoken to the daughter about the feeding tube. Since the nurses and nurses' aides had differing opinions, this only confused the daughter. While she valued their opinions, she felt that some of them had exceeded their professional roles in telling her what to do.

Nurses. The nursing staff on the unit, especially the aides, said that they had been taking care of Mr. M. for several years and knew him better than his own family. They felt that they should be included in the decision-making process and allowed to express their opinions.

One group of nurses who had cared for Mr. M. since he was admitted to the home said that he would never want to be dependent on a feeding tube. They spoke of his strong drive to be independent. Prior to his stroke, he took pride in the things he could do for himself and became frustrated when he needed assistance. In his more lucid moments he commented that he did not want to become bedridden like some of the other residents on the unit.

Other unit nurses expressed a personal view that they were ethically and morally opposed to removing a feeding tube. They believed they would be starving Mr. M. to death by withdrawing the feeding tube and that it was against the law and a violation of professional nursing ethics that required them to preserve life. They believed that he would experience great pain and suffering if the tube were withdrawn. The difficulty in the case, for one nurse, was that Mr. M. was not dying from a terminal illness nor in a persistent vegetative state.

Social Worker. The social worker had a list of her own concerns. First, Mr. M. had no advance directives or health care proxy. She was concerned with the need to substantiate Mr. M.'s views on what he would have wanted if he were able to make the decision for himself. Since there were no documents prepared, this information would have to be gathered from Mr. M.'s previous statements and life style. Comments from family, physician, staff, and others would be important. She was concerned that the family members might be making decisions reflecting their own views and not those of their father.

Second, she was concerned that the conflict between the brother and sister and the members of the health care team be resolved. She wanted to encourage the son to see his father and to meet with the physician and his sister prior to any final decision being made. It was important to have consensus between the sister and the brother since they would have to live with this decision for the rest of their lives. She was also concerned about the liability of the nursing home if the dispute could not be resolved and the decision was made based on the opinion of only one of the children.

Third, the social worker was concerned about the staff's need for involvement in decision making and also for education in end-of-life decisions, including medical, nursing, ethical, and legal issues. She wanted a meeting to be held wherein the staff and family members could discuss their views. She was concerned that individual nurses were sharing their opinions with the daughter in an informal method. She believed that staff who were opposed to the decision should not have to care for Mr. M. if the tube were withdrawn.

Physician. Once the resident's condition had changed because of stroke, the physician believed that there was no chance of improvement and no way to restore Mr. M.'s health or function. She believed that the tube feeding was nonbeneficial and was actually burdensome to him since he had to be restrained not to pull out the tube. If the tube were to remain, the alternatives were to sedate him sufficiently so that he would not pull out the tube or to surgically insert a gastrostomy or jejunostomy feeding tube.

She believed that artificial nutrition and hydration were forms of medical treatment that could be discontinued when they no longer produced improvement and that as a physician she was not required to continue futile treatment.

* * *

Discussion Question

1. What recommendations should the ethics committee make regarding the decision maker? the care plan? the withdrawal of the feeding tube? the involvement of the staff?

Chapter 4

Management of Long-Term Care Organizations

Seth B. Goldsmith

The management of long-term care organizations presents a unique challenge in the field of health care administration. This uniqueness results from the particular circumstance that long-term care organizations are both social and clinical institutions in which residents, and to a lesser extent families, are totally immersed as full-time members of an organic community. For the residents, the nursing home is the place where they live, work, play, grow older, and, in time, die. For the nursing home manager, the job is a 24-hour-a-day commitment that encompasses all the facets of running a labor-intensive and expensive medical institution plus those of managing a housing complex and a social services program. This chapter explores the role and function of management in nursing homes by first defining management and then developing a challenge for management. Next, there is an examination of the functions of management, followed by an analysis of the special challenges of management in nursing homes. Then the chapter looks at what is expected of managers and concludes with an analysis of ideas that prospective nursing home managers might consider in deciding whether to enter the critical field of long-term care management.

DEFINING MANAGEMENT

Virtually every textbook dealing with management at some point offers the reader a definition of the subject. For example, in 1947, Cornell answered the question, What is management? by noting, "The work of management is to plan, direct and control the organization and to weave together its various parts so that all factors will function properly and all persons cooperate—that is, work together efficiently—for a common purpose."[1]

In perhaps one of the grandest understatements, Drucker, in his best-selling book *Management*, suggests that "management is tasks, discipline, people and practice."[2] Management must be viewed as both an art and a science. On one hand, it deals with sharply defined areas, such as productivity and efficiency, that are exemplified best in current times by the operations research–management science approach to problem solving. On the other hand, it also deals with more diffuse areas, such as leadership and motivation.

THE MANAGERIAL CHALLENGE

For a manager, this sets up the following challenge: How does a manager construct or reconstruct an organization so that it maximizes efficiency and effectiveness for its various external constituencies and simultaneously minimizes stress, disaffection, and unhappiness for its internal constituencies? It should be recognized that this statement of the problem or challenge is value laden, as are most definitions of management and concepts of the manager's role. The emphasis in this statement is on satisfying external constituencies, performing efficiently in economic and financial terms, being effective, and, finally, respecting the human dignity of workers. If, for example, workers are considered drones, peasants, or simply inputs for a resource system, the challenge might be restated to eliminate concern for disaffected workers. Indeed, the manager's concept of the meaning of work can dramatically shift his or her perspective.

A management approach based on a value system—and all approaches are based on a value system to some degree—must examine that system if it is to be responsive and continue to function as a mechanism of achieving organizational goals.

THE FUNCTIONS OF MANAGEMENT

The specific activities of management vary from one organization to another, as well as from time to time in the same organization. The sum total of management in an organization tends to be relatively stable, however; the same managerial functions are carried out in all organizations, although circumstances, organizational needs, and personalities dictate which of these functions predominates at any given time. The most often cited management functions are planning, organizing, staffing, directing, controlling, coordinating, and representing.

Planning

Planning involves those activities associated with setting objectives, making policy, and creating strategies for attaining the objectives within the organizational policy framework. It is considerably more difficult to identify objectives, particularly in the health field, than it appears at first glance. Organizational objective setting is a process that requires global vision, diplomatic skill, and considerable good fortune. Planning normally results in an output—a written plan. Such a document can cover time frames that vary from rather short periods, such as six months or a year, to periods as long as five or ten years. An effective plan results in a positive outcome for the organization; a bad plan has the potential to destroy an organization.

Because of their size and organizational depth, most free-standing nursing homes, as opposed to those belonging to a for-profit or nonprofit chain, do not have a full-time planner. Rather the responsibility for planning is in the hands of the owner, board planning committees, and, quite clearly, management. The actual development of a plan or plans may be a group activity involving the aforementioned people and groups and, with increasing frequency, consultants. The role of a consultant in the planning function is to introduce into the planning process a level and range of expertise not available in the organization. However, the value of the consultant's work is significantly related to the quality of input the consultant receives from the nursing home's management. Indeed, it is an illusion to think that top management can delegate the responsibility or authority for planning to a planner or consultant.

In the best of situations, a plan functions as an organizational control device. With a plan, management can continually identify expectations (goals) for people, programs, or projects and measure the progress and the rate of progress being made toward these goals. In some cases, a manager will prefer to utilize the lack of a plan as a control device for the organization; the only plan is what is in the manager's head. In this way, the manager maintains total control and great flexibility but reigns over a situation that may often be close to disaster.

Organizing

Organizing is a second function commonly associated with management. This is the function of determining what activities will be carried on by the nursing home, how these activities should be grouped, and who shall have the authority and responsibility for carrying out these activities. The organization chart is the graphic representation of the decisions made regarding this function.

In nursing homes, legal and fiscal constraints, including Medicaid and Medicare reimbursement formulas, may dictate the most cost-effective organizational structure. For example, during a two-year period, I observed a staff member shifted to three different units as the result of an administrative search to find a way to get a state Medicaid program to pay her salary. Tradition and a sensitivity to professionalism will often dictate a particular configuration, as evidenced by the fact that nursing directors rarely report to anyone other than the chief executive or chief operating officer. Similarly, it would be a rare nursing home where a director of food services reported to the head of nursing.

Although organizing and reorganizing seems to be in the blood of managers, it should be recognized that reorganizations are often not the solution to deep-seated organizational problems. Indeed, shifting mediocre staff members to new organizational boxes usually provides the illusion but not the substance of positive change. To have the substance of change, nursing homes, which are like most other health care organizations in being basically labor-intensive, must not merely change the organizational structure but also focus on getting the right people the first time. And that is the task of the staffing function.

Staffing

Staffing is perhaps the most obvious and most critical of management functions. Basically, it involves getting the right people for the jobs and developing them. To be most effective in this managerial area, the executive and his or her staff must be adept at using personnel management tools such as job descriptions and specifications, be fine judges of character, and be master detectives capable of ferreting out what is between the lines of a letter of recommendation.

For any organization, the cost of each new hire is extremely high. This cost involves all expenses related to recruiting, training, and turnover. Fortunately, a nursing home will sometimes find superb people who easily fit into the organization and develop with the job. Occasionally, however, much time, money, and energy will be expended on someone who must be terminated, with all the attendant costs and ill will.

The unfortunate reality is that for many people nursing home jobs are viewed as second choice positions in the health field. The challenge that management must accept is to convince potential recruits of the importance and indeed excitement of a position in long-term care, plus the possibility of a fulfilling career.

However, if employees are to avoid dead-end jobs and management is to make good on its promises, management must take a number of important steps. First, it must be philosophically committed to the professional development of each employee. Second, it must provide financial support for a broad range of development activities, such as taking academic courses, attending in-service training, and going to professional meetings. Finally, management must be prepared to support an employee's advancing career, which may mean giving hiring preference to internal candidates, developing clearly defined career ladders, and encouraging excellent but underemployed staff to leave the organization and develop their careers in a different organization.

In sum, staffing is a process that begins with the identification of an organization's staff needs and continues through staff development. The job of management is to avoid mistakes and develop potential. Mistakes can most often be avoided if managers pay as much attention to process and requirements as they pay to "feel" or "intuition." Too often people are hired because of a good interview that has not been confirmed by a review of credentials, recommendations, or second interviews. Once the "right" decision has been made, the new employee, if he or she is to be most valuable to the organization, must be supported in the development of his or her potential.

Directing

Directing is the function most often associated with management. Indeed, in many instances the title of the most senior administrator is Executive Director.

Directing is also the function most associated with the image of managers as individuals who sit in their offices, no doubt quite removed from any part of the operation, and bark out orders to a compliant group of employees. Except in rare cases, this is a fantasy. Managers may like to view themselves as the captain of a ship, but their word is no longer the law. Rather, they must use their position to guide, persuade, or coach subordinates. Even in highly bureaucratic organizations, such as universities or hospitals, management is by consensus, and the effective manager must shepherd subordinates toward agreement.

In practice, directing an organization is not giving orders or commanding staff, it is closer to pointing out a direction or goal and leading employees toward the goal by coaching, training, encouraging, and occasionally commanding and threatening.

Controlling

Controlling is based on the measurement of performance against predetermined standards. Two elements must come together if the manager's control is going to be effective: There must be standards, and there must be information systems to indicate the progress that is being made toward meeting those standards.

Standards can range from performance indicators to budget indicators. For example, assume a manager has set standards for the marketing representatives, such as 25 confirmed and signed contracts with deposits by a given day. The goal is clear and both the manager and marketing representatives are able to measure progress toward the goal. A more ambiguous target, "Do the best you can," results in confused expectations as well as the possibility of unfair managerial practices.

Setting the standards against which an employee's or unit's performance will be measured is difficult in long-term care because of the complexity and diffuseness of mission of most long-term care organizations. If, for example, the goal is to enhance the quality of care given to residents, how does one measure success? Is it merely the amount of care given? A decrease in complaints? An increase in resident or family satisfaction? A decrease in bedsores, falls, or medication problems? Unfortunately, the waters are a bit murky when it comes to quality of care and quality of life issues.

On the other hand, managers can exercise a considerable amount of control through the budgetary process. In this process, usually after a complicated and protracted negotiation, a unit can project its revenues and expenses and be given the funds to meet its goals. When this occurs, management's job is to track progress toward the goal and follow up on deviations from the budget plan. Finally, management is responsible for decision making to solve or mitigate mid-budget problems.

Coordinating

Coordinating is one of the least important functions. Traditionally, a coordinator has plenty of responsibility and little authority—analogous to the carpenter who is given wood and nails but no hammer. It appears that the most successful coordinators are those with real or apparent authority, a total commitment to the program, or extraordinary skills as a persuader. To put it differently, important managerial problems are often too deep-rooted to be solved through coordination. They must be "managed" in an affirmative manner.

Representing

The seventh traditional function is representing—being the spokesperson for the unit, organization, or industry. A department head represents the department and its case on the division level, and the director represents the organization to the government, a foundation, or even the board.

Representation is a critical managerial function. Those at the top of each component usually represent the component to those at the next higher level. Representation is a time- and energy-consuming function that requires a political sensitivity to the needs of a constituency (or unit) and a similar sensitivity to the needs of those to whom the constituency is being represented. Presentation, debate, analysis, and articulation skills are critical, since they can help to influence the opinions of those who are listening to the presentation.

SPECIAL CHALLENGES OF NURSING HOME MANAGEMENT

Nursing home management has its own special set of challenges that are related to the mission of nursing homes, their relatively small size, and the particular situation of nursing home residents.

The first of these challenges is a function of the complex mission of long-term care organizations—providing quality of care services and quality of life services to the elderly. The two goals are difficult to quantify and are often elusive. For management, whether dealing with a board of a nonprofit facility or the owners of a proprietary home, this apparent diffuseness of mission consistently presents problems. For example, how does one argue for more resources such as an additional staff person in the activities department when the person is not required under state law and you can only hypothesize that an increased staffing level will enhance the quality of the residents' experience?

Equally problematic for managers is the issue of the "bottom line" and its relationship to mission. Virtually every decision is likely to have an impact on the profitability of the home, and the balancing act between money and mission is a delicate one. Consider again the decision whether to hire an additional activities staff person. The cost of hiring, perhaps $20,000, can represent a significant part of a proprietary home's annual profit or require considerable fund-raising activity for the nonprofit home.

A second issue that differentiates nursing home management from other areas of health care administration is the size of nursing homes, which tend to be small and intimate and have a small but quite consistent set of clients. The manager of a typical 100-bed home might have to work with 85 employees organized into three shifts. Additionally, the residents are likely to have an average length of stay of two and a half to three years. This means that residents (and their families) inevitably become knowledgeable about the home and often quite demanding about what happens in it. The administrator also becomes an intimate friend and counselor to residents and families, a role absent from a hospital, where a patient's total stay is usually five or six days.

A third challenge relates to the government oversight of nursing homes. For a host of reasons, some legitimate, others questionable, nursing homes are simply not trusted by society. The result of this is myriad regulations and inspections. For the manager, this means a constant flow of outsiders evaluating the home and causing disruption and periodic ruffled feathers. The manager is responsible for representing the home—dealing with deficiencies, correcting what needs to be corrected, and sometimes challenging the findings and conclusions of the outside experts. The manager must also show constant vigilance in trying to detect changes on the horizon that could affect the organization, such as reimbursement formulas or eligibility criteria for admission. Vigilance allows the manager to plan and organize political activity to help the home and its residents.

A final crucial challenge is dealing with a staff that must work on a daily basis with people who are getting older and sicker and dying. Additionally, the staff members themselves are aging and perhaps becoming less physically able to deal with the constant demands of assisting residents with their activities of daily living.

Thus, in a sense, the nursing home manager functions as the mayor of a small community who is called upon to perform an extraordinarily broad range of functions. As often happens in small and intimate organizations, management operates in the proverbial fishbowl. Indeed, in most nursing homes, there are few secrets and little that escapes the scrutiny and evaluation of staff and residents. Additionally, because of the visibility and accessibility of managers, they are not insulated from the impact of their decisions.

To effectively deal with these challenges, management must act in a manner that is consistent and equitable. To not act in such a way is to court disaster by demoralizing the staff and residents. Yet, although the balancing act in management is difficult, the rewards are high. Nursing home management is perhaps the one type of health care management that presents opportunities for a single administrator to have a dramatic impact on an organization. Indeed, in many nursing homes the administrator wields a significant amount of power, often substantially more than a hospital's administrator might wield. This power, which may be related to the lack of a medical staff or the relatively small size of the management team, means that nursing home managers have the opportunity to truly manage their organizations.

EXPECTATIONS FROM MANAGERS

What should be expected from a manager? In answering this question, two dimensions must be considered: behavior and values.

Both fiction and reality present a picture of managers as "organization men." Their loyalty is to the organization, and the most important professional person in their lives is their boss. The image is of a tight hierarchical structure and operations that respond to that structure. Regardless of the theoretical "flatness" of an organization, there is always someone on the top who has the authority and responsibility to represent the organization and negotiate in its interest—at least that person's conception of its interest.

A clear example of this is the attempted takeover of McGraw-Hill by American Express. This takeover was viewed as an anathema by McGraw-Hill's chairperson, Harold McGraw, Jr. Because of his personal view, he waged a relentless and successful campaign against the invasion. He stated in a letter to the chief executive officer of American Express that American Express lacked "integrity, corporate morality and sensitivity to professional responsibility." He went on to criticize the management and behavior of American Express. All of this was done with the express approval of stockholders, many of whom clearly stood to gain by such a merger.[3]

A different perspective on management is presented by Michael Blumenthal. During his tenure as Secretary of the Treasury, he prepared an article for *Fortune* titled "Candid Reflections of a Businessman in Washington."[4] In it, he contrasted his experiences as a senior government official in charge of an agency employing 120,000 people with his experiences as chairperson and chief executive officer of the Bendix Corporation. Control, he suggests, is related to the ability to "hire and fire," and he identified his problem in government thus: "Out of 120,000 people in the Treasury, I was able to select twenty-five, maybe. The other 119,975 are outside of my control."[5]

It was noted earlier that top management is involved in setting goals and organizing activities that allow the goals to be attained. The contrast between the private sector and the public sector is highlighted in Blumenthal's article by his comment that the senior executives in industry can control who is and who is not involved in policy development and implementation, but that in the government, because of the plethora of official and nonofficial interest groups, many of whom have influence and power, the policy process is considerably more complex.

A final point is that management in industry does most of its business in private. Government executives and, to a lesser extent, managers of nonprofit community organizations, however, must function under the spotlight of the press. How then do performance expectations for health care managers differ from those for industrial managers? In a magazine article about the recipient of the Young Hospital Administrator of the Year Award, it was pointed out that the award winner had "superior administrative capability," which was demonstrated variously, including by the hospital's quality of care, physical and programmatic growth, financial health, and positive professional image. As if that were not enough, the article continued with a description of the administrator's activities as a local and national leader and ended with a statement regarding his "positive spirit." An analysis of this article suggests that, to be successful, at least in the eyes of one professional organization, managers must be joiners and innovators, accept their organization's goals as their own, and invest their spiritual and physical energy in building the organization.

Among the essentials of management are technical skills and the ability to recruit and retain able subordinates. Technical skills are often underemphasized, but they contribute substantially to a manager's credibility and value to an organization. For example, can the manager accurately forecast the utilization of services based on a high-quality assessment of needs, likely demands, and competition? Can the manager develop an appropriate strategic plan or budget for the organization? This is not to suggest that the manager must write the budget personally, but he or she must plan, organize, and review the budget before it is placed in the hands of the board or the owners. Mistakes, conceptual or mechanical, are earmarks of a careless or technically unskilled manager, particularly at the beginning of a career. Indeed, if there is one shortcoming of new managers, it may be an over-reliance on the importance of their image as managers and an under-reliance on the technical tasks that constitute the essence of their job.

Since few managers, even workaholics, have the time and ability to do everything themselves, they must rely on subordinates for their own success. A manager's ability to find people who will be supportive and complement his or her own skills is crucial. Some managers view high-quality subordinates as threats and respond by hiring sycophants. Others view subordinate managers as tools to carry out unpleasant jobs and hire "hatchet men." A third group view subordinates as key colleagues, and they attempt to surround themselves with the best people available. One problem with the "best and brightest" is that they tend to move on if new challenges are not forthcoming. However, for the manager who is comfortable with talented subordinates and invests in their growth and development, the rewards are significant.

ENTERING MANAGEMENT

In his book *Management*, Drucker identifies six common mistakes in designing managerial jobs.[6] These mistakes are (1) designing "the job so small that a good man cannot grow"; (2) designing jobs that are not really jobs; (3) designing jobs that do not combine work with managing; (4) designing jobs that require continuous meetings and continuous cooperation and coordination; (5) giving out titles rather than jobs; and (6) creating "widow-maker" jobs, that is, jobs that are simply impossible to do. Drucker's advice is particularly useful for a chief executive officer who must establish or reorganize an organization. However, it is also useful for a manager who must decide whether to accept a new position. So with apologies to Drucker and acknowledgment of him as the source, following is a list of six ideas to consider when entering or shifting positions on the managerial ladder.

❦ *Take a job in which you can grow.* In the field of nursing home administration, growth is both a function of the job and the organization. In selecting a position, consider the growth potential. What will you learn on this job? What challenges and opportunities are associated with this job? How, in three to five years, will you be better off as a result of having had this job?

❦ *Do not be a gofer for another person.* Nonjobs are particularly common in the health industry and are well described by Drucker as positions whose title includes "assistant to." A manager's performance should be observable by the total organization, and his or her position should not depend on the good will of the manager next in line. In small health care organizations, particularly at the entry level, this kind of dependency is difficult to avoid. Some managers attempt to avoid it by continually defining and redefining their positions in writing (via a series of memos). If there is good will and if those higher in the organization feel secure, there are few problems with this method. If the junior manager is simply another tool in the senior manager's bag, all the memos in the organization are insignificant compared with the opinion of the "boss." To the extent possible, then, the job should represent a commitment from the organization, not from the manager next highest in the chain of command.

• *Take a job in which you work and manage.* No one can suggest that management is not hard work, but quite clearly there is a tendency for young managers to ensconce themselves in pleasant offices, deal only with those who seek them out, respond only to those higher in the hierarchy, and "play the manager role." Periodically, however, managers should get their hands dirty. For the physician manager, this might mean seeing patients occasionally. For the nonphysician manager, it might mean handling special projects or observing certain operations. Managers must continue to develop their own competencies and periodically test them. Such development and testing can have positive effects in terms of self-esteem and respect from colleagues and subordinates. An analogy with academia might clarify this concept further: A dean should not only administer the school but should also work by teaching and doing research. In one nursing home I visited, the executive director spent at least several hours per week helping out on the resident units and directly delivering care—clearly she was both working and managing.

• *Avoid a position with a great deal of nonproductive time.* Most people are measured by their output or the outcomes of what they do, not the processes used to attain the outcomes. Although processes are critical for reaching goals, it is easy to forget that a process is not, in fact, an outcome. For example, meetings can become more important than the decisions reached and the implementation of the decisions. All positions include some nonproductive time, but new managers must look for positions in which it is either minimized or can be controlled. Many new managers look back over their first few years on the jobs and realize they have spent most of their time in meetings and have done few things that have had much effect. Organizations want the bases touched but also want runs scored.

Get your objectives straight. Knowing what you really want is extremely difficult, because there is a strong current impelling managers toward accepting the objectives of the organization as their own. Soul-searching is often tiring and time consuming, but it is necessary if managers are to understand what they really want from their position. Is it power, prestige, security, glamour, intellectual stimulation, money, or a combination of these and other objectives? A manager who has come to grips with his or her personal objectives is in a much stronger position to make career choices. Not only that, but the manager will be less likely to suffer from unnecessary and possibly debilitating anxiety.

❧ *When in doubt, maximize your potential for success by taking proven jobs.* Managers should not risk their future on a widow-maker job, a job that others have tried and failed at. The payoff for being a hero is high, but when other qualified people could not handle the job, new managers must be careful not to slip on their own egos. A proven path is a more sensible choice and less fraught with uncertainties and danger. Here, again, objectives come into play, since some people find a well-constructed ladder less appealing than a greased flagpole.

CONCLUSION

Managers of nursing homes play an absolutely crucial role in the lives of hundreds of employees and residents. The tone they set for the organization reverberates throughout the facility. They have the power to create a cold, stressful, indeed unhealthy environment. They also have the power, fortunately, to construct a warm, caring, and productive organization—the type of place where most of us would choose to work or, if necessary, live.

NOTES

1. W.B. Cornell, *Organization and Management in Industry and Business* (New York: Ronald Press, 1947), 46.

2. P. Drucker, *Management* (New York: Harper & Row, 1973), xiii.

3. *Fortune*, In the News (February 12, 1979), 16.

4. *Fortune*, Candid Reflections of a Businessman in Washington (January 29, 1979), 36–49.

5. Ibid.

6. Drucker, *Management*, 405–410.

Case Study 4-1

Death at Bondville

Seth B. Goldsmith

On a cold Tuesday morning in January, probably between the hours of midnight and 3 A.M., Max Morse, a resident of the Bondville Geriatric Center, left his room, went outside of the home, and died of exposure in the frigid night air. Mr. Morse's body was found between 8 and 8:30 A.M. after the morning shift discovered that Mr. Morse was missing.

On the Monday evening before this incident, at approximately 5:30 P.M., Richard Albertson, the home's administrator, left work after checking with the evening supervisor on the overnight (11:00 to 7:00) staffing pattern, which called for a total of two aides and one nurse for the 200 residents in the three-story building. At approximately midnight, one of the aides put Max Morse to bed. The nurse's records indicated that the side rails on Morse's bed were put up and that he was checked every two hours and passed an uneventful night.

* * *

Discussion Questions

1. With regard to Max Morse's safety, what was the duty of the night supervisor? of the Administrator?
2. How could this incident have been prevented?
3. Was there any staff negligence?
4. Was there any criminal behavior involved in this case?

Case Study 4-2

The Dietary Dilemma

Seth B. Goldsmith

For a man seldom thinks with more earnestness of anything than he does of his dinner.

—Samuel Johnson

On June 15, just seven months after he had been hired, Ian MacLean, the director of food service at the 200-bed Hebrew Home for the Aged of the Dakotas (HHAD), was asked to meet with Benjamin Jonas, the home's director. For Jonas, who himself had been hired less than a year ago, this meeting was a difficult one because its purpose was to ask MacLean to resign, and if MacLean would not sign a letter of resignation, Jonas was prepared to discharge him.

Jonas began by saying, "Ian, I'm sorry that things have come to this but I think, in light of the problems in food service, it would be best for all of us if you resigned. I warned you last month that this would happen unless the department was straightened out."

MacLean replied, "Resign? Are you kidding? I'm just getting into the rhythm of this place. I know that I've made some mistakes but I think that I am now getting things under control. Are you just angry about my kashruth mistake at the board dinner last week? This kashruth business is a pain and I've worked very hard to get your Jewish dietary laws down, but the whole business about what meats and seafood can't be eaten and the laws against mixing meat and milk aren't second nature to a Scotsman like me."

"Ian, please listen to me carefully," Jonas implored. "The kashruth at the board meeting was clearly a problem. But after being here as long as you have, plus your agreement to study the rules of kashruth, there really is no excuse for order-

---

Fictitious names of both the organization and individuals are used to ensure anonymity.

Source: This case and related notes are taken from the long-term care management case study collection found in *Cases in Long-Term Care Management: Building the Continuum,* by Donna Infeld and John Kress, published by AUPHA Press and used with permission.

ing the staff to put sour cream on the tables when the dinner is going to be roast beef. You know perfectly well that we never serve dairy and meat at the same meal. By now you should know that all of that cream for the coffee and whipped cream are really non-dairy substitutes. So while I acknowledge that I am annoyed by your putting the sour cream on the table, fortunately Louis [Louis Isaacs, Assistant Administrator] saved the day by checking the dining room out before the board came in and taking the sour cream off the tables. But I think there is something more important. Did you ever wonder why Esther, Max, Julio, and Jill didn't say anything to you since they certainly know better? I'll tell you why: They don't trust or respect you."

"Wait a minute," MacLean interrupted. "I think there is another explanation and that is they were trying to undermine me. I took over a 30-person department that had never had a manager, that was run by the senior cook, and that the state inspector said didn't meet the requirements for proper food handling. You hired me to set up a new tray delivery system and you yourself said I did an outstanding job of that."

This time Jonas interrupted, "Look Ian, you did a great job setting up the tray system, but that is history! I need someone who can manage the department. Last week when we went out to the Jewish Community Center to discuss the senior citizens feeding project, you couldn't even justify our bid of $3.37 per meal, which is probably considerably under our real costs. I've got a million dollars tied up in your department, one-sixth of my budget, and I need someone who can control what is going on in there."

In a pleading voice Ian MacLean then went on to ask Mr. Jonas for another opportunity to manage the department. Jonas replied that his decision was final; MacLean could resign or be fired. MacLean agreed to resign and Jonas agreed to let him phase out over the next 30 days.

THE HISTORY OF HHAD'S FOOD SERVICE PROBLEMS

Ben Jonas's agreement to have MacLean stay on for another 30 days was largely due to his own uncertainty about what to do about food service. When he had accepted the administrator's position ten months earlier, he recognized there was a food service problem but he did not know how serious it was. What was obvious from the outset of his tenure was that the food served at the home lacked variety. The standard joke was, "If it was fish it must be Wednesday." A far more serious problem that emerged shortly after Jonas's arrival was a state inspection report (Exhibit 4-2-1) that found the food service deficient. The problem was the food handling procedure in which food was delivered in bulk form to the six resident units and then portioned out by the nursing and dietary staff. The state

Exhibit 4-2-1 Statement of Food Service Deficiencies

Date of Inspection: August 25–26, 19___

1. Sanitation—Stewed prunes and applesauce were stored, uncovered.

2. Disposable glasses and cup liners were used at the breakfast and evening meals.

3. Sufficient numbers of trained personnel were not available to serve and prepare food (e.g., nurses were observed preparing and serving breakfast on the units on two consecutive days of visit). Standard not met.

4. A current diet manual was not readily available at one nursing station.

5. Sanitation/preparation—Food was observed being served in the hallway; the floor was being washed at the same time. Nurses on all units were observed serving food without hair nets. Standard not met.

6. Menus/nutrition—There was no indication that recommendations by the dietitian regarding iron-rich foods for patients with hematocrit levels below normal were brought to the attention of the attending physician. Standard not met.

7. Instructions (place cards) for the serving of special diets were not available at the breakfast meals. A patient on a 2-gram sodium diet received highly salted corned beef; a patient complained that his wife, also a patient, never received her low-sodium diet; nurses, not trained dietary help, serve meals.

8. Of ten patients interviewed, six complained about the food. They said the food was overcooked, that steak was never served, and that the temperatures are better now (implying that the food had been cold).

inspectors also evinced concern about a lack of attention to the dietary restriction orders of the physicians.

In response to these problems, in particular the report of the state inspectors, Mr. Jonas asked David Axelrod, president of the home's board, to appoint an ad hoc committee on food service. Because the solution to these problems seemed at the time obvious but expensive, Jonas wanted to make certain that the board was supportive of his first major personnel decision and capital expenditure. After three meetings during a two-month period, the board agreed to fund a new position, director of food services, and allocate $25,000 per year for the director's salary. Secondly, they agreed to allocate $75,000 for a new tray delivery system.

Finding an appropriately qualified food service director turned out to be more problematic than Jonas had anticipated. The response to his blind advertisements in the local and regional papers was disappointing. None of the candidates had experience in managing medium-scale kosher institutions. Almost all the candidates were in assistant manager or shift manager positions at local institutions, particularly schools. Only Ian MacLean stood out as a person who, despite a lack of kosher catering experience, had the experience with systems to implement the tray delivery service. When the HHAD hired MacLean, he was a freelance food service consultant on implementation of new systems. His references all agreed that he had the technical skill to get virtually any size new system up and running on a reasonable schedule. He was called "hardworking," "loyal," and a "nice person." In the two months prior to the tray system installation, MacLean worked 70–80 hours per week and never requested any overtime pay or compensatory time off. He was at the home evenings and virtually every Sunday.

The implementation of the new system was technically flawless. The food arrived at the units in the correct amount, residents received the diets their physicians had ordered, and the food was appropriately warm or cool. The system proved to be a boon for the nursing staff who no longer needed to spend over two hours per shift delivering meals, cleaning up, and dealing with the patient discord about portions or flavor.

REACTIONS TO THE NEW TRAY SYSTEM

Despite Jonas's educational effort before the new system was implemented, an effort that included a letter to both the residents and their families about the system, within a week of its installation the complaints about it were overwhelming the administrator. The first problem encountered was a petition from the residents council, an organization of residents that normally confined itself to deliberations about refreshments for various social events. The petition read as follows:

PETITION

Whereas the Residents of the Hebrew Home for the Aged of the Dakotas must consume almost all their meals on the home's premises; and,

Whereas the Residents have selected the home for its kosher food as well as other services; and,

Whereas there has for many years been a tradition of food being served in a family style that helps in maintaining a home-like atmosphere at the home;

It is respectfully requested that the former style food service be reinstituted.

Duly made, seconded, and passed by a vote of 14 to 3 of the residents council, April 1, 19___.

_____

s/ Molly Goldberg, President
Residents Council

Next, Jonas heard from several board members who, in reaction to complaints from relatives who were residents of the home, brought the problem to Jonas. In response to these complaints, Jonas met with the residents council and sent the following letter to the residents' families:

Hebrew Home for the Aged of the Dakotas
1818 N.W. Chai Street
Fargo, North Dakota

May 1, 19___

Dear Friends:

As you are aware from my earlier letter on this subject, on April 1, 19___ we installed a new food service system at the home. A major overhaul of our food service system was essentially dictated by the state at a recent inspection. Specifically, they found our bulk food delivery system to be unsatisfactory in terms of both sanitary and dietary standards. They were particularly concerned about being unable to respond properly to physician's dietary orders under the bulk system.

After much deliberation, the board and administration selected the Simcha tray system, which ensures that your loved ones get their food promptly and properly. So far the system has been in operation for one month and we are pleased with the results.

Change is difficult but, as in this instance, quite necessary. I hope this letter has clarified what is happening with food service. If you would like more information, please feel free to contact either me or Louis Isaacs.

Sincerely,

Benjamin B. Jonas
Executive Vice-President

The letter seemed to work. After its mailing, the complaints decreased but food service still had problems. The old problems of variety and quality were joined by the new problems of cost and personnel.

INADEQUATE FOOD SERVICE COST ACCOUNTING

The need to prepare a bid for the Jewish Community Center's senior citizens feeding project was what brought the cost problem to the fore. The bid required that the home provide detailed data on food costs, preparation costs, transportation costs, and profit margins. As this process was being carried out, it became obvious that cost data for food service were sparse.

The problem of obtaining accurate data was not limited to food service nor was it totally unexpected. It was clear to Jonas from his first day that the home, while having many strengths such as its physical plant and strong community support, had serious weaknesses in management. Problems he identified at the outset included a total lack of a management information system or a purchasing program. Both programs were unsatisfactory and had been under the direction of Assistant Administrator Irwin Brown for many years. As part of his review of costs, Jonas examined the food service cost data sent to the State Commission for Nursing Home Rates. Subsequent discussions with the home's outside accountant and Brown led Jonas to the conclusion that the food service costs were primarily based on trends from data of the previous year. Further, Jonas concluded that the true costs were unknown and that the present accounting systems could simply not account for the costs. For example, each of the resident units had a nourishment station at which were stored tea, coffee, bread, crackers, peanut butter, jelly, juice, and soda. Twice weekly food service restocked these supplies, but the expense of this operation was not included in the food service costs.

Finding data about food service was part of Jonas's larger agenda—to develop a state-of-the-art financial management and management information system. To implement this item on his agenda, Jonas proposed at the February 15 board meeting that the board fund a new position for a certified public accountant with both nursing home and computer experience and fund the purchase of a computer system. The board agreed to this proposal but, because of the home's $500,000 deficit, asked Jonas to delay the acquisition of the new staff and system until July 1.

PERSONNEL CONFLICTS

Dealing with the personnel problems was one of Lou Isaacs's responsibilities (the other major one being purchasing). Isaacs, who took over from Brown on January 1, was a recent graduate of the master's program in long-term care administration at the University of Lake Wobegon. His experience in health care management was limited to a one-year administrative residency at the Jewish Home in Lake Wobegon. Before entering the field, he worked for six years as a home contractor in Vermont following two years as a Peace Corps volunteer in Colombia.

Shortly after MacLean began as food service director, the personnel complaints started coming to Isaacs. Within months, at least half of the food service workers had come in at least once to criticize MacLean's management of the department. For example, Max the cook complained, "Ian didn't like the way I cooked the chicken so he complained loudly in the kitchen. It was very embarrassing." Esther complained about his harassing her about productivity: "Lady, why does it take you so long to clean up? You're slower than a mule." Julio also complained about the way MacLean treated him, "I think he's racist. I was on my morning break and meditating and he comes up to me and tells me that we don't allow siestas here." Probably the most crucial problem, however, was the rumor of a union drive that might attract the food service employees, most of whom, until the beginning of the MacLean regime, were thought to be very loyal to the home.

THE DIRECTOR'S OPTIONS AND FINAL DECISIONS

Soliciting MacLean's resignation was difficult for Jonas for both personal and professional reasons. From a personal perspective, he disliked discharging people and he was genuinely appreciative of MacLean's excellent job in implementing the new system. Also, he found MacLean to be charming and engaging. Both Jonas and MacLean were outdoorsmen who shared a passion for skiing and fly fishing, and on a couple of occasions had spent several hours together fishing.

From a professional perspective Jonas had two problems. First, he felt that MacLean was one of his earliest and most visible recruiting decisions and only months later he was discharging this person. After thinking this through, Jonas decided that the embarrassment of admitting a poor decision was outweighed by the damage that was likely to be done if MacLean continued as food service director.

The second professional problem was what to do about the food service department as a whole. Jonas identified several options: (1) Allow food service to be managed the way it was before his arrival; that is, the scheduling of employees and departmental management would be done by senior cooks and the assistant administrator would be actively involved in the department (he would essentially function as the part-time food service director), (2) Hire a new food service director, (3) Contract out the food services to a contract caterer.

The first option would require the continued active involvement of Louis Isaacs in the management of the department. While Jonas thought that his assistant had a good sense of catering and food service management, it was clear that he was not a food service professional. Additionally, Jonas worried that Isaacs would burn out if he attempted to manage food service as well as carry out his other responsibilities. Finally, complaints from some board members about Isaacs' performance and personality were starting to reach Jonas, who was beginning to think that he might need a more seasoned deputy.

After dismissing the first option, Jonas decided to pursue the other two options simultaneously. To develop a pool of candidates for the food service director's position, he contacted the administrators of other nonprofit nursing homes in the region and placed advertisements in local and regional newspapers.

FOOD SERVICE DIRECTOR
Nursing Home and Geriatric Center

Must be experienced in tray systems
and kosher food service. Salary open
based on experience and qualifications.
Send resume to Box 3131, *Fargo Gazette.*

The third option involved using an outside contract caterer. Based on his earlier experience and information he gathered from administrators of other Jewish homes, Jonas invited three firms to make bids on the food service problem. Each company made a two-day survey of the institution and presented Jonas with a formal proposal. All three companies were asked to incorporate the following assumptions into their bids:

1. There will be 72,000 patient days and 216,000 meals per year.
2. The day-care program has 24 participants a day, 237 days a year, which requires an additional 5,688 meals.
3. There will be congregate meal services (The Jewish Community Center Program) serving 21,000 meals.
4. Free meals are to be served to an estimated 70 persons per day.
5. Subsidized meals are served to approximately 60 staff per day.
6. Food service costs for unit nourishment stations are to be calculated at $.30 per patient day or $21,600 per year.
7. Food service costs for the coffee shop are to be calculated at $5,895.

The problem now facing Jonas was what to recommend to the board. He received 12 resumes, of which five were in the acceptable category (Exhibit 4-2-2). Three persons were selected for an interview. Additionally, he received three proposals (portions of each appear in Table 4-2-1). Descriptions of the companies that submitted them are given in Exhibit 4-2-3. Evaluate the exhibits and decide what you would do if you were Jonas.

Exhibit 4-2-2 Sample Resumes of Applicants for Position of Food Service Director

---

Juan Domingo
1314 Green St.
Nashua, New Hampshire

Education
BS (1974)   Michigan State University
             School of Hotel and Restaurant Management
             E. Lansing, Michigan
             Major: Institutional Catering

1970–1972   Naval School of Hospital Administration
             Bethesda, Maryland
             60 BS credits through Abraham Lincoln University

Professional Experience
1955–1967   Hospital Corpsman—attained rank of Chief (E-7) in August 1966

1967   Selected for commissioning as Ensign, Medical Service Corps, U.S. Navy

1967–1970   Assistant Personnel Officer
             Naval Hospital, Adak, Alaska

1974–1978   Food Services Officer
             Naval Hospital
             Newport, R.I.

1978–1980   Director of Food Services
             Naval Medical Center
             Portsmouth, Virginia

1980–1984   Manager
             Admiral Sparky's Seafood Emporium
             Norfolk, Virginia

1984–   Director of Food Services
             Nashua Hospital
             Nashua, N.H.

Personal
             Divorced
             Two children: Juan, Jr., 23 and Ilana, 19
             Fluent in Spanish and Portuguese

---

continues

Exhibit 4-2-2 *continued*

William C. Weeks
917 Crescent Street
Lake Wobegon, Minnesota

Employment:

Since 1985 I have been Manager of the dietary department of the Jewish Nursing Home of Lake Wobegon. The home has 110 residents and a day care center of 10 clients. My department has 11 employees and a budget in excess of $500,000.00. Under my direction, labor turnover has been lessened and productivity increased. The number of resident complaints have decreased significantly. I have introduced a variety of innovations, including New York Deli night, lox and bagel breakfasts, and special holiday meals. Additionally, as part of our activities programs I have taught cooking to the residents and allowed them to come work in our kitchens and prepare their own specialties.

From 1980 to 1985 I was assistant director of food services at the Lake Wobegon Medical Center, a 200-bed general hospital. In this job I managed a staff of 35 and was involved in the implementation of a tray delivery system.

From 1975 to 1980 I was employed by the Royal Catering Company as a marketing representative in the Lake Wobegon and Fargo area. This job involved my working with various institutions that hired the company to provide in-plant catering services. My job involved sales and troubleshooting.

From 1971 to 1975 I was an undergraduate student at Johnson and Wales College, Providence, R.I., majoring in Hotel and Restaurant Management. I graduated in 1975 with a BS and a GPA of 3.4. At the college I was Vice-President of my fraternity, a member of the school choir, and active in the Toastmaster's Club.

I am married to the former Jean Phillips, who is a registered nurse, and have two children, Tim, 6, and Becky, 9.

S. Gorbaniphar
P.O. Box 514
Fargo, N.D.

Experience:

1987–Present	Consultant	Gorbaniphar and Associates Fargo, N.D.
1985–1987	Manager	The Lake Wobegon Inn Lake Wobegon, Minn. Salary: $29,000 per annum
1983–1985	Night manager	The Fargo Hilton Fargo, N.D. Salary: $27,500 per annum
1979–1983	Group Manager	The Cyclops Computer Corp. Minneapolis, Minn. Salary: $34,000 per annum

continues

Exhibit 4-2-2 *continued*

1974–1979	Student	University of Massachusetts School of Engineering Major: Computer Systems Degree: BS
1972–1974	Student	University of Teheran School of Engineering No degree

Personal:

Married
One child: Avraham, age 4

References:

1. Professor Maxwell Smart, Chairman, Department of Computer Sciences, University of Massachusetts.
2. Mr. Adolph Bijou, Owner, Lake Wobegon Inn
3. Mr. Joseph de Coates, Manager, Fargo Hilton

Mary Anne Davis, R.D.
Dietitian
Fargo Lutheran Hospital
Fargo, North Dakota

Professional Licensure: Registered Dietitian #01659

Present Position: (since 1984)	Dietitian at Fargo Lutheran Hospital Responsibilities include supervision of three assistant dietitians and seven aides. Work closely with Manager of Food services in preparation of therapeutic diets and supervision of staff. Served as acting director of food service in absence of manager.
Previous Position: (1981–1984)	Assistant Dietitian at Fargo Lutheran Hospital This position involved working with patients and physicians on selecting the most appropriate therapeutic diet. A major part of the job involved monitoring the diets and encouraging patient compliance. Work involved both inpatient and outpatient activities.

EDUCATION

M.P.H. 1981 (Honors)	University of Minnesota School of Public Health Minneapolis, Minnesota Thesis: The cost benefit of therapeutic diets in nursing homes
BA 1979 (Magna Cum Laude)	University of Minnesota School of Home Economics Department of Human Nutrition

---

continues

Exhibit 4-2-2 *continued*

Gloria Robertson

Job Objective: To secure a senior-level food service management position in a progressive and high-quality long-term care facility that will encourage innovative developments and innovative management.

Background:

1. I have a BA from Smith College in Northampton, MA. At Smith I majored in Art History and minored in Economics.

2. After graduating from Smith in 1975 I entered a new joint degree program at Columbia University between the School of Business and the School of Human Nutrition, receiving both an MBA and an MS in Human Nutrition in 1978. In 1969 I received my R.D. certification.

3. From 1978 to 1981 I was a marketing representative in New England for Pillsbury. This position involved working with wholesale grocers on the introduction of new products. I resigned from this position in order to travel for one year in Europe.

4. From 1982 to 1985 I worked as Assistant Director of Market Research for the Quest Corporation based in Minneapolis. Quest is a nonprofit research center jointly owned by several food manufacturers that does market research on changing eating habits of the population. My particular project involved eating patterns of the institutionalized elderly.

5. Since 1985 I have been a food service consultant for the Chanin Group. The Chanin Group owns 56 nursing homes through the midwest, ranging in size from 45 beds to 300 beds. My job involves consulting with contract dietitians and food service managers on improvements in both meeting dietary standards and innovations in systems.

References:

Professor Mary Wolfe, Smith College, Department of Economics

Dr. James McGee, President, University of Minnesota, Minneapolis, Minnesota

Walter Johnsonn, Former Mayor, City of South Minneapolis, Present address: c/o 545 Rio Piedras Drive, Ponce, Puerto Rico

Ms. Diane White, Vice-President for Planning, Rocky Mountain Medical Center, Denver, Colorado

Table 4-2-1 Summary Proposals

	B. Spoke	Pepper	St. Cloud	Current Actual
Food cost	$423,953	$481,316	$417,330	$466,800
Salary	48,000	73,464	104,258	—
Tax/fringe	11,040	20,422	26,065	—
Direct expenses	43,200	88,100	63,447	84,000
Nonmanagement salary	329,518	343,816	400,063	546,005
Tax/fringe	75,789	75,639	88,013	120,121
Management fee	36,000	40,000	50,000	—
Subtotal	967,500	1,122,757	1,149,176	1,216,926
Credits				
Cafeteria	20,000	20,000	20,000	20,000
Coffee shop	13,100	13,100	13,100	13,100
Other	5,000	5,000	5,000	5,000
Total cost	$929,400	$1,084,657	$1,111,076	$1,255,026
Cost/patient day	$12.91	$15.06	$15.43	$17.43

Exhibit 4-2-3 Overview of Companies Submitting Bids

1. B. Spoke Company

   The B. Spoke Company is the largest company devoted to food service management in Jewish nursing homes. Presently, it has 15 homes under contract. In addition to the Jewish homes, B. Spoke has another 75 nonkosher nursing home facilities throughout the country and is a division of a corporation that is the fifth largest industrial caterer.

2. The St. Cloud Company

   The St. Cloud Company is the largest dietary management firm in the health care field presently having in excess of 400 clients. At present it has a total of four Jewish hospitals and seven Jewish nursing homes under contract and is interested in expanding its nursing home operations in the Fargo area. At present, St. Cloud has the catering contract with Fargo Lutheran Hospital and several other institutions within a 100-mile radius of Fargo.

3. The Pepper Corporation

   The Pepper Corporation is a regional food service firm based in St. Paul, Minnesota. Its primary business is industrial catering, but for the past ten years it has been trying to develop a nursing home contract management division. At present it has ten nursing homes under contract, one of which is a 75-bed kosher proprietary facility in Minneapolis.

Chapter 5

The Role and Function
of Governing Boards

Seth B. Goldsmith

Governing boards are a fact of life for managers of nonprofit nursing homes. State statutes set a host of requirements for these boards, ranging from the number of members on the board to voting requirements. These same statutes then invest the board with the legal responsibility and authority for the operation of the enterprise, and in some instances they even limit the liability of the board for its decisions if a prudent decision process has been followed. The board in turn normally delegates a significant amount of its power to a full-time managerial staff headed by a paid chief executive officer.

BOARD FUNCTIONS

In discussing board functions, Heen identifies eight areas of board activity:

(a) policy decisions with respect to products, services, prices, wages, labor relations; (b) selection, supervision and removal of officers and possibly other management personnel; (c) fixing of executive compensations, pension/retirement, etc., plans; (d) determination of dividends, financing and capital changes; (e) delegation of authority for administrative and possibly other action; (f) possible adoption, amendment and repeal of by-laws; (g) possible participation, along with shareholders, in approving various extraordinary corporate matters; and (h) supervision and vigilance for the welfare of the whole enterprise.[1]

Although a few of these functions are not applicable to nonprofit homes, most of them are central to the responsibilities of health care organization board members.

The problem of board effectiveness and involvement is common to all organizations. For example, when the famous bankruptcies of W.T. Grant, Lockheed,

Eastern Airlines, and hundreds of banks and savings and loan associations occurred, who claimed to be uninformed? The board! Does it seem possible that board members of major industrial concerns, the elite of America's business establishment, could be so unaware?

Drucker, in his book *Management*, titles a chapter "Needed: An Effective Board." He argues that boards, because of their very nature, the ambiguity of their mission, and the divergence of interest of their members, are programmed for failure.[2] It is a common experience in health care to find executives whose performance is excellent in business but who cannot function effectively on the board of a nonprofit organization. This can be partly understood by considering the composition of boards—health care or industrial. Data from a Heidrick and Struggles study of directors indicate that most board members are well into middle age (the average age being 57), that most are selected for their personal or professional stature, that functional area of expertise is a second but significantly less important reason for selection, and that availability is a considerably less important reason in selection.[3]

This is a pattern seen almost universally in the health care field. A review of a typical board's membership (with the exclusion of community-based programs such as neighborhood health centers) is like reading the who's who of the local area. Boards generally are not representative of any group other than the upper middle class of the community. The justification for this skewed representation is that such a group is likely to bring greater financial and intellectual resources to a board. Addressing the issue of board composition in an amusing article, Chandler suggests (somewhat backhandedly) that a balanced board must be the goal and that various criteria must be used, "from the subjective—candor, enthusiasm, manner of presentation (articulation and appearance), willingness to serve community, cooperativeness; to the more objective—age, occupation, standing in the community, place of residence, etc."[4]

Indeed, my own work with nursing home boards throughout the country supports these observations: Few board members are under 35 years old; most boards are male-dominated; board juntas, cliques that are on a board for life, are common; and virtually no boards have community representatives (i.e., elected and voting resident or family representatives).

BOARD–MANAGEMENT RELATIONS

For the nursing home administrator, the fundamental question is, How can a manager have an effective relationship with a board? At one extreme, the manager must cope with a necessary evil; at the other, the manager is able to utilize the resources that a board can offer. Many managers view their relationship with their board as adversarial. This was well articulated by J. Peter Grace, the chief executive of the multi-billion-dollar W.R. Grace conglomerate, when he said,

> Do you mean to tell me that if I work 100 hours a week for 4.3 weeks a month on average so that I'm working 430 hours a month, some guy is going to come in and in three or four hours outsmart me? I mean that's crazy! No matter how smart you are, if I work 100 times harder than you on a given subject, you have no way of catching me.[5]

As a reflection of his perspective, Grace's board room does not have the traditional conference table but rather is arranged more like a college classroom. In dealing with his board, Grace keeps them fully informed. For example, for one monthly meeting he provided board members with a report over 400 pages long.

Is this typical? Based on the Heidrick and Struggles study, it seems most companies provide their directors only with minutes of the previous meeting, some financial data, and an agenda for the next meeting. In most cases, no summaries of board committee meetings subsequent to the last board meeting, no marketing data, and no data to support agenda items are provided. It can be concluded that only those board members who are involved with committees, which is usually the group making critical decisions, or those who are extremely well informed about agenda items, can offer much of worth at a given meeting. Going back to the Grace example, it must be recognized that without an independent staff or a major investment of their own time, board members would find it impossible to digest or evaluate critically the 400 pages sent to them. Management, then, through its control of information given to the board, has the potential to have a major impact on the effectiveness and value of the board.

The issue of the relationship between management and the board is a recurring theme in the literature. For example, in a 1980 review article on governance, Umbdenstock noted that,

> for hospital trustees, administrators and physicians, many of the same issues in hospital governance remained in the forefront throughout the 70s. What are the board's proper roles and responsibilities? What are the proper relationships with management and the medical staff? What about the board's need to represent the community? Who ultimately directs the institution and how do trustees ensure the quality of care provided in the hospital?[6]

Several years earlier, the U.S. Chamber of Commerce, in its 1974 publication *A Primer for Hospital Trustees,* cautioned the trustees about their balance of involvement.[7] The advice given was to set policy but stay out of implementation. The administrative perspective and concerns are perhaps best identified in a 1973 document from the American College of Hospital Administrators titled *Principles of Appointment and Tenure of Executive Officers.* In it, the authors noted that "some board members in some hospitals cross over into line management, consciously or unconsciously."[8] When that occurs, directors become potential adversaries. As a preventive medicine measure then, the behavior suggested by Grace is almost a necessity for survival.

In 1974, the Macy Foundation produced its landmark study on the governance of voluntary teaching hospitals in New York City. Nelson, the former president of Johns Hopkins Hospital, found the major teaching hospitals in New York City facing many serious problems, some of which related to the board and most of which still plague the nursing home industry:[9]

- There is confusion of authority among governance, management, and medical staffs resulting from the duality of mission of the teaching hospital, which faces toward the medical school in the performance of its teaching and learning functions and toward the community and its doctors' patients in the performance of its service functions.
- Boards of trustees are predominantly white, male, and business-oriented, and there is only token representation of other interests.
- Board leadership is concentrated in small, entrenched groups complacent about the quality of their leadership.
- Except for leadership groups, board members are poorly informed about hospital goals and problems and uninformed about outside forces impinging on hospitals.
- Trustees are frustrated by the lack of information and involvement but nervous about getting involved in financial and medical problems.
- Chief executives lack the authority and backing required for effective negotiation with outside forces and effective control of medical affairs.
- Administrative staffs are generally strong at the top level but lack depth of expertise in finance, law, medical staff orientation, and other specialties.
- Communities are mistrustful of institutional goals and critical of institutional services.
- There is a lack of any standards of performance for hospital trustees or methods of evaluating quality and effectiveness of governance.

The picture of boards painted by Nelson and the others is gloomy indeed, and unfortunately, two decades later, little has changed. Who or what is responsible for this state of affairs? Among the causes might be that board members are sometimes picked on the basis of bad reasons—a person who has the prestige but lacks the time might be selected over someone with the time but limited prestige.

Potential wealthy contributors may be considered more important than those with expertise and interest.

Of course, some managers may want a weak board (and an uninformed board is weak). This is perhaps understandable, yet a strong board can offer dramatic leadership. Individually and collectively, board members can represent and promote the organization's interest; can serve as a sounding board or as a review and comment mechanism for innovation; and, with proper development, can serve as the major organizational evaluation mechanism.

KNOWLEDGE AND UNDERSTANDING OF DIRECTORS

Several years ago, while conducting an executive education program, I met with a group of 26 senior health administrators and asked them what they thought was most important for directors to know or understand about the health system and the role of the manager. Responses to the question varied widely. Some managers wanted their boards to be focused on national affairs, looking at the broad legislative and policy issues and planning alternative health systems; others were more interested in having directors focused on the role their own organization might play in a community or in developing quality services. To put it in conceptual terms, some managers view the board as an external reporting and sounding panel, whereas others see it as part of the internal drive mechanism of the organization.

When this same group of managers considered what they wanted the directors to know and understand about the manager's job, there was considerably less variance. Virtually all wanted their directors to know more about management and fiscal problems and issues. Additionally, a number of managers felt it was important that board members understand the importance of delegating authority and responsibility—a particularly troubling option considering that many board members do not appear to delegate authority in their own organizations.

THE BOARD IMPERATIVE

During a recent visit to a large midwestern geriatric center, I met with the newly elected board president and the center's chief executive officer. Both were successful and competitive men in their midforties, and each was trying to dominate the other as well as the organization. Several months after the meeting, the CEO was unemployed and the organization was in chaos (and fortunately later rescued by a very competent new CEO).

Could the firing have been avoided? Could the period of chaos and its long-term effects have been prevented? Perhaps none of this would have happened if the board's role was less ambiguous. It is absolutely imperative that a board be properly structured, operate within clear guidelines, be focused on the organization's mission, and periodically step back and examine its own performance.

Proper structuring requires a clear delineation of the authority and responsibility of the board and its managers, plus an implementing mechanism. In practical terms, this means the board must meet regularly, have a committee structure that functions, have clear lines of communication with the administration, and have a structure that supports its policy orientation and precludes any drift in the direction of micromanaging the institution.

The board must operate within clearly understood guidelines. For example, it must have its own internal rules about attendance, participation, and conflicts of interest. Individuals should be appointed or elected to the board because of their capacity to serve the organization, not because of a desire to be served. Nothing is more detrimental to the continued health of an organization than having board members who serve for the wrong reasons, such as enhancing their status in the community or, worse yet, using the power of the board to garner business from the organization. Guidelines should also deal with the role board members should have in dealing with staff and programs. Board members must limit the sharing of their expertise to the board room. Administrators need to be assured that their management team will not be undermined by board members who do end runs around administration by cultivating staff for "inside information."

Of paramount importance to any board's future is its ability to keep focused on its mission, which includes constantly re-examining that mission. For this reason, the mission must be clearly articulated and written down, and important decisions should be consistent with the mission statement. Management is responsible for ensuring that decisions reflect the organization's mission and for preparing the ground work for a re-examination of the mission through periodic mission-focused retreats.

CONCLUSION

A board can be a valuable asset of a long-term care facility, but only if it is properly selected and nurtured. Membership selection is crucial. Here, myth must be distinguished from reality. For every story about a board person who gave a building, there are a hundred other stories about someone who "we thought" would give a building but died and gave nothing." Organizations should approach the selection of directors with considerable seriousness and select only those people who will enhance the value of the organization because of their expertise, availability, and, yes, in some cases, prestige. One way to approach the possible selection of a candidate is to ask this question: If time and effort are invested in this person, will there be a return on that investment? A negative answer suggests that the search process should be continued.

Once an appropriate new board member has been selected, the administrator must invest time and energy in educating the new member. First, the administrator should learn as much as possible about the new member, including his or her experience, profession, or business. This first phase should include an assessment of the new member's strengths, weaknesses, and interests. Doing this diagnostic workup demonstrates an interest in the board member's personal and professional development while simultaneously permitting an evaluation of how and where the new director might best fit into the organization. Second, the board member must be educated about the major issues and problems facing the long-term care industry and how those issues and problems are affecting the nursing home. Third, the board member needs to be routinely informed about the big picture (i.e., developments in long-term care) and the smaller picture (i.e., the nursing home). Finally, the board member must be asked to work for the good of the nursing home through service on committees, representation functions, or other appropriately useful activities. Most board members do not want to feel like proverbial bumps on a log.

In sum, a board that is tuned into and committed to the mission of the organization can make an invaluable contribution to the success of the manager and the organization as a whole.

NOTES

1. H.G. Heen, *Handbook of the Law of Corporations* (St. Paul, MN: West Pub. Co., 1970), 415.

2. P. Drucker, *Management* (New York: Harper & Row, 1973), 627–636.

3. Heidrick and Struggles, *The Changing Board* (New York: Heidrick and Struggles, 1975), 5.

4. R.L. Chandler, Filling Empty Board Seats, *Hospital and Health Services Administration* 25, no. 1 (Winter 1980):85.

5. Peter Grace's Love-Hate Relationship with His Board, *Forbes* (May 15, 1976), 76.

6. R.J. Umbdenstock, Governance: A Decade of Steady Growth, *Trustees* 33 (1980):17.

7. U.S. Chamber of Commerce, *A Primer for Hospital Trustees* (Washington, D.C.: U.S. Government Printing Office, 1974), 25.

8. American College of Hospital Administrators, *Principles of Appointment and Tenure of Executive Officers* (Chicago: ACHA, 1973), 4.

9. The Macy Foundation, *The Governance of Voluntary Teaching Hospitals in New York City* (New York: Macy Foundation, 1974), 8–9.

Firing the CEO

Seth B. Goldsmith

On the morning of November 1, 1991, Paul Blackman, administrator of the Crescent City Nursing Center, received a call from Roger Johnson, former president of the home's board, who told him that on behalf of the other former presidents of the board he was asking for his resignation by the end of the year. Blackman was stunned by this call and immediately telephoned Angela Fisher, the home's board president, and received assurances from her that despite the fact that he had no employment contract his job was secure.

The Crescent City Nursing Center is a 250-bed skilled nursing home that has a reputation for being the finest home in the region. Since its founding shortly after World War II, the home has been under the direction of a 24-member self-perpetuating board of trustees. The original board comprised a number of people who were instrumental in the founding of the home, including members of the Johnson family, who were not only involved in the home's founding but also provided close to $3,000,000 of the home's total $5,000,000 endowment. The most important of the Johnson family members were two brothers, Roger and William. The 24 members of the present board consist of seven former presidents and at least ten other people who have been involved with the home for over 15 years. The board is now dominated by Roger's son Kenneth and William's son John. In addition, five other Johnson family members are on the board, along with several board members who have significant business involvement with the Johnson family businesses.

Since the home opened, there have been three administrators. The first administrator also served as director of nursing and held the job until 1958 when she was replaced by Mac Davidson, who administered the home for the next 30 years. Davidson's training was in social work and he came to the home at a crucial time in its evolution. He was responsible for its growth from a 100-bed, old-age home to the high-quality home it is today. Davidson and his wife Leslie were intimately involved in all the functionings of the home. Although Leslie was only a part-time receptionist, she still made her presence felt throughout the home by being there a significant part of each day, visiting the residents daily, participating in the various resident shows, and socializing with many of the volunteers and board members. Mac Davidson also kept a very high profile in the home through various means, including early morning rounds of all the resident units, close contact with family members, and an active series of social engagements with many of the board members—in particular, the Johnson clan. In contrast, Paul Blackman has spent more time in his office and less time visiting with residents or socializing with the board. Mrs. Blackman, who is an accountant with a certified public accounting firm, has also been quite uninvolved with the home, in sharp contrast to Leslie Davidson.

The last few years of Davidson's tenure were both professionally and personally difficult for him. On the professional side, he faced a broad range of difficult challenges, including an attempted unionization at the nursing home, a decrease in the home's ability to raise funds, and a decrease in income from residents due to a declining private pay census as well as Medicaid cutbacks. On the personal side, Davidson had a series of medical problems, including a heart attack, bypass surgery, and a bout with prostate cancer. After enduring these problems for three years, the board prevailed upon Davidson to retire. Because of Davidson's health problems, he retired in January and his long-time assistant, Alvin Jones, who for 27 years was the home's personnel manager, took over as the acting administrator.

The board recognized Jones's limitations and agreed among themselves to increase their supervision of the home, particularly in the area of finances. The increased supervision provided the board with some unexpected and unpleasant information about the facility's fiscal health. Specifically, the board learned that in 1989 the home would run a deficit of close to $1,000,000. They also learned that the home was overstaffed and that the salary and benefit structure at the home was exceedingly problematic.

The board decided to find a new CEO to solve the problems and bring the home's finances into line. After a six-month search, they hired Paul Blackman, a 39-year-old, experienced nursing home administrator with an MBA in health administration. On January 1, 1990, Blackman took over the job and set about identifying the problems and rectifying them. The first of these problems involved low morale among the staff, which was largely due to Davidson's long history of favoritism that resulted in inequitable pay and fringe benefits for employees. For example, in the food service department, a cook with 20 years of seniority was paid less than another cook who had been with the home only 7 years. Also, the 20-year veteran was only entitled to three weeks of paid vacation, whereas Davidson had negotiated a four-week vacation package for the new cook after 5 years of service. The food service example was not an isolated case. There were numerous inequities throughout the organization, many of which apparently resulted from Davidson's desire to control staff through a series of private negotiations in which the individual staff member would become beholden to Davidson because the administrator bent the personnel rules to accommodate the employee's desires.

Other problems to be faced included the huge deficit resulting from overstaffing and state Medicaid cutbacks. Blackman dealt with these problems by undertaking a thorough review of personnel policies and actions as well as staffing levels. In addition, Blackman decided to replace a number of senior management personnel with people loyal to him. In one conversation with Angela Fisher, he stated that the home was still full of Davidson loyalists who ran to him with every complaint or controversy. A further problem was that many of those who were likely to lose from Blackman's policies had cordial relationships with the board—another legacy of the Davidson years when the CEO often hired people at the suggestion of board members, particularly the Johnson family.

In pursuing his policies, Blackman felt considerable pressure to get things in order as soon as possible. He also felt that every change he made reflected poorly on his predecessor and that frequently either Davidson or one of his friends on the board would react to any proposed change with the question, "How come we never had this problem when Mac ran the home?"

Blackman's analysis of the situation was that Mac Davidson was an out-of-touch and manipulative manager who ran the home by keeping the board in the dark and the board was complicit by choosing to stay in the dark. John and Kenneth Johnson, both former board presidents, viewed Blackman as the key problem. From their perspective, Blackman was doing a respectable job of dealing with the home's fiscal problems but was making a mess of the staff situation. Specifically, they believed he was wrong to fire or force into retirement so many top management staff, including the director of nursing, the director of the physical plant, the food service director, the personnel manager, and the purchasing agent. In addition, while they applauded his efforts at developing a more equitable system of wages and benefits, they were concerned about its costs as well as its potential for labor strife. Other matters that concerned these board members included Blackman's activities outside the home, such as his active participation on the state nursing home association's board of trustees, as well as his lack of time to socialize with the residents.

Angela Fisher found herself in the middle of this dispute. On the one hand, she personally liked Paul Blackman and respected what he was trying to accomplish. On the other hand, she felt that he should probably spend more time at the home and perhaps be more diplomatic about board relationships.

Her main concern, however, was how to deal with the powerful group of former board presidents who had announced that they were firing Paul Blackman.

* * *

Discussion Questions

1. Is there a problem with the structure of a self-perpetuating board?

2. How does this board's behavior differ from that of an "ideal" board?
3. Is Blackman's action of replacing Davidson loyalists a good strategy?
4. What appear to be the strengths and weaknesses of this board?
5. What appear to be the strengths and weaknesses of Mr. Blackman?
6. Assume that the board has decided to offer Mr. Blackman a written contract: What should be the key provisions of that contract?

Chapter 6

Role of the Medical Director in the 1990s

Steven A. Levenson

Limiting factor: $100-$150 /hr.

In 1974, for the first time, the Department of Health, Education, and Welfare (HEW) required every skilled nursing facility to retain a full- or part-time medical director. However, the only guidance offered was the inclusion of a medical director's potential job description. In 1977, the American Medical Association (AMA) issued a booklet of articles about the position of medical director, but since then it has given scant attention to the role of that position in the nursing home.[1] There was little further in-depth discussion of medical direction in the literature until some articles and books began to appear in the mid to late 1980s.[2]

In the 1990s and beyond, the role of the nursing home medical director is certain to expand. The current legal foundation for that role, and the strongest impetus to its further evolution, has come from the extensively revised federal nursing home regulations ("Conditions of Participation for Medicare and Medicaid"). These are known as the OBRA '87 regulations, because the law mandating their revision was part of the 1987 federal Omnibus Budget Reconciliation Act (OBRA).

The OBRA '87 regulations require that there be a medical director in all the nation's nursing facilities (former skilled and intermediate facilities). The only explicit regulatory duties of a medical director are to oversee the medical care and to coordinate the facility's resident care policies. However, other accompanying guidelines also imply that the medical director is obligated to help the facility apply appropriate professional standards and to take action when clinical care is inconsistent with those standards.[3]

This chapter will explore the required and optional responsibilities of the nursing home medical director, including the potential for the medical director to help improve the care of the institutionalized elderly.

THE CHANGING MEDICAL SITUATION IN LONG-TERM CARE

The nursing home has become a primary site for managing advanced old age and the health problems associated with aging. There are currently more people

(1.5 million) in nursing home beds than in acute care hospital beds in the United States.[4] Most nursing home residents are over age 65 (mean age, 80 years or older), predominantly female (approximately two-thirds), physically disabled with respect to basic activities of daily living, and cognitively impaired.[5]

One-fourth of those reaching age 65 will spend some time in a nursing home before they die. Because of shorter lengths of hospital stays under prospective payment reimbursement, nursing homes are receiving sicker patients and providing more medical care than before. More nursing home residents are dying within 30 days of admission, including more terminally ill patients transferred to nursing homes just prior to death.[6]

The nursing home population is very diverse. Facilities and attending physicians must manage a broad spectrum of age groups, illnesses, functional problems, and goals of care. Nursing home residents range from those who enter extremely ill and have a life expectancy of less than six months to those who have a mix of physical and cognitive impairments and will remain for many years.[7]

Thus, nursing homes are changing their functions and relationships, shifting from a predominantly social model providing personal care to a health care model managing illnesses and dysfunctions. Simultaneously, the roles of caregivers within nursing homes are changing, too.

THE PHYSICIAN'S ROLE

More than ever before, nursing home residents need quality medical care. Yet, many facility administrators and nursing directors wonder about the medical director's role in their facilities and how physicians might help them provide and improve care to the elderly population under their custody.

The diversity of the nursing home population requires medical flexibility. The management of a short-stay rehabilitation resident differs significantly from that of a short-stay terminally ill resident or of a long-term ambulatory but cognitively and functionally impaired resident. Many problems of nursing home residents are not medical in nature. If they are medical, they may be only partially treatable by physicians and the tools of modern medicine.

Attending physicians in the nursing home must coordinate their management of diseases, including their orders, with the plans and activities of other staff providing care (e.g., social workers, dietitians, nurses, nurse's aides, and physical and occupational therapists). Others impacting care include families, administrators, regulators, ombudsmen, and lawyers. Also, there are greater expectations for the residents' participation in care decisions. The medical director has a responsibility to encourage attending physicians to respect this interdisciplinary approach and to pay attention to the information provided by other staff.

Medical directors can also help improve clinical care by helping attending physicians and other caregivers manage acute and chronic illness more effectively in the nursing home. Nursing home residents have many potentially remediable medical conditions, including malnutrition, dehydration, depression, and infections. Apparently, many such problems could be treated successfully in their earlier stages in the nursing home, thus preventing costly and traumatic hospital admissions.[8]

There are important differences between providing care in acute and long-term care settings. Whereas acute care focuses on treating a medical disease or condition, long-term care focuses on restoring and maintaining functional capabilities, supporting maximal autonomy and quality of life, providing comfort and dignity for those who are dying, managing chronic medical conditions, and preventing and recognizing acute medical and iatrogenic illnesses.[9]

The extent to which the medical problems of a nursing home resident should be treated depends on the available therapies, the prognosis, and the wishes of the resident and family. An effective system to ascertain those wishes must be combined with good communication between and policies and protocols for cooperative management by physicians and other caregivers. Thus, a medical director should possess and promote a broader understanding of the meaning and implications of clinical care in the nursing home, including but not limited to the medical management of acute and chronic illness.

THE MEDICAL DIRECTOR'S REQUIRED AND OPTIONAL ROLES AND FUNCTIONS

In 1988, a group of medical directors met to develop a comprehensive enumeration of roles, functions, and tasks for nursing home medical directors.[10] Exhibit 6-1 lists these major administrative functions.

Only the first three (performing administrative functions, such as coordinating policies and procedures; organizing and ensuring adequate medical coverage; and overseeing care) are required by OBRA '87 regulations. Exhibit 6-2 lists some specific medical director activities relevant to regulatory compliance.

Table 6-1 illustrates the potential depth and breadth of medical director activities. Additional functions represent a broader, more activist physician role that many people believe could help improve the quality of care in nursing homes. It remains to be seen to what extent improvements will occur. The rest of this chapter considers the various tasks associated with these medical director functions.

Exhibit 6-1 Major Medical Director Functions

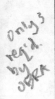

- Participate in administrative decision making and recommend and approve policies and procedures
- Organize and coordinate physician services and services of other professionals as they relate to patient care
- Participate in the process to ensure the appropriateness and quality of medical and medically related care
- Participate in the development and conduct of education programs
- Help articulate the facility's mission to the community and represent the facility in the community
- Participate in the surveillance and promotion of the health, welfare, and safety of employees
- Acquire, maintain, and apply knowledge of social, regulatory, political, and economic factors that relate to patient care services
- Provide medical leadership for research and development activities in geriatrics and long-term care
- Participate in establishing policies and procedures for ensuring that the rights of individuals are respected

Source: J.J. Pattee and T.M. Altemeier, Results of a Consensus Conference on the Role of the Nursing Home Medical Director, *Annual of Medical Direction* 1, no. 1 (1991):5–11.

MAJOR TASKS AND FUNCTIONS

Administrative Decision Making and Policies and Procedures

Typically, the medical director of a nursing home is the primary or only medically oriented person with administrative responsibilities. These responsibilities concern both the medical staff and the rest of the facility.

Administrative Staff

The medical director should work closely with the facility's departmental and professional leadership (i.e., the administrative staff).

The primary administrative decision makers in the nursing home are the administrator and the director of nursing. The medical director should meet regularly with them, using such meetings to discuss clinical issues and problem prevention and resolution, explain the medical staff's needs to the administrator and the director of nursing, listen to their concerns and needs regarding medical care, review the current status of previous problems, and provide medical input into

Exhibit 6-2 Examples of Medical Director Functions To Comply with OBRA '87 Regulations

---

Admission Rights
- Help create admission policies that clarify the process for approving and accepting prospective residents based on medical and psychosocial needs

Change in Resident Condition
- Help create policies about notification of physicians of incidents and accidents, changes in resident condition, or death
- Help ensure an effective system for evaluation and triage of significant changes in condition and timely transfer of residents out of the facility for further assessment or treatment in case of serious illness
- Review unexpected deaths and unanticipated discharges as part of quality assurance monitoring

Infection Control
- Work with other facility staff to establish appropriate policies and procedures for prevention and management of infections and the spread of infections
- Help establish policies and procedures for vaccination, isolation, universal precautions, and surveillance
- Establish policies and procedures for physician involvement in the assessment, prevention, and management of infections and infectious outbreaks
- Review all infection reports and analyze pertinent data for trends or potential or actual problems as part of the quality assurance/risk management process
- Participate in relevant infection control committee meetings

Medical Director Oversight of Care
- Ensure that physicians are aware of applicable professional standards
- Communicate and distribute pertinent information about geriatrics and related care standards from the clinical literature
- Help educate attending physicians to understand and apply those standards for care
- Review attending physician performance through quality assurance activities based on those standards
- Create appropriate medical policies and procedures
- Oversee the implementation of other clinical policies and procedures, coordinating the medical and nonmedical aspects
- Evaluate questions and concerns about the care of individual residents and discuss findings with residents, families, staff, and attending physicians, as pertinent
- Observe care on rounds and through record review
- Actively advocate for realistic improvements in the overall quality of care
- Document personal efforts to improve care, especially as part of the quality assurance process
- Ensure timely attending physician visits and follow up
- Keep records of discussions or correspondence with individual attending physicians regarding care of residents and with physicians who have significant problems complying with regulations and policies

Physician Staffing
- Create a system (bylaws, policies, etc.) that gives attending physicians a clear understanding of their regulatory responsibilities and their facility obligations and privileges
- Help the facility handle situations of significantly noncompliant attending physicians
- Provide the facility, residents, and families with guidelines for selecting or changing attending physicians

Source: S.A. Levenson, *Medical Direction in Long-Term Care,* 2d ed. (Durham, N.C.: Carolina Academic Press, 1993).

Table 6-1 The Medical Director's Roles and Functions

Planning	Organizing	Managing	Leading
		FUNCTIONS	
Help plan facility programs and services	Organize medical services	Participate in administrative decision-making process	Demonstrate appropriate geriatric medical principles through patient care and consultation
Plan for medical staffing and support needs	Establish bylaws and policies and procedures	Create and modify clinical policies and procedures	Advise facility of medical staff need for assistance and support
Plan for research and education activities and programs	Establish quality assurance program	Ensure appropriate and timely quality medical care	Participate in overall quality assurance program and quality improvement process
		Ensure physician compliance with laws, regulations, and policies	Represent the facility to the community
		Investigate and resolve medical staff problems	Participate in an employee health program
		Coordinate medical and other patient care services	Help ensure promotion of residents' rights
		Perform medical quality assurance oversight	Attain and apply knowledge of regulatory, legal, economic, and social factors affecting care
			Participate in research and education activities and programs
		TASKS	
Planning activities	Organizational activities	Physician facilitation and oversight; medically related problem solving	General systems facilitation and problem solving; physician and nonphysician education and training
		SKILLS	
Organizational	Organizational	Clinical	Clinical
Conceptual	Conceptual	Informational	Informational
		Interpersonal	Interpersonal
		Problem solving	Problem solving
		Communication	Communication
			Conceptual
			Decision making
			Teaching

pertinent decisions. This is an excellent opportunity to emphasize the importance of clinical and administrative coordination in providing good care.

The medical director should also establish effective communication with other professional staff leadership. This may include meeting with them individually or collectively and exchanging information about individual cases or about general issues or problems in the facility.

The medical director may find it helpful to prepare a periodic (e.g., quarterly or annual) report to the administration in order to make known the medical staff's activities and perspectives, summarize medical quality assurance and other activities, and ensure that the administration is aware of the medical staff's concerns and questions.

Admissions

Increasingly, nursing homes take residents with multiple medical, cognitive, behavioral, and functional problems. Therefore, some medical input into the development of general admissions criteria and into the decision process for individual admissions is desirable.

The medical director should advise the facility on appropriate medical criteria for admissions based on knowledge of the facility's goals and mission and the residents' conditions and problems. Also, the medical director should help the facility determine the staffing, services, and programs it needs to care for individual admissions. Related activities might include serving as an advisor to a facility admissions committee and recommending which medical information should be collected in a facility's preadmission assessment process.

Committees

Under the OBRA '87 regulations, the medical director must oversee the resident care policies. The OBRA '87 regulations require only a quality assurance committee. Also common in nursing homes are pharmacy and therapeutics, medical records, and infection control committees.

Committees are an important part of interdisciplinary communication and policy formulation in any nursing home. The medical director must work effectively with committees so that they will support the care.

The medical director and other key staff should decide together on an efficient way to hold these meetings. A combined meeting, in which the same key staff participate in handling several functions consecutively (medical records, infection control, risk management, etc.), can save time and be highly efficient. Many facilities are finding the quality assurance committee to be a valuable focus for solving and preventing problems and for obtaining critical interdisciplinary participation.

Financial Issues

Part of the medical director's role is to help ensure adequate facility resources for patient care. Decisions made by the administrators, owners, and board through the budgeting process determine the priorities for acquiring, distributing, and using these resources.

The medical director should participate in the facility budget process to help ensure that such resources are available. Often the medical director will have little input into anything other than his or her own compensation. In other cases, the medical director will be responsible for certain services, programs, or personnel, such as dues and travel, office supplies, staff physicians, support staff, consultants, or technicians.

Wherever possible, the medical director should be involved in certain steps in the medical budget process. This process begins with the preparation of departmental or medical staff objectives and goals based on current medical activities, a description of accomplishments during the past year, plans for the coming year, and the relationship of these activities and programs to the facility's goals and objectives. Based on these projections and on the medical staff's portion of the facility's revenues and expenses, a medical budget should project revenues and expenses for the coming year and justify any significant changes.

Medical Direction

Every medical director should have a written job description. Writing the description is best done after reviewing medical direction requirements and assessing the facility's desire or need for additional roles and responsibilities.

A physician's time commitment to medical direction will vary with a facility's size, its programs and services, the complexity of the residents' medical problems, and the expectations of the administrator and director of nursing. It also depends on the extent to which the medical director is new to the job or is organizing a new medical staff system, as opposed to improving or refining an existing system. Once a medical director establishes an effective system, ongoing management will take less time.

A medical director's contract should specify responsibilities and approximate time expectations; terms of the relationship (employee, contractor, etc.); compensation and benefits; secretarial support; and any financial support for education, meetings, and acquiring journals and other reference materials. Also, it should ensure that the medical director will receive adequate administrative support and authority to do the job properly.

Given the growing complexity of residents' medical problems, and the expanded responsibilities under OBRA '87, medical directors will probably need at least four to eight administrative hours a week per 100 beds to meet basic requirements effectively. Less than an hour a week is almost certainly insufficient.

Medical Records and Documentation

Though not a requirement, the medical director should help evaluate and improve the quality and consistency of the clinical information available in the nursing home and the quality of the systems for collecting, storing, retrieving, analyzing, and reporting that information. In the future, such systems will be needed not only for patient encounters but for management decisions and regulatory compliance.

Current medical records systems in health care are often inadequate for dealing effectively with complex patient care, especially with high volumes of regulations and standards, and where there is substantial variability in a staff's knowledge, skills, and performance. Poor quality, inaccurate, and inconsistent information should be considered a significant risk factor for the facility and its practitioners, since it contributes to errors of omission and commission. The reliability of sources of clinical information in the nursing home is hampered by the many cognitively impaired residents with a limited ability to give an accurate history and the often limited number of caregivers with adequate assessment skills to gather good quality clinical data.[11]

Partly because of pending requirements to record minimum data set information in a computer-usable format, many facilities are beginning to realize the value of computerizing clinical as well as financial information. The nursing home industry will need to use computers and other technologies creatively to meet growing expectations for quality care for a growing population. The OBRA '87 interpretive guidelines explicitly allow for computerized medical records, provided there are certain safeguards.

Some developments in the computer field that will likely impact significantly on nursing home practice in the next five years include much cheaper and more portable computers, reductions in the cost of linking users in effective networks, growing interest by vendors in nursing home software, and improved voice and handwriting recognition capabilities. Computers and other modern information technologies also offer great possibilities for staff and patient education, staff communication, and collection and use of information for multiple purposes, including clinical care, quality assurance, and regulatory compliance.

Also, "applied intelligence" software is becoming more widely used in many areas of government and industry. This software guides moderately skilled individuals to collect and input data, which are then interpreted by the software according to rules based on the accumulated knowledge, judgment, and experience of experts in the field. This kind of software has the potential to revolutionize the care in nursing homes by allowing modestly trained and skilled individuals to benefit from expertise not immediately available in their facility.

Medical directors should become more knowledgeable about information management and the potential uses for computerized information systems in long-term care. The needs of all caregivers, including the attending physicians, must be taken into account as facilities consider and then reorient toward the creation and future automation of effective clinical information systems that help provide high-quality patient care and meet regulatory and documentation requirements.

Patient Care

The medical director has an important role in helping to establish and achieve overall patient care goals for the facility and to ensure adequate physician participation in the care planning process.

Besides trying to ensure the best possible medical care for facility residents, the medical director should also encourage attending physicians to help the facility satisfy several major regulatory expectations: that treatments and medications are "medically necessary," that negative outcomes are "medically unavoidable," and that residents are able to attain the "highest practicable" levels of function and quality of life.

Policies and Procedures

In any complex system, such as the one delivering care to nursing home residents, policies and procedures are essential guides to performance. Effective policies and procedures are the ground rules that guide a collection of individuals of diverse experience and background toward common standards and expectations and that help ensure a more consistent understanding of essential goals and objectives.

Policies may be defined as officially interpreted general goals, objectives, and expectations. Managers or directors of businesses, departments, facilities, or organizations establish policies for those who work with or for them. Procedures are the specific steps or mechanisms for achieving these goals or objectives.

The medical director is specifically responsible for implementing resident care policies, including policies in such areas as admissions, transfers, and discharges; infection control; physician privileges and practices; emergency care; resident assessment and care planning; accidents and incidents; ancillary services such as laboratory, radiology, and pharmacy; use of medications; use and release of clinical information; utilization review; and overall quality of care.

The medical director should help create and coordinate effective policies and procedures to guide clinical care and related processes. These policies and procedures should incorporate social, medical, and economic information and advances and reflect good care standards. Some will be physician-specific and others will concern general clinical issues requiring physician participation and input. The medical director may share the responsibility for writing and implementing them.

Several references now exist to provide medical directors with comprehensive medical policies that can help them and their attending physicians fulfill their responsibilities under OBRA '87.[12]

For example, when, why, how, and how urgently should nurses notify physicians of changes in a resident's condition? Such changes appear to be a common source of physician-nurse disagreement in many nursing homes nationwide. Nursing home staff need a timely physician response to notification of changes in condition, and physicians desire an effective system to distinguish emergency problems from routine ones. Thus, protocols and policies for notification are important communication and clinical tools.

Regulatory guidelines note that a medical director is expected to help monitor and improve the actual care, not just write and approve policies. Like other managers in the nursing home, the medical director should understand the relationship between quality care and policies and procedures.

Surveys and Inspections

The medical director should help the facility interact with outside regulatory agencies and represent the medical staff at health department and other licensure and certification reviews.

During the actual survey process, surveyors match their evaluation of a facility's care to the OBRA '87 rules and guidelines. Before the licensure survey, the medical director can help improve overall physician compliance with physician-centered regulations such as visit requirements, and he or she should encourage attending physicians to support care by talking to staff and patients and coordinating their orders with staff care plans. The medical director can also recommend to the facility's administration and staff ways of improving general clinical care, communication, information management, and documentation systems.

During and after the survey process, the medical director can help by answering general or case-specific questions on medical care, requesting clarification of citations regarding clinical care, helping to draft corrective actions, and communicating with health department physicians who might understand better the nuances of disputed complex medical issues.

If done fairly and objectively, the survey process is a potentially useful opportunity for getting and giving feedback to confirm and improve care. Based on the results of such surveys, the medical director may want to revise medical or other clinical policies and procedures and help the facility institute or modify quality assurance activities to deal with the issues raised.

Organizing and Coordinating Medical Services

The medical director must ensure adequate and timely medical coverage for the facility's residents. This may be accomplished by

- organizing medical coverage
- helping ensure staffing to meet the facility's needs and goals
- helping ensure the quality, timeliness, and appropriateness of medical care
- credentialing the medical staff
- helping ensure medical staff compliance with facility, federal, state, and local requirements
- ensuring that the medical staff executive committee or its equivalent performs its appropriate functions
- developing and reviewing policies and job descriptions for midlevel practitioners such as physician assistants and nurse practitioners

Typically, nursing facilities have used any of several different physician staffing arrangements. Most still use open staffs of community-based attending physicians. Especially in larger nursing homes (more than 200 beds), some medical directors are turning to closed staffs, sometimes hiring full- or part-time salaried physicians, using nurse practitioners and physician assistants to provide primary care, or using fewer attending physicians, each with more patients.

More medical directors realize the importance of at least some organization of attending physicians. They have found it hard to exercise their responsibility without a system enabling them to assert some authority and fulfill quality assurance oversight functions. Attending physicians must know the regulations, policies, and expectations that determine what constitutes adequate performance.

Bylaws

More medical directors are using bylaws (also referred to as practice agreements) to organize attending physicians and to create a foundation for medical care. Bylaws describe the legal foundations and the structure and functions underlying medical staff activity, establish a broad general framework of expectations for physician performance, create a mechanism for enforcing responsibility, and establish ground rules for the medical staff to carry out its responsibilities to the residents and the facility. They establish the medical staff as a self-governing entity and define its relationship to the governing body, which is ultimately responsible for the care delivered in the facility. Sample nursing home medical bylaws are available from the American Medical Directors Association and elsewhere.[13]

Since the nursing home medical director typically serves the functions of the chief of staff and medical executive committee in an acute hospital, nursing home medical staff bylaws can be simpler than those for a hospital medical staff. These bylaws should at least obligate practitioners to acknowledge that they understand the regulatory and clinical requirements that contemporary nursing homes must meet, are willing to cooperate with the medical director and facility staff to provide good geriatric medical care and help meet those requirements, and are receptive to the medical director's suggestions, based on medical quality assurance activities, about ways to improve care.

Consultative and Emergency Coverage

As much as possible, the medical director should ensure that the facility has access to needed consultants and that such consultants respond in a timely fashion. This objective may be hindered by the limited availability of consultants in many areas of the country. Also, the medical director may need to educate consultants about the special aspects of nursing home residents and long-term care so that they will understand the special problems of prescribing in the facility and in carrying out complicated orders for residents who may not be able to participate in their care.

The medical director should ensure that the facility has access to essential medical coverage, including for emergencies, and that attending physicians and their backups respond in a timely fashion to urgent or emergent problems. Also, the medical director should help ensure that equipment, drugs, and supplies are available in the facility for emergencies. This may include reviewing the emergency cart, the interim medication box, supplies, procedures for resuscitation, and protocols for deciding when to notify attending physicians of new problems or changes in a resident's condition or status.

Outside Affiliations

The medical director should help the facility attain and maintain certain outside affiliations. For example, the medical director might be given the job of initiating, analyzing, and supporting links with hospitals and universities, serving as medical liaison with other facilities, or helping obtain ancillary services (such as lab and x-ray services).

Since most medical directors with nursing home patients are also on the staffs of local hospitals, they have an opportunity to try to improve hospital care of the elderly, which can in turn help the nursing home meet its care responsibilities. Many acute care hospitals and their medical staffs have yet to realize they can play a role in helping nursing homes give better care. Examples of possible improvements include reducing placement of indwelling urinary catheters in nursing home residents who are hospitalized, reducing development or worsening of pressure sores in nursing home residents who are hospitalized, and improving the documentation and discharge instructions regarding ongoing care when hospital patients are transferred to the nursing home. Possible approaches to improving support may include informal discussions and presentations at grand rounds or other medical meetings.

Trainees

Increasingly, the nursing home is an important site for health professional students and trainees to learn about the problems of the elderly and about the practice of geriatric medicine and other health professions.

Students and postgraduate trainees from many different schools who may rotate through teaching nursing homes must be monitored and supervised. The medical staff or medical director will often have some responsibility for these trainees. The medical director is at least indirectly responsible for monitoring trainee activities that might impact on the physical or psychological well-being of the residents. Training programs work best when those being trained and those responsible for them understand each other's needs and problems and make accommodations accordingly. Trainees must appreciate that they are learning within a residence and must not let their presence interfere with the operation of the facility or infringe on the rights of the residents.

The medical director should collaborate with directors of various training programs to ensure that supervision is adequate and appropriate and that the programs are educationally worthwhile. This may necessitate creation of program policies and procedures that describe qualifications, requirements, supervisory responsibilities, other responsibilities, prerogatives and limitations, liability, and conditions for termination of assignment.

Ensuring the Appropriateness and Quality of Medical and Medically Related Care

The OBRA '87 regulations mandate physician participation on a facility quality assurance committee. Most likely, the medical director will serve as the physician member. To function effectively the medical director should have some role in setting up the monitoring systems; deciding how to collect data; reviewing and analyzing the data; identifying high-risk, high-volume, and problem-prone areas; and educating attending physicians based on analysis of the data.

The Joint Commission on Accreditation of Healthcare Organizations has recommended a ten-step process for quality assurance activities.[14] This process includes

1. assigning responsibility
2. defining the scope of care
3. considering the important aspects of care
4. developing key indicators
5. creating evaluation thresholds
6. collecting and organizing data
7. evaluating care
8. taking problem-solving actions
9. assessing the results of those actions
10. communicating relevant information

In some form, these principles apply to all disciplines.

The quality assurance process should focus on education rather than disciplinary action, which should be reserved for the most flagrant and persistent offenders. Education activities may include providing education materials to help staff improve the quality of care, monitoring and evaluating the effectiveness of education programs, providing quality assurance feedback to staff and recommending ideas to improve performance and decrease problems, and ascertaining the national standards for quality care and helping the facility translate these into internal standards.

Medical Staff Quality Assurance

The medical director has a major role in helping establish standards and indicators for quality medical care and physician performance.

The goals of medical quality assurance in the nursing home are to safeguard good care already being provided, recognize opportunities to improve care, and identify and resolve problems. Briefly, a successful medical quality assurance program in a nursing home involves the following steps. The medical director and attending physicians should identify important aspects of care and collaborate in establishing appropriate policies, medical care standards, and quality indicators (criteria for reviewing specific aspects of care). The medical director, perhaps assisted by other medical staff, should then ensure a mechanism for collecting pertinent data, review the data when collected, analyze problems or seek areas for possible quality improvement, provide feedback to attending physicians (both quality assurance information and education), and follow up to see if education and policy making improve care and prevent subsequent problems.

Though responsible for evaluating data and taking follow-up actions, the medical director can rely mostly on data that others already collect or report for other purposes. Medical directors typically evaluate care and identify care problems by reviewing accident and incident reports, pharmacist reports, change of patient condition reports, and infection control reports; by making observations while delivering care and on rounds; by attending quality assurance committee meetings; by helping design special studies and ongoing audits; and by offering consultation and guidance to other caregivers regarding the management of individual residents.

Medical directors may respond to identified problems with care by communicating with individual physicians (orally or in writing), communicating with the medical staff about care problems in general (not pertaining to a specific resident), communicating with nonphysician staff regarding clinical care, participating in facility in-services to correct general care problems, and preparing written reports of actions taken.

Facilitywide Quality Assurance Program

Defining quality care in a nursing home is a complex task, since nursing homes provide both personal and medical care.[15] Demonstrating quality care is also difficult.

As a leader in the nursing home, the medical director should understand and advocate for tactics and systems that help both physicians and nonphysicians work more effectively. According to one perspective, professional and facility leaders must take the lead in seeking continuous quality improvement, promoting a vision of the health care system as capable of continuous improvement, and using modern technical and theoretically grounded tools to improve care processes. It is also important to get physicians to join in the efforts to achieve continuous improvement.

Although the value of the concept of continuous quality improvement in the nursing home remains to be proven fully, it appears that an effective system is critical to providing good care. The medical director should at least encourage and help attending physicians to understand their role in a common effort to improve care instead of seeing themselves primarily as isolated practitioners treating disease in individual patients.

In relation to the facilitywide quality assurance process, the medical director can help

- ensure the relevance of programs and standards to quality patient care
- ensure adequate quality review in areas mandated by laws and regulations
- draft policies and procedures that correct and prevent problems
- establish and monitor factors related to quality of life in the facility
- discuss quality of care issues regularly with other key administrative staff
- establish basic standards and criteria for quality medical care and physician performance

- incorporate new knowledge and quality assurance findings into the patient care–planning process

Risk Management

Risk management may be defined as the preventive arm of a quality assurance program. Risk management activities seek to reduce or eliminate potential problems that may impact negatively on care or on those providing care.

The medical director's role in a facility's risk management program may include reporting pertinent observations (e.g., about safety hazards or potential sources of clinical errors or miscommunications) to the director of nursing and the administrator; becoming involved in the employee health program; and educating physicians to help reduce risks (e.g., by responding quickly to nursing notification of changes in condition, ensuring adequate alternate coverage in case of unavailability, and reducing the use of medications that may increase functional problems such as dizziness and falling).

Utilization Review

The medical director should work with the medical staff to help the facility ensure appropriate, cost-efficient use of beds and services, ensure that patient admissions and placement are consistent with established criteria, and ensure that patients receive the programs and services they need based on the comprehensive assessments and other pertinent findings. The medical director should participate in the utilization review process to monitor delivery of care within economic and social constraints. Although there is no longer a formal utilization review committee requirement for skilled nursing facilities, there may still be state and Medicare requirements.

Developing and Conducting Education Programs

The medical director may play an important role in helping educate the administration and board about care issues in the facility, including appropriate programs, necessary support, realistic expectations, quality of care issues, the medical role in long-term care, and the medical director's responsibilities. The medical director should also update the facility on clinical issues by providing current information gathered from attendance at meetings and conferences and from the medical literature.

An important part of the education process lies in the medical director's individual interactions with staff, administrators, patients, and families. Both formal and informal education should occur regarding clinical, ethical, regulatory, and legislative issues. Patient care rounds are also an excellent opportunity for teaching other staff.

The medical director also represents an important resource for the community. The medical director's role might include

- educating the community about long-term care and the facility
- making speaking appearances
- helping outsiders understand and have more realistic expectations of the facility and of long-term care generally
- educating patients and families about relevant clinical issues
- producing various written materials, such as handbooks, to assist facility staff in dealing with complex ethical and clinical issues

Educating the medical staff might involve

- informing attending physicians about changes in policies, procedures, laws, and regulations
- keeping medical staff informed about medical staff activities
- providing summaries of reports and meeting minutes
- keeping medical staff informed about pertinent policies, procedures, laws, and regulations

Promoting Employee Health, Welfare, and Safety

Employee Health

Employee health is an important but sometimes overlooked part of any facility. There are many areas in which medical input can be of assistance. Overall, the medical director should recommend ideas to decrease legal risks and prevent problems that could adversely impact patient care and the general safety of employees, staff, patients, and visitors. The medical director could play an important role in employee health by

- developing and participating in a pre-employment screening process
- helping to monitor and evaluate employee injuries and illness
- promoting employee wellness programs and ways to prevent job-related injuries and disease
- helping to foster a sense of self-worth and professionalism among employees
- establishing appropriate health maintenance screens and procedures, such as TB testing

- identifying community resources for employees with psychological or social problems
- planning and determining the scope and policies of medical services
- providing overall medical direction for the physical examination program, including initial and ongoing assessments, and determining the scope of the examination
- evaluating the physical capacity of employees to perform their jobs
- discussing and interpreting findings with employees when health problems are found and making appropriate referrals
- evaluating employees' ability to return to work
- helping to establish programs to assist in the employees' return to work after an injury or illness
- reviewing reports from employees' outside personal physicians
- making periodic tours of the physical plant to become familiar with the physical requirements of the various jobs
- helping to ensure employee compliance with infection control requirements
- helping the facility minimize workers' compensation losses
- contributing to a program to monitor, evaluate, and prevent injury and illness
- contributing to the activities of a safety committee
- encouraging proper use of assistive devices by employees
- developing a modified work program for injured employees

Representing the Facility in the Community

Traditionally, nursing homes have a bad reputation among physicians and other professionals. The medical director can help play a role in enhancing the facility's reputation among local professionals, including physician colleagues, by

- participating in pertinent activities of professional organizations, hospitals, and so on
- meeting regularly with other long-term care professionals in the community
- identifying issues and negotiating solutions to problems involving outside institutions and programs
- helping to handle problems with outside organizations or agencies (lab, x-ray, other hospitals, outside physicians, etc.)
- serving as liaison between the facility medical staff and other local medical staffs

- providing grand rounds, conferences, and other information about the facility and long-term care

Programs and Systems

The medical director may also participate in health care planning, including helping the facility develop innovative and cost-effective alternative health care programs and integrating those facility programs with others in the continuum of long-term care. This may involve

- networking with community groups and long-term care organizations
- helping others understand the systems approach to health care
- evaluating and correlating admission patterns relative to community trends and needs

Applying Knowledge of Social, Regulatory, Political, and Economic Factors

The medical director should keep abreast of political, regulatory, legal, and economic developments that could affect care in the facility, such as new mechanisms for long-term care reimbursement and changes in state and federal rules and regulations. Possible applications of such knowledge might include

- suggesting reasonable cost-containment measures (contracts, lab usage, formularies, etc.)
- recommending ways to improve the efficiency and productivity of facility staff
- giving feedback to legislators, policy makers, and local decision makers on existing and proposed rules and regulations

Promoting Research and Development Activities in Geriatrics and Long-Term Care

Most medical directors do not consider research to be a major responsibility. Those involved in research may do the following:

- evaluate and review the feasibility and goals of research projects
- solicit funding for research activities
- learn about basic research methodologies

- ensure proper safeguards for patients involved in research projects, including informed consent protocols
- serve as chairperson of the institutional review committee

Even for a medical director who does not have an interest in formal research, it is worthwhile to try to foster appropriate facility attitudes toward investigation and change by applying a rational problem-solving approach and pertinent research findings from the medical and related literature.

Ensuring That the Rights of Individuals Are Respected

The OBRA '87 regulations heavily emphasize residents' rights. The medical director should be familiar with those rights, ensure that the attending physicians help protect and enhance those rights, and help the facility do likewise. The medical director can assist in the protection of general patient rights by

- helping ensure rights of privacy and confidentiality
- ensuring application of the patient bill of rights
- facilitating choice of physicians
- helping the facility monitor for and handle patient abuse
- becoming knowledgeable about pertinent legal precedents

Ethical Issues

Many elderly people now expect a say in decisions about their care and about the initiation, discontinuation, or withdrawal of treatment. Legal and regulatory guidelines have expanded the rights of recipients of care.

Medical ethics involves clarifying or selecting values and evaluating to what extent treatment options are consistent with specific values and beliefs.

In fact, individualization and selectivity are key values in the care of the elderly. Broad ethical and clinical goals are directed to maximize individual benefit. Not everyone should have to make the same treatment choices, just as not everyone with heart failure should receive the same medications. However, adherence to a consistent process will allow better individualization of outcomes.

Although the physician can best present medical facts (e.g., "These are your options and the likely benefits and risks"), the elderly individual or an appropriate substitute decision maker should evaluate the options and make choices under the guidance of the physician and other caregivers. It helps to remember that making a medical choice is not purely a scientific matter but also has personal, social, and philosophical dimensions.

In geriatric medicine, especially in the nursing home, ethical considerations should be included routinely in the clinical decision-making process. Problems can be reduced or prevented by following appropriate procedures consistently and by presenting information thoughtfully, documenting prudently, and involving residents and families in the decision-making process, as appropriate. All parties should view the use of guidelines as a way to improve geriatric medical practice and to enhance the well-being of residents, not just as a way to avoid being sued.

The medical director's responsibilities may include

- ensuring that patients have a say in their own care through appropriate documents and expression of wishes
- helping establish a program to manage ethical issues
- developing policies and procedures to deal with limited treatment plans
- developing a mechanism for transferring information regarding patient choices through the spectrum of care sites
- participating in an institutional biomedical ethics committee

THE FUTURE OF MEDICAL DIRECTION

The future of long-term care medical direction looks bright. With current regulatory requirements and the rapidly growing elderly population, medical directors will have greater responsibility for organizing medical care and coordinating it with other programs and services, creating and refining policies and procedures, and overseeing medical and general clinical care. Most of all, medical directors can perform a major service to facilities and their residents by helping ensure effective compliance with the expectations for improved quality of life and quality and thoughtfulness of the clinical care, as described in the OBRA '87 regulations and guidelines.

Undoubtedly, the extent of medical director participation and influence in individual facilities will vary widely. The full potential impact of the medical director on clinical care remains uncertain. It will be important to study the effect on outcomes and quality of care of the time that medical directors spend on activities such as quality assurance; employee health, education, and training; and research and development.

Some medical directors feel handicapped by a shortage of attending physicians, the lack of cooperation or interest on the part of some attending physicians, the relative lack of facility support, the quality and skills of nonphysician personnel working in nursing homes, regulations, limited reimbursement, and paper work. However, a substantial minority of medical directors do not appear to face any significant impediments to improving physician or nonphysician care in their facilities.

Currently, a number of nursing facilities have satisfied and effective attending physicians because of effective collaboration between these physicians and their medical director as well as effective collaboration between the medical director and the other facility staff and the administration. Nursing home administrators should encourage and support physicians who are considering serving as medical directors and attending physicians in the nation's nursing homes. In the nursing home of the future, there will be few professionals more valuable than a skilled and committed medical director.

NOTES

1. American Medical Association, *The Medical Director in the Long Term Care Facility* (Chicago: American Medical Association, 1977).

2. S.R. Ingman et al., Medical Direction in Long-Term Care, *Journal of the American Geriatrics Society* 26 (1978):157–166; J.J. Pattee, Update on the Medical Director Concept, *American Family Physician* 28, no. 6 (1983):129–133; W. Reichel, Role of the Medical Director in the Skilled Nursing Facility: Historical Perspectives, in *Clinical Aspects of Aging,* ed. W. Reichel, 2d ed. (Baltimore: Williams and Wilkins, 1983); S.A. Levenson, *Medical Direction in Long-Term Care* (Baltimore: National Health Publishing, 1988).

3. U.S. Department of Health and Human Services, Health Care Financing Administration, Part 483 Requirements for Long Term Care Facilities, *Federal Register* 56, no. 187 (September 26, 1991):48867–48879.

4. AMA Council on Scientific Affairs, American Medical Association White Paper on Elderly Health, *Archives of Internal Medicine* 150 (1977):2459–2472.

5. J.G. Ouslander, Medical Care in the Nursing Home, *JAMA* 262 (1989):2582–2590.

6. AMA Council on Scientific Affairs, White Paper on Elderly Health.

7. Ouslander, Medical Care in the Nursing Home.

8. AMA Council on Scientific Affairs, White Paper on Elderly Health.

9. Ouslander, Medical Care in the Nursing Home.

10. J.J. Pattee and T.M. Altemeier, Results of a Consensus Conference on the Role of the Nursing Home Medical Director, *Annual of Medical Direction* 1, no. 1 (1991):5–11.

11. Ouslander, Medical Care in the Nursing Home.

12. S.A. Levenson, *Medical Policies and Procedures for Long-Term Care* (Baltimore: National Health Publishing, 1990); J.G. Ouslander et al., *Medical Care in the Nursing Home* (New York: McGraw-Hill, 1991).

13. Levenson, *Medical Direction in Long-Term Care;* J.J. Pattee and O.J. Otteson, *Medical Direction in the Nursing Home* (Minneapolis: Northridge Press, 1991).

14. Joint Commission on Accreditation of Healthcare Organizations, *Quality Assurance in Long-Term Care* (Chicago: Joint Commission, 1989).

15. S.A. Levenson, Quality Care in the Nursing Home—Defining and Providing It in a New Era, *Geriatric Medicine Today* 8, no. 8 (1989):29–40.

Case Study 6-1

A Prescription for Change

Seth B. Goldsmith

After reading an article in a medical journal on medication problems in nursing homes, Myra Quinn, MD, the newly appointed medical director of the Wayside Home, a 200-bed skilled nursing facility, decided to undertake an evaluation of the drug usage situation at Wayside. Her study involved a review of drug and medical records of all the residents, most of whom are not her patients.

The results of her research were only slightly better than that reported in the literature: Close to 40 percent of the residents received at least one inappropriate medication. With these findings in hand, Quinn decided to embark on an educational program and sent the following letter to each physician on the home's medical staff.

Wayside Skilled Nursing Facility
Snowville, State

Dear Colleague:

As you can see from the enclosed article, there is a serious problem with inappropriate drug-prescribing behavior in nursing homes. In response to this article, I reviewed the drug and medical records of each of our 200 residents and I am sorry to report that we are doing about the same as the 12 homes reported in the study. What this means in practice is that we all need to be more careful about our prescribing habits. My research indicates that about 40 percent of our residents are getting drugs that they simply should not be receiving.

It would be appreciated if you would review the enclosed article and also review your prescriptions for your patients in the home and make any adjustments as appropriate.

Thank you for your attention to this matter.

Sincerely,

Myra Quinn, MD /s/
Medical Director

The reaction to Quinn's letter was swift. Within hours the home's administrator, Robin McNeil, received eight phone calls from medical staff. Their response to the Quinn letter was overwhelmingly negative, with comments such as "Who the hell does she think she is?" "What business does she have reviewing my medical records without my permission?" and "I want her fired."

McNeil was stunned by these responses and felt he needed to respond to the enraged medical staff as well as the legitimate concerns about the quality of care raised by Quinn.

* * *

Discussion Question

1. What strategies could McNeil follow to achieve the goals of supporting Dr. Quinn in her new position, the medical staff in its involvement with the home, and a commitment to high quality care for the residents?

Chapter 7

Nursing in the Long-Term Care Facility

Joan Marie Culley and Janet Courtney

This chapter is designed to give administrators of long-term care facilities a brief guide and overview of nursing as it can be organized and delivered in the long-term care setting. Nursing provided in this setting and to the elderly population is very different from nursing in the acute care facility, free-standing clinic, outpatient clinic, or the home. This chapter focuses on the development of the department of nursing and the selection of a nursing model to be used as a guide for delivery of care to our elderly population in the long-term care setting.

OVERVIEW

In replacing the term *nursing home* with *long-term care,* the central mission of a long-term care facility may be obscured. This mission is easily articulated by family members or residents of long-term care facilities: It is *nursing care.*

Most people enter long-term care facilities to receive the type of care offered by the facility's nursing department. Reduced ability to perform activities of daily self-care, loss of cognitive skills for self-care and home management, and difficulty moving about in the physical environment are the most common problems that lead an elder and his or her family to seek nursing home residence. The long-term care administrator needs to appreciate the centrality of the nursing care function in the facility and organize the operations of the facility to support that function.

Support for nursing begins with designating the director of nursing as a top management position in the organization. Selection of a director of nursing who is educationally and experientially qualified for the position is the next major step. In a majority of long-term care facilities, the director of nursing has a direct line relationship with the facility administrator and is the second in charge of the administrative aspects of the facility. Because of the importance and scope of responsibilities, the director of nursing should be educationally prepared at the master's level in nursing and should be experienced in the care of the elderly. Experience with the elderly is an extremely important requirement and cannot be overemphasized. (See Appendix 7-A for qualifications and a suggested job description.) A good working relationship between the long-term care facility administrator and the director of nursing is essential for successful institutional management. Indeed, the director of nursing and the administrator frequently share on-call responsibilities.

The responsibilities of the director of nursing in the long-term care setting include

- implementing extensive and complex federal and state regulations
- operationalizing the concept of resident instead of patient
- operationalizing the concept of home
- developing services with the capability of caring for elderly persons, whose presentation of illness is unique and very different from younger persons'
- focusing on residents' potential capabilities rather than limitations

The long-term care setting is unique and demands the use of skilled caregivers who are knowledgeable about and experienced in long-term care. Although many acute care skills may be applied, the long-term care setting requires a nursing leader who clearly understands the differences between acute and long-term care and is able to administer a department responsive to the differences.

The director of nursing should be involved in the development of the philosophy and goals of the facility. The philosophy and goals of the department of nursing complement and enlarge upon those of the long-term care facility. Nursing is viewed by most residents and family members as the major focus of the delivery of care and services. Residents and families judge the quality of the facility by the care delivered at the bedside.

Bureaucracy often seems to engulf long-term care, making it easy to lose sight of the caring and nurturing environment that should determine outcomes and set the course for the services that are delivered to residents. In attempting to meet the many demands of both federal and state regulations, a facility may become obsessed with the tasks to be accomplished rather than with outcomes. Time, energy, personnel, and resources are required to manage the documentation and forms that must be completed.

Residents entering long-term care facilities and their families view the bureaucracy through their own personal set of glasses. They frequently report seeing numerous personnel hustling and bustling around in expensive suits and dresses, carrying paper back and forth between departments, but only two or three actual caregivers on each residential unit. To them, this means a system that is top-heavy with administrative personnel and inadequately funded to provide enough direct care to the residents. They wonder how the money they are spending on long-term care placement translates into direct caregivers and time spent at the bedside.

Speech therapy, occupational therapy, physical therapy, recreational therapy, dietary counseling, social services, psychiatric services, pastoral services, financial counseling, and physician services are all critical services in the inpatient facility. Nursing services differ from these in that nursing is provided on a continuous basis to each and every resident 24 hours a day, 7 days a week, 52 weeks a year, year after year.

Nursing staff are there when Mrs. Yoke is having a nightmare and needs someone to talk with, to ask for some warm milk, to rub her back, and to walk her in the hall until she is calmer. They understand that providing a sedative to Mrs. Yoke causes disorientation and agitation, and thus they have designed a plan for Mrs. Yoke that prevents these upsetting side effects.

Nursing staff are there to plan the celebration for Mr. Brown's 93rd birthday. Mr. Brown is all alone because his friends and relatives have died. They understand that, in order for a resident like Mr. Brown to complete the psychological development tasks of the older adult, related to integrity rather than despair, reflection about the past is essential. They therefore make time to listen to Mr. Brown reminisce about the past. Each night, a nurse finally tucks him safely into bed, remembering to place the urinal within easy reach. Mr. Brown has urinary urgency and needs to have the urinal within easy reach to prevent falls from his attempts to get to the bathroom. The nursing staff know how upset Mr. Brown becomes when he is incontinent and that such "accidents" prevent him from sleeping the rest of the night. A plan has been developed to prevent the incontinent episodes. Now that the urinal is always placed within reach, Mr. Brown only rarely has episodes of incontinence, sleeps well, and has had no further falls at night. In developing such a plan of care, the nursing staff reduced the risk of falls and the number of patient care hours required to change Mr. Brown's bed. Mr. Brown's quality of life has been greatly enhanced by the plan as well.

Nursing staff are there to carefully dry between the surfaces of Mrs. Hernandez's toes so that she will not develop an infection between her toes again. Five months ago Mrs. Hernandez had a foot infection that prevented her from wearing shoes for two weeks. She enjoys walks outside each morning with the nursing assistant but could not take these walks until the infection was cured. When the elderly are restricted in their activities and less mobile, the chance of such complications as thrombophlebitis, pneumonia, and renal problems increases. These complications affect the quality of life for residents, often result in acute care admissions, cost the facility and health care system money, and increase the number of patient care hours needed.

As can be seen from these illustrations, nursing is the focus in the long-term care setting. The ability of the nursing department to perform assessments, establish priorities, develop appropriate plans of care, and deliver and monitor care (making adjustments when necessary) ensures that the long-term care facility will be able to manage resources and productivity effectively, reduce the risk of liability from negligence, and, most important, provide a quality of life for older persons that is respectful of their capabilities.

The director of nursing has the responsibility of organizing the department. The critical elements of this task include (1) the establishment of the philosophy of the department, (2) the development of a nursing care practice model, (3) the development of patient care standards, (4) the development of policies and procedures, and (5) the selection of personnel. Each of these topics is discussed below.

PHILOSOPHY OF THE DEPARTMENT OF NURSING

When defining the philosophy of nursing care that is to be delivered in any institution, it is necessary to delineate the expected outcome of that care. Historically, many long-term care facilities have adhered to a custodial rather than restorative philosophy of care.

With the custodial philosophy, the focus is on providing services to residents, who are viewed as passive recipients of routine assistance with daily living activities. The goal is protection through watchful vigilance. With a restorative philosophy, the focus is on working with the residents, who are viewed as participants capable of reaching their maximum potential. This approach to caregiving is not in conflict with the needs of the terminally ill or cognitively impaired resident. Even terminally ill residents can be regarded as participants capable of determining how their care should be managed. Cognitively impaired residents can be assessed for potential strengths, which can then be used to achieve maximum development of capabilities. Custodial care focuses on weaknesses, not on strengths. It is human nature to focus on problems or disabilities, but an environment becomes nurturing when the focus is switched to the actual and potential capabilities of the individual.

The choice of either the custodial or the restorative approach will be reflected in all services and care provided to the residents. Federal guidelines on reimbursement currently mandate that a restorative philosophy be implemented in long-term care facilities.

For example, although it may seem easier and more efficient to simply diaper Mrs. Ortiz as a way of dealing with her urinary incontinence, it may not be in her best interest. If the restorative goal is to increase her self-esteem and maximize her independence by making her capable of continence, then specific alterations in her environment and care delivery could probably be planned to achieve this goal. Once a thorough assessment of the continence problem is completed, the incontinence might be controllable without diapering by moving furniture in Mrs.

Ortiz's room so that she has a direct path to the bathroom, placing a raised commode seat on the toilet, carefully selecting clothing that Mrs. Ortiz can remove quickly to expedite toileting, and educating and supporting staff in this plan of care.

SELECTION OF THE PRACTICE MODEL

The organizational framework for delivering care to residents operationalizes the restorative philosophy of care. Features of this framework include (1) decentralized authority and responsibility; (2) accountability to the resident and the resident's family; (3) decision making as close to the resident as possible; and (4) staffing the institution with the proper mix and numbers of licensed nurses, certified nursing assistants, and qualified personnel, giving each staff member the appropriate responsibility and authority for completing the required tasks. (See Appendix 7-A for detailed job descriptions for the personnel assigned to the department of nursing.)

Decentralization provides flexibility and promotes greater participation in decision making at the level at which decisions should take place. The role of nursing as the principle provider of care 24 hours a day and as responsible for identifying, treating, and monitoring the physical sequelae of illness places nurses in the position of being managers of care. The nurses, as a result, are accountable for the quality of health supervision and care in the long-term care facility. It should be noted that the role of manager of care may be new to nurses whose clinical experience has been primarily in acute care hospitals, where physicians are usually the managers of care.

In the long-term care setting, it is often nursing that identifies the need for other available health services and intervenes to ensure that the services are provided in a comprehensive, well-organized manner. Nursing is the maestro that orchestrates the harmonic delivery of care.

The restorative philosophy of care requires the proper mix of personnel possessing the expertise to assess resident needs, develop interdisciplinary plans of care, implement care, evaluate the outcomes of care, and make changes in the plans of care when indicated. Long-term care recipients "on the average have four or more chronic illnesses and frequent episodes of acute illnesses."[1] Care must therefore be developed to respond to residents' needs dynamically. This requires a carefully balanced ratio of residents to staff. In other words, it may not be cost-effective in the long run to staff units with mostly unlicensed personnel. Although federal and state authorities provide regulations that guide minimum staffing patterns, it may enhance productivity to place greater numbers of licensed staff at the bedside. Licensed staff have the ability, authority, and responsibility to make decisions and perform assessments quickly, reduce incidents such as falls and skin integrity problems, and enhance the residents' ability to toilet and dress themselves so that they can be more active participants in their own care. When residents' capabilities are utilized and falls and skin integrity problems are prevented, the institution saves time and money.

The environment in a long-term care facility can become much more productive and stimulating if nursing staff are responsive to the residents' feelings of being valued as individuals capable of making decisions, participating in their own care, and reaching their maximum potential. All personnel in the department of nursing must have a clear understanding of the goals and must share in the interdisciplinary approach that is characteristic of a decentralized model. In particular, the director of nursing must demonstrate an attitude toward nursing assistants that is respectful of the important role they play in providing direct care to residents. This includes recognizing their contributions and involving them in interdisciplinary meetings, end-of-shift reporting, and staff development activities. One of the most valuable resources in the long-term care setting is the quality of the direct caregivers—the nursing assistants.

SELECTION OF PATIENT CARE STANDARDS

Standards provide norms for assessing a department of nursing's performance. They serve as a framework for departmental evaluations and as the yardstick by which liability is judged in a court of law. The standards most frequently cited are set by the federal government in regulating long-term care facilities. These are used by survey teams in evaluating long-term care facilities and serve as a reference for analyzing both the organizational structure and direct care services.

In addition to the federal and state written standards, the American Nurses' Association (ANA) has established standards for geriatric nursing practice and organized nursing services in long-term care facilities. Unlike the federal and state standards, the ANA standards do not reflect the minimum level of quality but the optimum level. A long-term care facility must also comply with the standards set by the Joint Commission on Accreditation of Healthcare Organizations (Joint Commission) or it may not be eligible for government funds. *No*

The ANA's Standards for Organized Nursing Services state that the department of nursing must (1) have a philosophy and structure that ensures the delivery of high-quality nursing care, (2) have a qualified administrator who is a member of the corporate administration, (3) have policies and practices that provide for equality and continuity of services, (4) use the nursing process to plan and organize care, (5) provide an environment that ensures the effectiveness of nursing practice, (6) ensure the development of educational programs to support high-quality care, and (7) initiate and utilize research for improvement of care.[2] These standards form the framework used by most nursing executives in the development and organization of their departments.

The departmental and organizational philosophies and goals of a long-term care facility form the basis for identifying what can and should be done. Standards are the articulation of this process. Once the organizational standards are developed and in place, the direct patient care standards are written. The purpose of these standards is to provide the highest level of care possible within the economic and productive capacities of the nursing department. Following are three examples of general resident standards of care:

1. Ninety percent of the time residents will receive pain medication within ten minutes of the request when the request is appropriate and orders are available.
2. One hundred percent of the time residents will receive the correct medication, at the correct time, in the correct dose, and by the correct route.
3. Ninety percent of the time the Minimum Data Set (MDA) will be completed by the interdisciplinary team within one month of admission for a resident.

The formulation of patient care standards can also be plugged into the level of care required for each resident. The standards then show the interventions required for care, identify the desired outcomes of the interventions, and assign cost. This allows the department of nursing to isolate better what is done for residents, how much it costs, and how it can be done more productively and economically.[3] The MDA is now required in long-term care facilities to assess each resident's level of functioning. Once the level of functioning is established, standards identify the interventions required for each area of functioning. A cost can then be assigned to each standard or unit of care.

Role of Quality Assurance and Risk Management

Quality assurance and risk management, although different in focus, work together to identify and solve problems in productivity, quality of care, and cost containment.[4] The object of quality assurance is to use the established standards of care to measure and evaluate the delivery of services at the prescribed productivity levels. Effective, well-stated, measurable standards provide not only a vehicle for the measurement of patient care outcomes but also the foundation for performance appraisals of employees.

The Joint Commission now requires all of its accredited facilities to have a program in place that ensures (1) identification of care and services given, (2) identification of indicators of care and services, (3) establishment of thresholds to measure care and services, (4) collection of data, (5) evaluation of variations of the thresholds, and (6) documentation of actions taken. This new process is called quality improvement. The focus has shifted from the illusive value of ensuring quality to vigilant improvement. Quality cannot be ensured without a concern for improving what is already in place.

Risk management focuses on the identification, prevention, and resolution of potential or actual problems to minimize or prevent damage or loss to the institution or the risk of liability. If proper standards are set and a quality improvement program is in place at the unit level to evaluate the actual outcome of care as compared to the expected outcome, interventions can be instituted quickly to identify potential problems and to prevent liability or loss. Quality assurance and risk management activities are a requirement of accreditation organizations and federal regulating agencies. With an aggressive quality improvement program in place, risk is controlled and liability is reduced.

If a standard of care states that each resident will have a skin integrity assessment completed within 24 hours of admission and an appropriate treatment protocol initiated if indicated, then the responsibility of risk management would be to evaluate (1) whether skin integrity assessments are being completed within 24 hours, (2) whether the appropriate skin protocol is being initiated, (3) whether the treatment plan is being properly implemented, and (4) whether the treatment protocol is resolving skin integrity problems. Note that the focus of quality improvement is ongoing assessment and initiation of changes in the plan when indicated. Retrospective analysis, while still a legitimate activity for certain aspects of the standards, now needs to give way to concurrent and prospective analyses.

SELECTION OF POLICIES, PROCEDURES, AND PROTOCOLS

Policies and procedures provide rules for guiding behavior and consistency in decisions and behavior in an institution. Policies are general directions or rules that create the legal and organizational framework through which the institution and nursing department carry out their goals. They specify the locus of authority and responsibility and the type of behavior needed to achieve a particular purpose. Procedures provide step-by-step instructions that direct individuals in how to proceed in carrying out activities or policies. Without such instructions, chaos might ensue and established standards would probably not be followed.

Imagine, for example, what might happen in a situation where a waste can fire was discovered by a janitor in a resident's room. Chaos might well result if a policy was lacking that clearly identified the evacuation plan, who to report to, who was in charge, the steps to be taken to prevent the spread of the fire, the responsibilities of other staff to protect residents and staff, and a schedule of drills that keep staff updated on their responsibilities and the location, for example, of extinguishers and emergency exits.

Policies and procedures standardize decision making and provide a mechanism for continuity and consistency in the way care and regulations are implemented. Each member dealing with the waste can fire cannot proceed with his or her own method of firefighting. Each must know specifically what his or her duties are and be trained in their performance. Policies are usually developed around such issues as accidents involving residents, staff, or visitors; admissions; autopsies; communicable disease; complaints; consents; deaths; discharge; doctor's orders; protocols for gerontological nurse practitioners; fire regulations; and documentation, to mention just a few.

Policies are developed when (1) there is confusion about the locus of responsibility that might result in neglect or malperformance, (2) residents' and families' rights must be protected, and (3) personnel management and welfare are at risk.[5] A policy manual is developed for the institution and for the nursing department. The manual then becomes a tool for orienting staff, a reference when unexpected problems arise, and a foundation on which to develop procedures and resolve conflicts or differences.[6]

Some nursing departments combine policies and procedures into one manual. Updating and revising this manual (or manuals, if there is both a policy manual and a procedure manual) is an ongoing responsibility. A committee is usually established to undertake this task. Policy and procedure manuals must be located on each nursing unit so that they are accessible to all staff for reference. The procedure manual must be correct, complete, up-to-date, and properly indexed.[7] The manual details such psychomotor skills as how to insert a Foley catheter, care for an intravenous catheter, or care for a deceased resident. Each procedure description comprises (1) a definition of the procedure to be performed, (2) a list of equipment needed to complete the procedure, (3) a statement of the desired outcome, and (4) a step-by-step outline of how the procedure is to be performed.

Procedures should be based on a review of the current literature in nursing and should reflect the most up-to-date findings and developments in the field. The requirements of regulatory agencies should be consulted so that the procedures are in congruence with their standards. Procedures are reviewed and approved by the appropriate nursing committee and medical advisory board. They are then used by all staff in implementing care and provide the standards by which liability and outcomes are assessed.

Procedures can of course be changed. Implementing changes on a trial basis through the use of miniresearch projects is one way to get staff involved in altering behavior and testing the effectiveness of the new techniques.

Protocols are plans of treatment that define specifically what is to be done for residents under specific conditions. Protocols are developed in consultation with the facility's medical director. Approval is gained from the patient care policy committee and each resident's physician. Review of each protocol should be done annually. Gerontological nurse practitioners usually work under protocols approved by the medical advisory board and by the resident physician of record.[8]

Practice Guidelines

One emerging trend is to replace policies, procedures, and protocols with practice guidelines. Policies, by legal definition, are "nonnegotiable" rules. With the development of technology has come increased litigation. Practice guidelines provide negotiable standards that allow for clinical judgment and expertise and truly promote collaborative practice among all health care providers. Practice guidelines are an alternative to care plans and can be used to streamline documentation, provide a basis for outcome-focused quality improvement (assurance), and demonstrate the integration of the nursing and medical plans of care.

The issue of policies versus practice guidelines can be elucidated by describing a common policy in acute and long-term care facilities related to the care of an intravenous (IV) catheter. Most policy manuals require the replacement of an IV catheter every 72 hours, or more frequently if indicated. Suppose, for example, that the registered nurse assessed the condition of an IV located in the right lower forearm of a frail elderly resident, Mrs. Dumas. Aware that the physician expects to discontinue the IV antibiotics tomorrow, the nurse notes that there is no redness, swelling, or obvious need to replace the IV catheter at this point, especially since the IV is scheduled for termination. The nurse is also aware that the staff have had tremendous difficulty locating an appropriate vein in the past and that the procedure of replacing the IV is always painful for Mrs. Dumas. Since the nurse cannot locate any veins that may be used to change the IV, she decides to allow the current IV to stay in place for one more day.

If Mrs. Dumas was to develop thrombophlebitis at the IV site subsequently, causing pain and the potential for more serious complications, Mrs. Dumas and her family could sue the facility for negligence in the management of the IV. The first document to be subpoenaed would be the policy and procedure manual. The nurse indicted in the incident would be questioned about her knowledge of the policy and procedure manual, would be asked if she was able to read, and would most probably be held liable for not following the policies and procedures outlined by the facility. After all, these policies have been approved by medical, administrative, and nursing authorities and been deemed acceptable health care practice. To deviate from the "rules" can be interpreted as negligence.

The corresponding practice guidelines, on the other hand, would describe the competencies of the health care providers responsible for caring for the IV; describe patient, staff, and administrative system outcomes; give indications for implementing the guidelines; define areas of responsibility for assessing, planning, evaluation, documentation, and teaching as well as for implementing actions to be taken if complications arise. The guidelines would provide a more flexible guide for care.

Use of Current Research in Developing Protocols

Following are three examples of the use of current research as the foundation for the development of protocols.

Skin Care

Changes in the skin of the elderly make them especially prone to skin pressure points, tears, and decubitus wounds. This is one of the most important and potentially expensive problems facing the administrator of a long-term care facility. Maintenance of skin integrity is a primary responsibility of nurses. The main focus of care is prevention of skin breakdown. The primary etiologic factor in skin breakdown is pressure combined with shearing force and friction. The daily routines of hygiene, turning, moving, and lifting residents must be carried out with an awareness of the potential of this factor to cause breakdown of the skin. When pressure sores do occur, the nurse is aided by having clear guidelines for assessing and staging the affected skin and implementing measures according to identified clinical criteria. A skin care protocol can provide consistent guidelines that promote continuity in the care of the individual resident. Elements of a skin care protocol include (1) a process for identifying residents who are at risk for developing pressure problems; (2) criteria for assessment and staging of pressure sores; (3) recommended dressing material, a specific treatment procedure, and a schedule for treatment for each stage of the wound; and (4) a time frame for evaluation and further referral.

Urinary Incontinence

Urinary incontinence is one of the major factors leading to the admission of elderly persons to long-term care facilities. The impact of incontinence on the self-esteem and social interaction of elders can be devastating, and the cost of care for incontinence can be substantial.

There are several types of incontinence common in older adults: stress incontinence, urge incontinence, and overflow incontinence. Functional incontinence occurs when advanced cognitive impairment, musculoskeletal disability, or effects of medication render an elder unaware of the need to void or unable to get to the toilet. Until recently, nurses have generally viewed incontinence as a single problem. Research has yielded clearer definitions of the etiologies and defining characteristics of incontinence problems.[9] Treatment modalities include medical interventions as well as a variety of nursing interventions that can reduce or elim-inate incontinence. It is now possible to identify the specific problem and develop specific protocols and treatment plans that can greatly reduce it. However, admin-istrators of long-term care facilities must first assign a high priority to dealing with incontinence and then develop protocols for nurses to implement.

Restraints

Maintaining safety for the long-term care resident has always been a nursing priority. This is one of the primary focuses of the OBRA '87 regulations. Too frequently the use of restraints has been a mainstay measure for preventing falls. The acceptability of this measure has come under attack as the negative physical and psychological effects of restraint use are better understood. Efforts are now directed toward developing alternatives to restraint. Cutchins describes a blue-print for care that involves changes in the environment and the operation of the facility and a reorientation of clinical practice that can give residents maximum protection in a restraint-free setting.[10]

SELECTION OF PERSONNEL

The scientific basis and specialized practice of nursing care of the elderly has developed. The long-term care facility is no longer a place where a nurse might work so as to get a rest from the hospital. No longer is it assumed that nursing skills necessary for acute care are easily transferrable to long-term care. The needs of elderly persons residing in long-term care facilities are unique. They and their families seek out long-term care facilities in the hope that dignity and self-esteem can be preserved in the face of tremendous losses—the loss of a spouse, for example, or the ability to walk or to ask for assistance. The nurse who accepts the care of these elderly persons as a professional responsibility deserves support and encouragement to pursue professional development in the field of geronto-logical nursing. The career development paths extend to formal advanced degree preparation (MSN) and roles as clinical specialists in gerontological nursing (CS) or gerontological nurse practitioner (MSN or C). For the nurse who does not wish to enroll in a formal program, recognition for specialized skills can be earned through the certification process as gerontological nurse (C).

Staffing Regulations

The provision of nursing care in any health care institution is regulated by the state's board of nursing (or the equivalent government regulatory body). This agency carries the responsibility for safeguarding the public and promoting high-quality nursing care. Each state has a nurse practice act that defines the scope of nursing within that jurisdiction. The licensure of nurses is regulated. In the United States, two types of licensure are currently identified, registered nurse (RN) and licensed practical nurse (LPN)/licensed vocational nurse (LVN). Since 1991, training and certification of nursing assistants has been carried out under federal OBRA '87 regulations for long-term care facilities. Specific job descriptions that define the role and scope of practice for RNs, LPN/LVNs, and certified nursing assistants and the expanded scope of practice for nurse practitioners and certified nurse specialists are provided in Appendix 7-A.

The director of nursing is responsible for knowing the regulatory mandates regarding the RN, LPN/LVN, and nursing assistant mix. The use of RNs and LPN/LVNs is constrained by the level of nursing care required by residents in a facility. This determines the staffing patterns in the institution. In general, there is a requirement for the around-the-clock, seven-day-a-week presence of a licensed nurse in the facility and for the availability of supervision by a registered nurse.

In addition to the direct-care nursing staff, the nursing department provides for specialized expertise in the areas of nursing management, direct care, and education. Appendix 7-A includes job descriptions for the types of nursing positions needed in a long-term care facility. The educational preparation for and responsibilities of each position are also described.

Infection Control

An infection control program is required for facilities that receive federal reimbursement as skilled nursing facilities. An effective program begins with an infection control committee composed of members from medicine, nursing, pharmacy, dietary, and housekeeping. The individual who implements the infection control program designed by the committee is usually a nurse. The role of this nurse is to collect data related to infection in the facility, to investigate episodes of infection, to educate the staff, and to develop policies and procedures related to prevention and control of infection. Elderly persons may not present the usual clinical signs and symptoms of infection. Subtle changes in an elder's level of awareness, the loss of appetite, or general complaints of "not feeling good" need to be carefully assessed to rule out the possibility of infection.

High Turnover Rates

Nursing administrators face the complex problem of high long-term care facility turnover rates for both nursing assistants and licensed nurses. Among the reasons for the high rate are "the difficult nature of the work and the residual stigma associated with nursing home work and the deterrents to practice in this setting; noncompetitive salaries compound the problem."[11]

About 8 percent of the RN population work in long-term care facilities, as compared with 67 percent employed in hospitals. Many licensed nurses who are hired by long-term care facilities have little educational preparation in the care of the elderly. They may be unfamiliar, for example, with the manager of care role. In addition, the ethical dilemmas posed by the setting are quite different from those common in acute care hospitals. Therefore, nurses will generally benefit from a strong staff development program that focuses on

1. strengthening the image of long-term care nursing as a specialized field
2. developing the nurses' management skills and leadership qualities
3. getting the nurses to perceive themselves as contributors to the interdisciplinary team caregiving process
4. changing the basis of practice from the medical model to a nursing model that emphasizes the physical, cognitive, and functional capacities of the elderly person
5. building awareness of how reimbursement issues influence long-term care

The nursing assistant's need for ongoing personal and career development must be addressed. Continuing education programs offered in the facility are needed for the renewal of the nurses' aide certification. In addition, programs preparing the nursing assistant for GED certification or offering child care assistance or facility-provided transportation may be added as incentives to promote recruitment and retention of staff.

As financial constraints continue to plague long-term care facilities, it is easy to give a low priority to staff development. Building and maintaining the competence of the nursing staff is an indispensable part of the facility's legal responsibility to the residents it serves.

LINKING LONG-TERM CARE WITH EDUCATION

Nurses who work in long-term care facilities may feel removed from the mainstream of the profession. They may find it difficult to keep current with advances in medicine and nursing. The administrator can assist in this area by promoting opportunities for the facility to link with educational resources in the community. Hospitals, community colleges, and universities would be natural partners in efforts to educate health professionals. There are several excellent models already established.

Currently a Kellogg Foundation–sponsored program, The Community College–Nursing Home Partnership, is in its dissemination phase.[12] Some community college nursing education programs are working with long-term care facilities to include care of the elderly in the clinical education of RNs. In the state of Washington, nurses at the Ida Culver House are collaborating with faculty at the University of Washington (Seattle) School of Nursing to provide a range of services to the elderly, including care in a 74-bed skilled nursing facility.

What these and other models of partnership share is the enrichment gained by each partner as nurses with various types of expertise come together to share knowledge and apply it to meeting the unique needs of elder persons. Advances in technology and knowledge have redefined many of the nursing problems seen in the long-term care facility and require that nurses change some of their traditional practices.

NOTES

1. E. Tagliarani et al., Participatory Clinical Education, *Nursing and Health Care* 12, no. 5 (1991):248.

2. American Nurses' Association, *Standards for Organized Nursing Services,* ANA Pub. No. NS-1 (Kansas City: American Nurses' Association, 1982).

3. B. Rutkowski, *Managing for Productivity in Nursing* (Gaithersburg, Md.: Aspen Publishers, 1987), 228.

4. Ibid., 195.

5. H.S. Rowland and B.L. Rowland, *Nursing Administration Handbook,* 2d ed. (Gaithersburg, Md.: Aspen Publishers, 1985), 101.

6. Ibid., 103.

7. Ibid.

8. Rutkowski, 213–214.

9. P. Turnink, Alteration in Urinary Elimination, *Journal of Gerontological Nursing* 14, no. 4 (1988):25–31.

10. C.H. Cutchins, Blueprint for Restraint-Free Care, *American Journal of Nursing* 91, no. 7 (1991):36–44.

11. C. Eliopoulos, *Caring for the Nursing Home Patient: Clinical and Managerial Challenges for Nurses* (Gaithersburg, Md.: Aspen Publishers, 1989), 241.

12. Tagliarani et al., Participatory Clinical Education; L.S.J. Trippett, Partners in Care, part of a panel presentation entitled "Partnerships in Gerontological Nurse Education and Practice" at the National Conference on Gerontological Nursing Education, Norfolk, Va., February 1, 1992.

Appendix 7-A

Job Descriptions

NURSING SERVICE PERSONNEL
JOB TITLES AND SCOPE OF PRACTICE

Nursing Service Director

Common Titles

Director of Nursing, Vice-President for Nursing, Vice-President for Patient Care, Assistant Administrator for Nursing, Chief Nurse.

Education, Training, and Experience

A baccalaureate degree in nursing is a minimum requirement, with a master's degree in nursing administration preferable. Current licensure as an RN by the state board of nursing in the state where the long-term care facility is located is necessary. Five years of administrative experience as a director or as a supervisor of nursing service and experience in care of the elderly are required. Demonstrated stature in the nursing profession and keeping abreast of changes in the profession are a must.[1]

Duties

Has 24-hour accountability for the department of nursing. A leader who interprets nursing both internally and externally and promotes and maintains harmonious relationships among nursing personnel, physicians, other administrators, residents, ancillary personnel, and the public. Is the role model and individual who establishes the professional environment in which efficient, productive, and caring services are delivered. Is able to organize and administer the department of nursing by establishing goals and objectives for the department; establishing the organizational structure of the department; developing, interpreting, and administering administrative policies; preparing and administering the budget for the department; selecting and appointing nursing staff; and directing and delegating the management of professional and ancillary nursing personnel. Also coordinates activities of the various nursing units, plans and directs orientation and in-service training programs, evaluates nursing and implements measures to improve care, and participates in community educational programs.

Assistant Nursing Service Director

Common Titles

Assistant Director for Nursing, Associate Director of Nursing.

Education, Training, and Experience

A baccalaureate degree in nursing is a minimum, with a master's degree in nursing desirable. Current licensure as an RN by the state board of nursing in the state where the long-term care facility is located is necessary. At least one year of management experience and two years of clinical experience in the care of the elderly are required.

Duties

Has 24-hour accountability for the department of nursing. Assists in organizing and administering the department of nursing as delegated by the nursing service director. Implements administrative policies and services by organizing appropriate committees and working directly with supervisors and department personnel. Coordinates and evaluates services to improve direct resident care. Structures an environment in which employees may grow and are rewarded for productive, efficient, and highly competent work. Writes job descriptions for the department and establishes performance evaluation or appraisal policies. Supervises and administers policies so that each individual employed in the department is held accountable for the job responsibilities outlined in his or her job description. Assists in review and evaluation of the department budget and in the implementation of the orientation and in-service programs. Assists in research and quality assurance activities.

Nursing Supervisor

Common Titles

Evening, Night, or Day Supervisor, Specific Unit Supervisor (Level 1 or Skilled Care Unit, Rehabilitation Unit, etc.).

Education, Training, and Experience

A baccalaureate degree in nursing is desirable, as is graduate preparation in gerontology. Current licensure as an RN by the state board of nursing in the state where the long-term care facility is located is necessary. Five years experience as a head nurse, demonstrated supervisory and teaching abilities, and demonstrated excellence in clinical skills in the care of the elderly are necessary.

Duties

Has either 24-hour or 8-hour responsibility for nursing service, depending on the definition and scope of responsibilities. Has the major portion of the responsibility of representing nursing at the unit level. Must be an excellent role model, must be diligent in supervising and providing guidance in direct patient care services, and must demonstrate leadership and excellence in nursing care. Supervises and coordinates activities of department personnel on the evening, night, or day shift so that continuity of care is provided on a 24-hour basis. Maintains direct contact with personnel and residents on the nursing units to ensure quality assurance and adherence to department policies and procedures. Delegates and supervises performance appraisals and any remedial actions to be taken. Works with the nursing service director and assistant director in establishing unit budgets and evaluating needs. Determines staffing needs for each shift. Is the administrative presence in the institution during the evening and night shifts and on the weekends and holidays and must be able to interpret administrative policies, make administrative decisions, and handle emergencies, as appropriate.

Director of Education

Common Titles

Director of Staff Development, In-service Education Coordinator, Director of Education.

Education, Training, and Experience

A baccalaureate degree in nursing is required, along with experience as a head nurse, supervisor, or nurse educator. Current licensure as an RN by the state board of nursing in the state where the long-term care facility is located is necessary. Must have a broad and thorough knowledge of nursing skills and be able to evaluate the quality of the nursing care given and the abilities of the staff administering care.

Duties

Plans, organizes, and implements educational programs for nursing staff and often for residents and families as well. May develop, implement, and evaluate nursing assistant certification programs that meet federal and state regulations. Works with nursing administration to evaluate quality assurance and plan remedial actions when necessary. Understands accreditation and federal and state regulations and ensures that the regulations are met. Keeps appropriate training records. Implements orientation and in-service programs and provides ongoing education and training of nursing assistants.

Head Nurse

Common Titles

Head Nurse, Clinical Nurse Manager.

Education, Training, and Experience

A baccalaureate degree in nursing is desirable, as is advanced preparation in the clinical specialty of gerontology. Current licensure as an RN by the state board of nursing in the state where the long-term care facility is located is necessary. Should have five years of experience as a professional nurse in the care of the elderly.

Duties

Usually has 24-hour accountability for nursing services provided on unit. Directly supervises the nursing staff and ensures compliance with policies and procedures on one nursing unit. Directly responsible for the provision of an environment where excellent nursing care may be delivered. Is the vital link between management, the nursing staff, and the residents and families. Is a resource to staff, develops and administers staffing schedules, and writes performance appraisals for staff on the assigned unit. Must be able to evaluate services delivered and to determine and implement appropriate remedial actions and rewards when indicated. This is the individual that most residents and families view as the key individual in the delivery of care on the unit. Therefore, the head nurse must have excellent interpersonal skills.

Staff Nurse

Education, Training, and Experience

Current licensure as an RN by the state board of nursing in the state where the long-term care facility is located is necessary. Education may include a baccalaureate degree in nursing, a diploma in nursing from an accredited hospital school of nursing, or an associate of science degree in nursing. Should demonstrate an interest in care of the elderly.

Duties

Has 8- or 12-hour shift accountability for nursing care provided on a specific unit. The scope of practice of the RN is defined by statutes of the state in which the long-term care facility is located. The long-term care facility may define duties that are narrower than those defined in the state's nurse practice act but may not exceed the duties and responsibilities spelled out in the statutes. Nursing at the RN level is generally defined as the "diagnosis and treatment of human responses to actual or potential health problems."[2] Professional nursing usually means (1) the performance for compensation of acts related to health maintenance, prevention, promotion, and restoration; (2) supervision and teaching of other personnel; (3) administration of medications and treatments prescribed by a licensed physician or dentist; and (4) the application of specialized judgment and skill based on knowledge and application of principles of the biological, physical, and social sciences.[3]

Assists in planning, supervising, and instructing licensed practical nurses, nursing assistants, and students. Develops, implements, and evaluates individual residents' plans of care. Maintains resident records, including the recording of nursing care given. Usually serves as the team leader for the group of personnel rendering care on a specific unit. Is responsible for the minute-to-minute direct service given. Has the responsibility to delegate, supervise, and administer nursing care commensurate with licensing regulations and personnel capabilities.

Most RNs perform activities and treatments such as the following: the administration of medications by mouth, injection, IV, and other prescribed routes and their evaluation; the provision of treatments involving equipment; the initiation, maintenance, and evaluation of IV infusions by peripheral, central line, and subcutaneous access ports; treatment of wounds as prescribed; the taking of temperatures, pulses, respirations, and blood pressures; the performance of physical assessment and implementation of appropriate actions when necessary; the administration and supervision of alternative feeding methods via a gastrostomy or jejunostomy tube; and the performance of other sterile procedures such as urinary catheterization and complex dressing as prescribed.

Licensed Practical Nurse/Licensed Vocational Nurse (LPN/LVN)

Education, Training, and Experience

The LPN/LVN is a high school graduate or has earned a GED and graduated from a recognized one-year practical vocational nursing program. Current licensure as an LPN by the state board of nursing in the state where the long-term care facility is located is necessary.

Duties

Has 8- or 12-hour shift accountability for nursing care provided on specific unit. The scope of practice of the LPN/LVN is defined by the statutes of the state in which the long-term care facility is located. The long-term care facility may define duties that are narrower than those defined in the state's nurse practice act but may not exceed those duties and responsibilities spelled out in the statutes. Works under the supervision of an RN. Is responsible for the minute-to-minute direct services given and for reporting significant changes to the RN. Participates in the assessment and planning of nursing care. Provides direct resident care (as assigned by the RN), which may include bathing; feeding; making beds; helping residents in and out of bed; taking temperatures, pulses, respirations, and blood pressures; collecting specimens; dressing wounds; using sterile procedures such as urinary catheterization; assisting with physical examinations by the physician; transporting patients; recording appropriate information in the resident's chart; and administering and evaluating medications given by oral, injectable, or other prescribed routes. *Note:* Some institutions, in accordance with their state's nurse practice act, train LPNs to start IV infusions, mix specified IV solutions, and discontinue IV infusions. Most LPNs are not allowed to manage the care of central lines or subcutaneous access ports, including the changing of tubing, aspiration of blood specimens, and changing of dressings; administer any drug by IV push; administer blood or blood products; administer chemotherapy; or administer hyperalimentation (TPA).

Nurse's Aide/Nursing Assistant

Common Titles

Certified Nursing Assistant, Nurse's Aide, Orderly.

Education, Training, and Experience

Federal regulations now require certification for all nursing assistants who are employed full time in a long-term care institution for more than four months. Certification is intended to protect the public by obligating nursing assistants to meet minimal classroom theory requirements and demonstrate skill competency.

A certified nursing assistant program requires approval by the state licensing authority. Certification requires (1) combined classroom theory and clinical skill instruction, (2) a supervised clinical experience, and (3) a clinical skills competency exam in which the examinee demonstrates safe practice in at least five of the required skills. Any long-term care facility can develop and administer such a program, but this is expensive and very time-consuming. Most long-term care facilities hire nursing assistants who have already completed an approved certification program sponsored by either private or state-supported sources. A list of approved certification programs may be obtained from the state regulating agency. Some certification programs do not include the clinical exam component. The clinical skills competency exam may be administered by any long-term care facility that has been approved by the state regulating agency. Most long-term care facilities apply for this approval and are then able to hire individuals who have completed the educational component of the certification process but still need to pass the clinical skills exam.

Note: Many nursing students are looking for part-time work and make excellent employees. Nursing students who have completed 75 hours of clinical instruction meet the educational requirement of the certification process, but they must still pass a clinical skills competency exam. Consult with the state regulating agency for specific requirements. Note that nursing students who are only part-time employees do not technically need to be certified.

Duties

Certified nursing assistants provide most of the care in a long-term care facility. This is one important difference between long-term care facilities and skilled nursing and acute care facilities, where most, if not all, of the care is delivered by licensed RNs and LPNs. It is therefore essential that the nursing assistants are chosen, trained, educated, and supervised with extreme care. Also, because of the minimal education and training received in a certification program, it is vital that ongoing training and education be conducted by the long-term care facility. The quality of care delivered is dependent upon the nursing assistants' insights regarding residents' needs and their ability to grow professionally and increase their skills. Most nursing assistants, if asked, will indicate their desire for ongoing training and supervision. Nursing assistants perform tasks delegated and supervised by either an LPN or RN. Such tasks usually include bathing and feeding residents; assisting with toileting; making beds; ambulating; helping residents in and out of bed; taking temperatures, pulses, respirations, and blood pressures; and collecting certain specimens.

Ward Clerk

Education, Training, and Experience

The following are required: high school diploma or GED; ward secretary certification if available; training in English, typing, spelling, and arithmetic. Ward clerks usually receive on-the-job training.

Duties

General clerical duties, including maintaining records on the unit; completing lab and other requisition forms; recording temperature, pulse, and respiration on residents' charts; keeping files of old records on the unit; maintaining inventory of supplies; ordering and replenishing supplies as needed; keeping records of residents transferred or discharged; answering the phone on the unit; and typing various records, schedules, care plans, or communications with physicians. It is often the ward secretary with whom the residents and families have first contact. The ward secretary must have excellent interpersonal skills and be able to answer the phone and greet people in a way that suggests the high quality of care provided in the institution.

SPECIALIZED ROLES AND TITLES

Clinical Nurse Specialist in Gerontological Nursing

Title

Registered Nurse, Certified Specialist in Gerontology (R.N., C.S.).

Education, Training, and Experience

Certified clinical nurse specialists have a master's or higher degree; have clinical preparation in a specialty such as gerontology, medical-surgical nursing, or adult psychiatric health; and have passed a certification examination developed by the appropriate professional society. The title RN certified specialist is reserved for individuals who hold credentials beyond degree preparation. Certification requires not only master's degree but certification and the demonstration of continued clinical competence and expertise. Clinical nurse specialists in gerontology are recognized as experts in the field. Current licensure as an RN by the state board of nursing in the state where the long-term care facility is located is necessary. Current evidence of certification should be kept on file.

Duties

The purpose of employing clinical nurse specialists is to place expert clinicians at the bedside. Clinical nurse specialists are usually put in staff rather than line positions. They do not have direct authority over other personnel and are typically responsible to the director of nursing. Clinical nurse specialists function as expert clinicians, administrators, teachers, researchers, and consultants. Clinical nurse specialists in gerontology have advanced knowledge and clinical skills in the care of the elderly, with a focus on the physical, psychological, and sociocultural dimensions of such care. Most long-term care facilities hire one certified clinical nurse specialist in gerontology to provide consultation.

Gerontological Nurse Practitioner

Title

Registered Nurse, Certified Gerontological Nurse Practitioner (R.N., C.).

Education, Training, and Experience

Gerontological nurse practitioners earn their specialized license and certification through (1) master's degree preparation or (2) a certification program that involves at least nine months (one academic year) of full-time study. Certification requires not only appropriate educational preparation but the passing of a certification examination and the demonstration of continued clinical competence and expertise. Gerontological nurse practitioners are able to practice in most states and are allowed an expanded scope of practice defined by state statutes. They have special nursing licenses that enable them to practice in this expanded role. Their licenses are renewed upon evidence of their meeting special requirements.

Duties

Gerontological nurse practitioners assume expanded roles in providing care to older adults. They possess in-depth knowledge of physical assessment and can manage stable, chronic, and minor acute illnesses or conditions. These practitioners collaborate with other health professionals to provide care. Their functions may include assessment of patient status, nursing diagnosis, goal setting, development of nursing care plans, implementation of care plans, and evaluation of progress.[4] They usually are put in staff rather than line positions. They do not have direct authority over other personnel and are typically responsible to the director of nursing. Protocols that gerontological nurse practitioners follow must be approved by the medical advisory board and the individual physician of record.

Most long-term care facilities hire one gerontological nurse practitioner to provide consultation. Long-term care facilities can be reimbursed under Medicare for services provided by gerontological nurse practitioners.

Gerontological Nurse

Title

Registered Nurse, Certified in Gerontology (R.N., C.).

Education, Training, and Experience

A nurse, in order to get this generalist certification, must have (1) an active RN license and (2) a minimum of 4,000 hours of practice as a licensed registered nurse in gerontological nursing practice (1,600 of the 4,000 hours must have occurred within the past two years). Certification requires not only appropriate clinical preparation but the passing of a certification examination and the demonstration of continued clinical competence and expertise.[5]

Duties

The purpose of the gerontological nurse certification is to recognize the skill and commitment of RNs who choose to work with the elderly as their primary focus. Gerontological nurses are able to identify and use the strengths of the elderly and to assist the elderly in maximizing their independence. These specialists encourage the elderly to be actively involved in the development of their plans of care. All RNs in the long-term facility who meet the educational and clinical requirements should be encouraged to seek this certification and be compensated for its achievement. Award of the certification indicates attainment of advanced and specialized knowledge and skill beyond what is required for safe practice.[6]

NOTES

1. H.S. Rowland and B.L. Rowland, *Nursing Administration Handbook,* 2d ed. (Gaithersburg, Md.: Aspen Publishers, 1985), 82.

2. ANA Board Approves a Definition of Nursing Practice, *American Journal of Nursing* 55 (1955):1474.

3. Ibid.

4. American Nurses' Association, Inc., Center for Credentialing Services, *1990 Certification Catalogue* (Kansas City: American Nurses' Association, 1990).

5. Ibid.

6. A.M. Rhodes and R.D. Miller, *Nursing and the Law,* 4th ed. (Gaithersburg, Md.: Aspen Publishers, 1984), 31.

Case Study 7-1

Private Matters

Seth B. Goldsmith

A few days after Barbara Miller began her position as director of nursing at the Bayview Nursing Home, she realized that she had a problem with a number of people who were privately employed by residents or their families to provide supplemental care for a particular resident. After checking with the floor supervisors, Miller learned that between 25 and 30 of the home's 150 residents had privately employed staff working for them. Ms. Miller found this situation disturbing and decided to discuss it with Jeff Isaacs, the home's administrator.

The meeting began with Miller indicating that she had never worked in a home with privately employed staff and that she was quite concerned about having so many people around who were not responsible to the nursing supervisor. She then asked Isaacs why it was necessary to have extra personnel at Bayview since the home had the best staffing ratio in the region. Isaacs replied that the use of privately employed staff had a history at Bayview dating back at least two decades when several residents received permission from the former administrator to hire employees to provide companionship and some basic assistance. He explained that in the last few years the use of private staff had escalated in response to staffing cutbacks and an increasingly debilitated health status of the residents.

Miller responded that she was philosophically opposed to the use of private staff because she felt that the home should provide all the necessary care. She was also troubled by what appeared to set up a two-class care system. In addition, she felt that it was intrusive to have so many people working in the home without any supervisory control. While Isaacs strongly sympathized with Miller's position, he also recognized that, in many instances, the private staff provided a significant amount of relief to the home's staff that would have to be augmented if the private staff were prohibited. Isaacs was also concerned about the strong negative response he would likely get from the home's board if he proposed prohibiting private staff. However, he was concerned enough about the issue to send Miller the following memo.

Bayview Nursing Home
Bayview, State

A Nonprofit Community Nursing Home

From: Jeff Isaacs, Administrator
To: Barbara Miller, Director of Nursing
Subject: Private staff in the home

This memo is written to follow up on our conversation concerning the use of private staff in the home. After giving due consideration to the points you raised, I think it prudent to continue the present practice of allowing families or residents to hire private staff to provide companionship and augmented care. However, I do think there are a range of problems with these staff and I would appreciate it if you and your staff would draft a memo that could serve as a manual for private staff. Specifically, I would like you to develop a scheme that would identify different categories of private staff, such as companions or registered nurses. How many categories should we allow? What responsibilities should the home have? For example, what rules should we impose on these people? To what extent should we get involved in the hiring and training of the staff? Finally, we need to consider how to inform residents and their families about our policies.

I look forward to hearing from you.

* * *

Exercise

1. Assume you are Ms. Miller and prepare a comprehensive response to Mr. Isaacs's memo.

The Case of Barbara Jones, RN

Seth B. Goldsmith

For the three years before having her license to practice nursing revoked, Barbara Jones had worked at the Clearview Nursing Center as a registered nurse. Some of the specific charges brought against Jones were that, for the three years she worked at Clearview, she had on 17 occasions failed to administer medication, treatment, and feedings to residents; 14 times she had made false entries into the residents' records concerning medications, feedings, and treatment; she had slept on duty; she had removed residents' call bells so that she would not be called in the middle of the night; she had abused patients, including the forced feeding of residents and hitting the stumps of two amputees against their bed rails; and she had failed to make rounds in accordance with the home's policies and the good practice of nursing.

After eight days of hearings a hearing officer recommended that Ms. Jones's license to practice nursing be revoked. The State Board of Nursing agreed and revoked Ms. Jones's license. Ms. Jones appealed the decision to the State Supreme Court, which upheld the decision.

A week after the State Supreme Court upheld the suspension, Ralph Robinson, the home's recently appointed administrator, was contacted by the administrator of a home in another state asking for a recommendation on Ms. Jones.

* * *

Exercise

1. Prepare a response for Mr. Robinson to send to the nursing home that asked for a recommendation on Ms. Jones.

Discussion Questions

1. Why would the egregious behavior of Ms. Jones be tolerated for three years?
2. Is it possible that the behavior of nurse Jones was unknown to her supervisor?

Chapter 8

Termination without Litigation: Practical Advice for Separating Employees

James E. Wallace, Jr.

In this era of exploding wrongful discharge and employment discrimination litigation, employers view even the most justifiable termination with hesitation and reluctance. Faced with the inevitable disruption caused by litigation and the potential exposure to awards of compensatory and punitive damages and attorney's fees, employers may allow unsatisfactory performance or unacceptable behavior to persist longer than is desirable or wise before taking the step of terminating employment. Some caution is prudent, of course, and it is certainly necessary to review the circumstances of a proposed termination before executing the decision. However, if an employer has been careful throughout the employment relationship, from hiring to termination, termination without litigation is still possible.

In most states, employment is "at will," meaning either the employer or the employee can terminate the relationship at any time and without notice, for any reason or for practically no reason at all. The right to terminate employment at will is not absolute, however, because that right may have been given up or modified by express or implied contract, and termination of employment in violation of specific laws, such as antidiscrimination statutes, is unlawful.

This chapter outlines the factors and considerations that should be reviewed prior to terminating an employee's employment, the goal being to reduce the risk of claims of breach of contract, discrimination, wrongful discharge, and related causes of action. (This chapter assumes that the employer is a nongovernmental employer with a nonunion work force. Issues particular to public employers or unionized work forces are beyond its scope.)

James E. Wallace, Jr., a partner in the Worcester and Framingham, Massachusetts, law firm of Bowditch & Dewey, is cochair of the firm's Labor and Employment Practice Group and represents management in discrimination and wrongful termination litigation. The writer acknowledges the contributions of Bowditch & Dewey attorneys David M. Felper and Karla J. de Steuben to this chapter.

THE NATURE OF THE EMPLOYMENT RELATIONSHIP

To properly assess whether problems may arise from ending the employment relationship, one must go back to the beginning of that relationship. The consequences of termination may flow from the very formation of the employment relationship.

Whenever termination is being considered, the following checklist should be reviewed.

I. Is there a written contract of employment (or an offer letter)?

   A. Does it specify a term of employment or require cause or notice for termination?

   B. Does it specify grounds for termination?

   C. Is the termination in accordance with the contract?

   D. Is there cause for termination? Does there need to be?

   E. Is termination pay specified?

II. If there is no written contract, is there an enforceable substitute for a written contract?

   A. Oral representations. In most states, a verbal promise of employment for more than one year is not enforceable.* But a verbal promise of employment for less than one year may be enforceable under the statute of frauds; likewise, an oral promise of lifetime or permanent employment may be enforceable since the employment could be performed within one year if the employee should die.

   1. Reliance or promissory estoppel. Oral representations of secure or long-term employment, if made to induce acceptance of employment, upon which the employee relies to his or her detriment (e.g., in accepting the offer of employment, the employee relocates or leaves secure employment), may be enforceable even though such promises would otherwise violate the statute of frauds. Thus wild promises or unauthorized offers (e.g., long-term or lifetime employment) must not be permitted. Employers should limit the number of people who are authorized to

---

*The Massachusetts Statute of Frauds, M.G.L. c.259 §1, is typical: "No action shall be brought. . .upon an agreement that is not to be performed within one year from the making thereof. . .unless the promise, contract or agreement upon which such action is brought, or some memorandum or note thereof, is in writing and signed by the party to be charged therewith or by some person thereunto by him lawfully authorized."

make offers of employment and ensure that all employees involved in the hiring process are trained.

2. Misrepresentations. Intentionally false statements on which the employee relies to his or her detriment may also be enforced.

B. Written representations.

1. A writing, such as a memorandum, may be sufficient to satisfy the statute of frauds and make what was thought to be an unenforceable verbal promise of long-term employment enforceable.

2. Personnel policy manuals or employee handbooks.

a) In some states handbooks or manuals may be considered implied contracts of employment that limit an employer's right to terminate at will. A court will consider the following factors as evidence that the manual should not be regarded as a contract:

(1) The employer reserves the right to amend or modify the handbook unilaterally.

(2) The handbook states that it is intended only as "guidance" or information.

(3) The handbook contains "at-will" and "no contract" disclaimers (see Appendix 8-A).

(4) The terms of the handbook were not negotiated prior to hiring.

(5) The handbook was distributed to the employee only after commencement of employment.

(6) The handbook was not signed.

(7) The handbook has in fact been amended unilaterally by the employer from time to time.

b) If these factors are not present and the manual is considered a contract, the employer's right to terminate may be limited if the handbook or manual:

(1) Contains representations to terminate only for cause and/or specifies the grounds for termination.

(2) Implies that termination after passing an initial probationary period can only be for cause by emphasizing that employment can be terminated for any reason during the probationary period (or promises "You'll always have a job here as long as you do your job").

(3) Requires notice for termination.

(4) Provides a discipline, grievance, or appeal procedure.

(5) Provides the opportunity to improve poor performance.

In such circumstances, termination of employment without following the policies or procedures spelled out in the handbook might be grounds for a claim of breach of contract by the employee.

3. Past practice may create "expectations" of treatment and an attendant need for justification of departures from that past practice.

PREPARING FOR TERMINATION

Obviously, since the employee was considered qualified enough to be hired, the reason for terminating employment arises during the employment relationship. Termination is usually the result of one of the following circumstances: misconduct, unsatisfactory performance, lack of work and need for a reduction in force, and reorganization or new management. It is rare that an employee is terminated for no reason at all. Whatever the reason, the following guidelines should be kept in mind:

1. Use written performance appraisals or evaluations on at least an annual basis. Be candid and honest in an evaluation, and review it thoroughly with the employee. Provide the employee the opportunity to comment on it, and have him or her acknowledge receipt of it.
2. Establish and apply uniform, progressive disciplinary standards. (But leave flexibility that allows you discretion to deviate when you decide it is appropriate.)
3. If business conditions allow it, afford the employee a reasonable opportunity to correct any deficiency cited in an evaluation before taking adverse action. Be as fair as you can.
4. Ensure that the rules and policies to which you hold employees accountable are reasonably related to legitimate business considerations and needs.
5. Ensure that all such policies are communicated and understood by employees. Reserve the right to amend, abolish, or add to such policies without notice and to deviate from them when you believe it is necessary or desirable.
6. Enforce rules and policies uniformly and consistently, and fully document in writing (with supporting evidence where possible) all violations. Make sure you know and follow your own rules.

7. Establish internal procedures to ensure that all adverse personnel actions, particularly terminations, are fully and fairly investigated. Use internal problem-solving procedures to give employees "due process." Advise the employee of the nature of the offense and, where appropriate, afford him or her the opportunity to be heard.

8. Use an exit interview to attempt to correct any misconceptions the employee may have about the termination and to uncover and defuse a potentially litigious situation. (You may even elicit an "admission" of misconduct or agreement with the decision.) Be candid about the reason for the termination but do not engage in a debate about the decision.

9. Conduct disciplinary or termination interviews in the presence of another management witness, who should take notes of what is said and done. You should both date and sign the notes. Be courteous and respect your employee as a human being; you'll gain nothing (and may lose much) by being rude or arrogant.

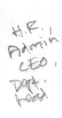

10. A member of senior management should be responsible for reviewing in advance all potential discharge cases to ensure that an offense was actually committed, that it was thoroughly investigated and documented, that all company rules and policies have been followed, that possible claims of discrimination and/or wrongful discharge have been identified and eliminated (see below), that the penalty (termination) is proportional to the offense, and that the penalty is consistent with past practice. (The same review should be done in cases of lesser offenses and discipline and regardless of the reason for termination.)

11. If there are any questions about the appropriateness of any disciplinary or termination decision, get competent legal advice. Your lawyer would rather take part in the decision-making process than read about the decision for the first time in a complaint.

12. Keep the reasons for an employee's discipline or discharge as confidential as possible and only discuss it with those individuals at work who have an absolute need to know of it. Do not make an example of the employee or use him or her to teach a lesson to the other employees. Claims of defamation and invasion of privacy are the inevitable result.

DISCRIMINATION AND WRONGFUL DISCHARGE

Every termination should be scrutinized to answer the following questions:

1. Is there a basis for a claim of discrimination (age, sex, race, color, national origin, sexual orientation, marital status, pregnancy, religion, or handicap),

failure to accommodate (religion or disability), or retaliation (e.g., sexual harassment)?*

- Is this employee being treated differently from other employees in similar circumstances? If so, why?
- Is there a legitimate, nondiscriminatory reason for termination?
  — Misconduct
  — Poor performance
  — Failure to meet standards
  — Reorganization
  — Reduction in force

Most cases of discrimination are not proved by direct evidence (e.g., a memorandum that states, "Let's terminate all employees over age 65"), because in most cases such direct evidence does not exist. A case of discriminatory termination is usually made out in the following way: The plaintiff (employee) presents evidence that he or she was in a protected category (e.g., black, female, over 40), that he or she was performing at a level that met the defendant's (employer's) legitimate expectations, that he or she was terminated, and that after the termination the defendant sought a replacement or replaced the plaintiff with a person not in the protected category. A plaintiff who presents such evidence makes what is called a prima facie case, and the defendant then must rebut the presumption of discrimination that is created by the prima facie case. The defendant does this by presenting evidence of legitimate nondiscriminatory reasons for the plaintiff's termination. The plaintiff then has the burden of proving that the explanation given by the defendant is pretextual, that is, is not true or is not believable (in other words, is a cover-up for a discriminatory motive). Failure to follow company policy or past practice, inconsistent or contradictory application of policy, and inconsistent or contradictory explanations of the reason for termination (e.g., a sudden finding of unsatisfactory performance when all prior written evaluations indicate excellence) may all be considered evidence of pretext. If the plaintiff convinces the judge or jury that the defendant's explanation is pretextual, the plaintiff wins.

---

*The most frequently invoked federal statutes are Title VII of the Civil Rights Act of 1964 (concerns discrimination on the basis of race, color, sex, religion, national origin, and pregnancy as well as harassment; applies to employers with 15 or more employees); Civil Rights Act of 1966 (42 U.S.C. §1981) (race, national origin; all employers); Age Discrimination in Employment Act of 1967 (age; 20 employees); Americans with Disabilities Act of 1990 (ADA), effective July 26, 1992, as to employers of 25 or more employees and July 26, 1994, as to employers of 15 or more employees; Civil Rights Act of 1991 (effective November 21, 1991, amending Title VII and ADA and adding new 42 U.S.C. §1981A). In addition, most states have antidiscrimination laws that parallel the federal laws.

2. Is there a basis for a claim of breach of the implied covenant of good faith and fair dealing?

   - Is the termination in *bad faith*—without good cause and intended to benefit the company financially at the employee's expense by depriving the employee of compensation earned for past services (e.g., commissions) or by preventing the imminent accrual of benefits (e.g., pension vesting)?
   - Is the termination *unfair*—without good cause and also not in bad faith or with ill motive but with the result that the employee would lose reasonably ascertainable future compensation based on past services?

   If the answer to either question is yes, the decision to terminate should be reconsidered or some monetary compensation should be considered.

3. Is there a basis for a claim that the reason for the discharge is contrary to public policy?

   - Is the employee being terminated for refusing to do something that public policy prohibits (e.g., refusing to commit perjury)?
   - Is the employee being terminated for doing something that public policy favors (e.g., filing a workers' compensation claim, taking time off to serve on a jury, reporting company violations of law [whistleblowing])?

   If the answer to either of these questions is yes, you are headed for trouble.

REDUCTIONS IN FORCE

Reductions in force (RIF) have their own distinctive characteristics and almost always run the risk of provoking claims of age discrimination. In age discrimination litigation, judges and juries must often decide whether the reduction in force was genuine or only a pretext to discriminate against older employees. The answer to that question usually means the difference between winning or losing the case.

Below is a checklist of factors that indicate whether an RIF is genuine or a pretext. If the factors listed in group 2 are present, the RIF may be in the danger zone.

1. Evidence indicating genuineness of an RIF

   - Written analysis of economic conditions necessitating reduction and a written plan to reduce costs by job elimination

- Objective evidence of adverse business conditions
- Exhaustion of alternatives to RIF
  — Attrition
  — Hiring freeze
  — Voluntary early retirement or incentive exit programs
- Objective, written criteria for determining which jobs or functions are to be eliminated
- Written instructions on how to implement the reduction
  — Criteria for selection of specific employees (seniority, qualifications or skills, performance, or evaluations)
  — Review by committee or higher levels of management
  — Documentation of reasons
- Plan showing consideration of impact on protected groups (e.g., statistical profile before and after reduction)

2. Evidence indicating pretext

- Replacement of plaintiff by or delegation of responsibilities to a younger employee of equal or lesser qualifications
- Failure to follow the RIF plan or guidelines
- Failure to follow seniority policies or practices
- Unclear seniority practices or RIF guidelines
- Hiring or job advertising soon after RIF
- Using high salaries as the main reason for selection
- Layoff of employees whose pension vesting is imminent
- Flawed performance evaluation used as the reason for selection
  — Unexplained or undocumented evaluation
  — Inconsistent application of standards or criteria
  — Subjective evaluation
  — Abruptly negative evaluation without prior warning
  — Uncorroborated or contradicted evaluation
- Undue encouragement of older employees to elect early retirement by reference to poor future business prospects, past poor performance, or tenuous future with the company
- Unjustified favorable treatment of younger employees
- Use of code words suggesting age ("youth movement," "deadwood," "young blood," "vigorous and aggressive")

SEXUAL HARASSMENT

Sexual harassment is a violation of Title VII of the Civil Rights Act of 1964 as well as the employment discrimination laws of various states. Sexual harassment occurs when an employee is asked or forced to submit to unwelcome sexual advances, requests for sexual favors, or other verbal or physical conduct of a sexual nature in exchange for some job benefit or to prevent some job benefit from being taken away. This is often referred to as "quid pro quo" sexual harassment. Sexual harassment also occurs when conduct of a sexual nature has the purpose or effect of "unreasonably interfering with an individual's work performance or creating an intimidating, hostile, or offensive working environment." This is often referred to as "hostile environment" sexual harassment.

Most lower courts have held employers strictly liable for quid pro quo sexual harassment engaged in by supervisory personnel regardless of whether the employer knew or should have known of the supervisor's conduct. In hostile environment sexual harassment cases, however, the employee has to show that the employer knew or should have known of the harassment and failed to take proper remedial action.

Sexual harassment may arise in the termination context in a number of ways. The victim, having complained about the harassment and having received no satisfaction from the company, may voluntarily leave employment and claim that she (or he) was constructively terminated because the working conditions were intolerable and she (or he) was forced to quit. The victim may be terminated in retaliation either because she resisted the sexual advances or complained about them. Finally, the alleged harasser may be terminated because the company believes the harassment occurred.

To decrease the risk of liability from sexual harassment claims, employers should adopt a specific written policy regarding sexual harassment that states such conduct will not be tolerated and that includes a description of the procedure for reporting and investigating any instances of sexual harassment. Once the policy is adopted, the employer should make sure that employees are aware of its contents by publishing it in handbooks, posting it on bulletin boards, circulating it periodically, and holding training sessions.

The following are the minimum steps for an effective investigation of the sexual harassment complaint:

1. Investigate promptly.
2. Treat complaints seriously and confidentially and discuss only with employees who have a need to know, making sure they understand the need for confidentiality. Stick to the facts and do not leap to conclusions.
3. Interview the complaining party. If the complainant wishes to remain anonymous, advise the complainant that you may not be able to investigate as thor-

oughly as desirable. Assure the complainant of freedom from retaliatory treatment.

4. Confront the alleged harasser, describe the information you have received, and obtain an explanation from that person. Warn against retaliatory treatment of the complainant even if the complaint is ill-founded.
5. Do not simply accept the alleged harasser's denial or explanation. Interview other employees who were or might have been in a position to observe the alleged conduct or aftermath (e.g., the victim crying or distressed), but do not disclose information to them unnecessarily.
6. If the harassment is admitted or substantiated, or if the complainant presents a believable story that the alleged harasser simply denies, take appropriate disciplinary action against the alleged harasser, including written warning, suspension, transfer, or termination if warranted. Respect the privacy rights of the alleged harasser, too.
7. If separation of the two parties is warranted, try not to put the burden of moving on the victim; do not "reward" the alleged harasser.
8. Report to the complainant what action is being taken.
9. Do not fail to investigate even if the complainant declines a formal investigation or withdraws the complaint.
10. Apply the investigation procedure and disciplinary policy consistently from case to case.
11. Document the steps of the investigation.

RELEASES OR WAIVERS

One way to reduce the prospect of litigation resulting from the termination of employment is to have the employee sign a release or waiver of claims. Employees who have signed releases or waivers are less likely to try to avoid the legal effect of that release by bringing litigation. However, in order to be valid and enforceable, a release must comply with the requirements of federal or state law. In particular, to be valid under the Federal Age Discrimination in Employment Act (ADEA), as amended by the Older Workers Benefit Protection Act of 1990, a release must have the following components:

1. The release must be part of an agreement between the employee and the employer that is written in understandable language.
2. The release must specifically refer to rights or claims arising under the ADEA.
3. The release may not waive rights or claims that may arise after the date the release is executed.
4. The release must be in exchange for consideration in addition to anything of value to which the employee is already entitled.

5. The employee must be advised in writing to consult with an attorney before executing the release.
6. The employee must be given at least 21 days to consider the agreement or, if the release is requested in connection with an exit incentive or other employment termination program offered to a group of employees, the employee must be given at least 45 days to consider the release.
7. The release must provide in writing that the employee has 7 days following the execution of the release to revoke the release, and the release may not become effective or enforceable until that 7-day period has expired.
8. If the release is requested in connection with an exit incentive or other group employment termination program, the employer must, at the beginning of the 45-day period mentioned above, inform the individual in writing as to (a) the group of employees covered by such a program and the eligibility factors and any time limits applicable, and (b) the job titles and ages of all employees eligible or selected for the program and the ages of the employees in the same job classification or organizational unit who are not eligible or selected for the program.

If you are not an employer covered by the ADEA (i.e., you have fewer than 20 employees), it is still advisable to structure the release so it complies with the first five requirements listed above. That will ensure its enforceability under most state laws as well.

CONCLUSION

No termination should be carried out without thorough analysis and preparation, and legal advice should be sought if any of the problem areas described above are encountered.

Such analysis and preparation can reduce the risk of claims of defamation, injury to reputation, invasion of privacy, intentional and negligent infliction of emotional distress, intentional interference with advantageous or contractual relations, and negligence (e.g., negligent supervision or evaluation) in addition to claims of breach of contract, discrimination, and wrongful discharge.

Consistency, common sense, caution, courtesy, and care, along with familiarity with the applicable laws, can enable you to achieve a most desirable result: termination without litigation.

Appendix 8-A

Suggested Disclaimer Language

Employment Application

I understand that nothing contained in this employment application or in the granting of an interview is intended to create an employment contract between the Company and myself for either employment or for the providing of any benefit. No promises regarding employment have been made to me, and I understand that no such promise or guarantee is binding upon the Company unless made in writing. I understand that no employer, manager, or other agent of the Company, other than the President of the Company, has any authority to enter into any agreement for employment for any specified period of time, or to make any agreement contrary to the foregoing. Any amendment to the foregoing must be in writing and signed by the President.

I certify that the information contained in this application is correct to the best of my knowledge and understand that concealment or falsification of this information is grounds for dismissal or nonhire. I authorize the references listed above to give you any and all information concerning my previous employment and any pertinent information they may have, personal or otherwise, and I release all parties from all liability for any damage that may result from furnishing same to you. I understand that my employment and compensation can be terminated, with or without cause, and with or without notice, at any time, at the option of either the Company or myself.

Employee Manual or Handbook

The contents of this manual are presented as a matter of information only and as guidance as to the Company's policies and are not to be understood or construed as a promise or contract between the Company and its employees. I understand that my employment and compensation can be terminated, with or without cause, and with or without notice, at any time, at the option of either the Company or myself.

The Company reserves its rights to modify, change, disregard, suspend, add to, or cancel at any time, without written or verbal notice, all or any part of the manual's contents at will, as circumstances may suggest.

Employee Acknowledgment

I have received a copy of the Employee Manual. I understand that any provisions of this Manual may be amended, revised, or cancelled by the Company at any time without notice. I also understand and agree that nothing in this Manual in any way creates an express or implied contract of employment between the Company and me. I also understand that my employment and compensation can be terminated, with or without cause, and with or without notice, at any time, at the option of either the Company or myself.

Case Study 8-1

Sexual Harassment

Seth B. Goldsmith

Shortly after Jane Jones started her new job as an accountant in the business office of the Green Tree Valley Nursing Home, she was approached by her supervisor, Bill Post, who asked whether she wanted to hear a joke. She agreed and Post told a short, but rather sexually explicit joke. Jones laughed politely and then went on with her work. The following Friday, Post again approached Jones and suggested that they have lunch together at a local restaurant. The luncheon conversation began with a discussion of the nursing home's cash-flow problems and continued with more conversation about several financial issues related to the employee benefits program. As they were concluding lunch, Post reached across the table, touched Jones's arm, and said, "How about continuing this conversation over dinner tonight and breakfast in the morning?" Jones said, "No, thanks. I have other plans." Post got quite angry and responded, "Jane, I hope you understand that I run this department and nobody is approved for a regular position unless I approve. I trust you remember that you are a probationary employee and that if you really want this job I need to give the word. So, let's not play games. You take care of my needs and I'll take great care of you." Jane glared at Post, got up from the table, and walked out.

Over the weekend she thought more and more about the conversation with Bill Post and decided that it was important that she meet with the nursing home's administrator of 15 years, Ms. Gail Page. Ms. Page responded to Jones's story by saying, "Look Jane, in this organization you have to learn to roll with the punches. Bill is a bit of a lecher, but he really is harmless and a terrific business manager. My best advice is just to ignore him and not go out to lunch with him anymore." Jones said nothing to Page at that time, but as she left the administrator's office she decided that her situation in the nursing home was simply untenable.

Exhibit 8-1-1 Definition of Sexual Harassment from Code of Massachusetts Regulations (151 B CMR 1.18)

The term "sexual harassment" shall mean sexual advances, requests for sexual favors, and other verbal or physical conduct of a sexual nature when (a) submission to or rejection of such advances, requests or conduct is made either explicitly or implicitly a term or condition of employment or as a basis for employment decisions; (b) such advances, requests or conduct have the purpose or effect of unreasonably interfering with an individual's work performance by creating an intimidating, hostile, humiliating or sexually offensive work environment. Discrimination on the basis of sex shall include, but not be limited to, sexual harassment.

Exhibit 8-1-2 Code of Federal Regulations

---

§ 1604.11   Sexual harassment.

(a) Harassment on the basis of sex is a violation of section 703 of title VII.[1] Unwelcome sexual advances, requests for sexual favors, and other verbal or physical conduct of a sexual nature constitute sexual harassment when (1) submission to such conduct is made either explicitly or implicitly a term or condition of an individual's employment, (2) submission to or rejection of such conduct by an individual is used as the basis for employment decisions affecting such individual, or (3) such conduct has the purpose or effect of unreasonably interfering with an individual's work performance or creating an intimidating, hostile, or offensive working environment.

(b) In determining whether alleged conduct constitutes sexual harassment, the Commission [the Equal Employment Opportunity Commission] will look at the record as a whole and at the totality of the circumstances, such as the nature of the sexual advances and the context in which the alleged incidents occurred. The determination of the legality of a particular action will be made from the facts, on a case by case basis.

(c) Applying general title VII principles, an employer, employment agency, joint apprenticeship committee or labor organization (hereinafter collectively referred to as "employer") is responsible for its acts and those of its agents and supervisory employees with respect to sexual harassment regardless of whether the specific acts complained of were authorized or even forbidden by the employer and regardless of whether the employer knew or should have known of their occurrence. The Commission will examine the circumstances of the particular employment relationship and the job functions performed by the individual in determining whether an individual acts in either a supervisory or agency capacity.

(d) With respect to conduct between fellow employees, an employer is responsible for acts of sexual harassment in the workplace where the employer (or its agents or supervisory employees) knows or should have known of the conduct, unless it can show that it took immediate and appropriate corrective action.

(e) An employer may also be responsible for the acts of non-employees, with respect to sexual harassment of employees in the workplace, where the employer (or its agents or supervisory employees) knows or should have known of the conduct and fails to take immediate and appropriate corrective action. In reviewing these cases the Commission will consider the extent of the employer's control and any other legal responsibility which the employer may have with respect to the conduct of such non-employees.

---

[1] The principles involved here continue to apply to race, color, religion, or national origin.

* * *

Discussion Questions

1. Would the action by Post constitute sexual harassment? (See Exhibits 8-1-1 and 8-1-2 for applicable regulations.)
2. What actions can be expected from Jones?
3. To what extent does Ms. Page's attitude affect sexual harassment in the organization?
4. If you were a consultant to the nursing home, what would you propose the home do to become a sexual-harassment-free facility?

Case Study 8-2

Firing at Sunrise Hill

Seth B. Goldsmith

A year after Francine Owen accepted a position as a staff nurse at the 100-bed Sunrise Hill Nursing Home, she was promoted to the position of assistant supervisor. Several weeks later she had an argument with her immediate superior, Barbara Jones, over the vacation schedules of aides on the night shift. At the conclusion of the argument, Jones said to Owen, "I feel that your arguing with me is disrespectful and I consider it insubordination. You are fired!"

After Owen recovered from the shock of being told she was fired, she went home and reviewed her records, including a copy of her employment application, which included the following statements:

> I understand that the first three months of employment will be considered as a period of probation and that my employment and compensation may be terminated with or without notice at any time, at the option of Sunrise Hill Nursing Home or myself.

> I understand that no representative, employee, or resident of the Sunrise Hill Nursing Home has authority to enter into an agreement with me for employment for any specified period of time or to make any agreement with me contrary to the foregoing.

Ms. Owen then took out her Sunrise Hill employee manual and reviewed the sections presented in Exhibit 8-2-1.

Exhibit 8-2-1 Sunrise Hill Nursing Home Personnel Manual (Excerpts)

INTRODUCTION

This manual was prepared so that all employees would know about their responsibilities and rights as employees of the Sunrise HIll Nursing Home.

In this manual we set forth our policies regarding employee behavior, the relationship between employees and residents, and the disciplinary procedures to be followed here at Sunrise Hill.

continues

PROBATIONARY PERIOD

To allow all employees to adapt to professional life at Sunrise Hill and to allow supervisors to make appropriate evaluations of your performance, *the first three months of employment are considered probationary.* During this three-month period you are considered a temporary employee and at the conclusion of that period you will be evaluated by your supervisor. If the evaluation is satisfactory you will become a regular employee and if not, your employment will be terminated.

DISCIPLINARY PROCEDURES

The rules and regulations of Sunrise Hill Nursing Home are designed to be fair yet ensure the efficiency and effectiveness of the organization and the ultimate well-being of the residents. Toward that end we have established three levels of employee offenses and appropriate disciplinary action for each offense:

Level I: Minor Offenses

    a. inappropriate dress or poor appearance
    b. loitering/wasting time/horseplay on job
    c. leaving work premises during working hours without permission
    d. absenteeism
    e. violation of common safety procedures, e.g., smoking in unauthorized areas
    f. failure to record work time activity
    g. negligence in performance of duty
    h. failure to report to work on time
    i. other minor offenses not included above

Disciplinary Action for Level I Minor Offenses

These offenses are normally corrected through discussion and a simple reminder. A brief notation of this offense will be placed in the employee's file. The seriousness of Minor Offenses comes with repeated occurrences of the same incident or multiple offenses of a minor nature. A fourth Minor Offense will be regarded as a second Major Offense.

Level II: Major Offenses

    a. falsification of any personnel record
    b. neglect of duties, insubordination, disobedience
    c. absence for three days without notification or reasonable cause
    d. fighting on nursing home property
    e. unauthorized use or removal of nursing home property
    f. discourteous treatment of resident
    g. use of any unauthorized drugs at work
    h. reporting to work under the influence of drugs or alcohol
    i. discriminatory action or harassment of one employee against another because of age, sex, race, physical disability, or religion
    j. other major offenses not included above

continues

Disciplinary Action for Level II Major Offenses

An employee found to have committed a Major Offense will receive counseling and formal written warnings which will be signed by the employee and department head. A copy of this document will also be sent to the Home's executive director.

A second Major Offense will result in a disciplinary suspension—the rest of the shift and up to five (5) scheduled work days upon approval of the executive director.

A third Major Offense will result in the dismissal of the employee.

Level III: Intolerable Offenses

 a. incompetency in resident care
 b. unauthorized possession of firearms, knives or explosives
 c. stealing from other employees, residents or others
 d. immoral or indecent conduct on Home premises
 e. conviction of a felony
 f. flagrant abuse of Home policies or standards
 g. repeated infractions of minor violations or as many as three (3) Major Offenses
 h. other Intolerable Offenses not included above

Disciplinary Action for Level III Intolerable Offenses

An Intolerable Offense is the most serious offense and results in *immediate temporary suspension* until the offense can be reviewed by the department head and the executive director. Dismissal without notice or severance pay is the penalty for Intolerable Offenses. However, dismissal is viewed as the last resort. The disciplinary review of an Intolerable Offense includes consideration being given to an employee's past record, to the circumstances surrounding the incident, and to the effects of the offense on the departments of the nursing home.

* * *

Discussion Questions

1. What responses should an administrator expect from nurse Owen?
2. Did nurse supervisor Jones handle this situation in accord with the personnel manual?
3. How can such problems be avoided in the future?

Chapter 9

Marketing for the Long-Term Care Organization

Linda J. Shea and Charles D. Schewe

INTRODUCTION

Health care administrators are recognizing the benefits that flow from applying basic marketing principles to health care organizations. As they struggle for long-term survival in this increasingly competitive industry, they are carefully analyzing competitive strengths, weaknesses, and growth opportunities, and they are conducting marketing research and positioning their organizations by zeroing in on target market segments. They are carefully designing promotion strategies to raise awareness and interest in their product-service mix and crafting pricing and other decisions to entice purchase. These, then, are some key activities of strategic marketing planning that administrators of the 1990s are finding essential for maintaining a healthy organization.

As the population continues to age over the next decade, the need for long-term care will increase enormously. Although only about 4 percent of the U.S. population live in institutions at any one time, nearly 25 percent will eventually spend some time in an extended care facility.[1]

The pattern of illness and disease for those over age 65 has altered since the turn of this century. Acute conditions have become less prevalent whereas chronic conditions are more frequent. The leading chronic conditions facing the elderly are arthritis, hypertensive disease, hearing impairments, and heart condition. Also, more hospital visits are for chronic conditions. Heart disease and circulatory difficulties, digestive and respiratory system problems, and cancer are the leading causes of hospitalization among those above age 65. Further, chronic illness is even more pronounced among women, who generally outlive men. Additional pertinent long-term health care facts about our 65+ market include the following:

- Between 15 and 20 percent of the elderly have serious symptoms of mental illness.
- A full 27 percent of state mental hospital residents are 65 or above.

- Whereas only 15 percent of people aged 65–69 report having difficulty performing one or more personal care activities, this rises to 49 percent for those 85 and above.
- Those 65 and over are hospitalized about twice as frequently as the younger population and stay 50 percent longer.
- The lifetime risk of institutionalization in a nursing home for those at age 65 is estimated at 52 percent for women and 30 percent for men.[2]

As our health care market continues its maturing, the importance of long-term care provision will only heighten. As competitors vie for a share of this growth market, those organizations best meeting the needs and preferences of long-term care consumers by soundly designing and effectively executing marketing plans will be the industry survivors.

This chapter focuses on the key components of a marketing plan. A marketing plan is directed by the overall organization strategy, which is the outcome of the strategic planning process. And that process begins by looking internally and externally to determine the strengths and weaknesses of the health care organization and the opportunities and threats lurking in the environment. The next section provides a description of the marketing concept. This is followed by explanations of (1) the uncontrollable environmental constraints that shape the organization's strategy and marketing activities, (2) the strategic planning process, (3) marketing research, (4) segmentation, and (5) positioning. Finally, the elements of the marketing mix, that unique, company-specific blend of activities that serve the market, are reviewed. These elements (product, price, distribution, and promotion) provide the foundation for guiding long-term health care managers as they make decisions about which services to offer, how to make them available when and where patients need them, and how services should be priced and communicated to current and potential patients.

Effective strategic marketing demands creativity and innovation. Although long-term health care has lagged behind in embracing marketing philosophy and action, many other health care providers have understood the rewards of implementing the practice of marketing. This chapter provides success stories from many corners of health care provision in order to breathe life into the conceptual material and, perhaps more importantly, provide a wealth of ideas for adaptation and adoption by long-term care organizations.

THE MARKETING CONCEPT: FOCUSING ON THE CONSUMER

The marketing concept is a philosophy. It guides the activities of the organization. The marketing concept means identifying consumer needs and wants and developing products and services to satisfy those needs. It realizes that consumers are the lifeblood of the organization; they are its reason for existence. Although the focus is on the consumer, two other elements are required for adoption of the marketing concept. First, the consumer orientation must be accepted and practiced by all members of the organization, not just the marketing department. Second, this marketing orientation must be accomplished while maintaining a profit or achieving nonprofit organizational goals.

The customers of a health care facility are the patients, and patient satisfaction is the primary focus of a marketing strategy. Several needs have been identified. Among those are cures from illness, information and education for self-help therapy and preventive medicine, a place to stay while getting well, and a place to wait while loved ones are helped.[3] Additional concerns for long-term care patients in particular might include comfort, reduction of fears and apprehension, preservation of personal independence, and provision of companionship and care. These additional concerns are examples of psychological *wants*. Often, psychological wants rather than physical needs make the biggest difference in the evaluation of health care facilities because patients cannot perceptually assess the quality of their health care. Recognizing this, one hospital created this motto: "People don't care how much you know until they know how much you care." Northwestern Memorial Hospital in Chicago designed "niceness training" seminars for doctors, nurses, orderlies, and staff. These marketing-oriented sessions encourage such psychological therapy as smiles and even fresh flowers served with dinner.

Identifying needs and wants is at the heart of the marketing plan. The marketing plan involves developing desirable products and services, pricing them according to patient ability and willingness to pay, designing effective promotional programs to gain attention and encourage usage, and making the services available at the right time and place. A review of the marketing environments will guide decision making in the development of a marketing plan.

ENVIRONMENTAL OPPORTUNITIES AND CONSTRAINTS

Truly understanding consumer needs and wants goes beyond knowing those articulated by current and potential health service users. It also requires knowledge about the uncontrollable environments that affect consumers' needs as well as the ongoing operation of health care facilities. Uncontrollable variables include political and legal issues, sociocultural trends, demographic changes, economic conditions, and the competitive environment. The intensity and direction of trends in these external forces must be monitored continuously and carefully and be reflected in the long-term health care provider's marketing plan.

Within the political and legal environment, changes in the Medicare and Medicaid programs, lobbying efforts by the American Association of Retired Persons, and the enactment of legislation regarding euthanasia are examples of events that could have an impact on a marketing program. The consequences of such events will guide changes in treatment and service offerings, pricing strategy, and other marketing decision areas.

Tracking sociocultural trends also provides direction for the marketing plan. One such trend is the increased social value placed on health maintenance and illness prevention over illness cures such as surgery. This emerging want indicates a greater need for such products as health education, self-help treatments, and preventive measures in the long-term care segment. In response, some hospitals offer educational seminars on stress management, clinics to stop smoking, and workshops on managing diabetes. St. Mary-Corwin Regional Center in Pueblo, Colorado, opened the Pueblo Senior Care Center to encourage independent living for the elderly. The program provides seminars on finding transportation, writing wills, handling insurance claims, taking prescription drugs, and getting help for psychosocial needs. The opportunities created by this sociocultural trend seem almost endless.

Demographic changes will continue to have the greatest impact on the marketing of long-term care. Currently, more than 50 million Americans are over age 55. Projections show that by the end of the year 2010, one-fourth of the U.S. population will be at least 55 years old, and one out of seven will be aged 65 or above. Further, by the year 2000, over half of the elderly population will be older than 75 years of age. The increase in the number of Americans above age 65 was ranked number one on a list of the top ten trends in long-term care for the 1990s.[4] To accommodate this trend, a shift is necessary from an acute illness to chronic illness orientation and toward increased ambulatory care for the diagnosis and treatment of elderly patients. Services to promote independent living for the elderly are also needed. Community Medical Center in Toms River, New Jersey, offers several programs for the elderly, including grandparenting classes, book discussion groups, and adult medical day care.

One major economic fact of the 1990s is the lack of federal funding to finance comprehensive long-term care proposals. Further, any recession is accompanied by increased payment difficulties facing older patients. To counteract these payment problems, Central DuPage Hospital in Winfield, Illinois, created the Patient Accounts Volunteer Experience (PAVE) program. PAVE allows patients to pay off delinquent bills by volunteering their services. Typical services include transporting patients in wheelchairs, providing room service, delivering flowers, and performing clerical work. About 600 volunteers contribute 90,000 hours a year.

In addition to national economic trends, hospitals and other care facilities must examine medical trends to predict the economics of future health care. For instance, cancer is expected to affect three out of four families and will account for over 20 percent of health care expenditures in the 1990s. This suggests the need to develop specialized cancer treatment facilities.

The competitive environment often has the most direct and dramatic impact on specific marketing decisions. Analyzing the competition in the long-term care industry will reveal which needs are currently being sufficiently met and which are not. The results will direct the type of health care specialties and services offered, the specific segments served, the location, and the communication and pricing structure.

Although environmental influences are uncontrollable and often viewed as constraints on the marketing activities of an organization, they should instead be regarded as "open windows" of strategic opportunity. During economic recessions, for example, some hospitals have attracted new clients by offering price incentives to cost-conscious patients. Waiving the deductible or offering reduced prices for checking in on weekends for elective surgery are examples. Looking for strategic opportunities is the first step toward developing an overall organizational strategy and ultimately a sound marketing plan.

CREATING THE STRATEGIC MARKETING PLAN

The importance of strategic market planning cannot be overstated. A recent study of 66 hospitals in both the for-profit and nonprofit sectors showed that the 51 with strategic plans had an average total profit margin of 3.16 percent, compared with –1.07 percent for the 15 without strategic plans. Within the for-profit segment, the difference is even more pronounced. For-profit hospitals with strategic plans earned 4.89 percent margins, compared with –6.4 percent for those without plans—and this was regardless of how the plans were implemented.[5]

Strategic planning addresses three questions: Where are we? Where do we want to go? How are we going to get there? The strategic planning process occurs at multiple levels in the organization. The marketing plan represents the implementation of the organizational strategy. The strategy follows the guidelines established as a result of the overall strategic planning process. Thus, the marketing objectives and strategies must be consistent with the objectives and strategies of the organization as a whole.

The first question addressed in the strategic plan suggests a situation analysis. Particular strengths and weaknesses of the health care organization must be identified, and matched with the opportunities and threats recognized in analyzing the environmental factors. Each long-term health care organization must have distinct competencies setting it apart from competitors. In-house data on occupancy rates, the number and type of scheduled surgeries or illnesses, and the composition of patients served may be used to help pinpoint possible strengths and weaknesses. For example, analysis of discharge forms led one Chicago hospital to begin advertising in Spanish to better serve its predominant customer base.

Another method for identifying strengths and weaknesses is through market share analysis. There are standard measures of market share, such as the number of patients served out of the total number or the share of the long-term care dollar, but an institution can look at market share from multiple perspectives. For instance, share can be calculated for several markets: share by geographic area, by type of illness, by pharmaceutical sales, by department, or by demographic group.[6] Analyzing market share with such scrutiny offers an enriched understanding of a long-term institution's strengths, weaknesses, and opportunities for improvement.

The situation analysis lays the foundation for strategic planning. It helps identify the businesses in which the organization competes and the businesses in which it should compete. Next comes establishing objectives. The objectives are based on the fit between the external opportunities and internal strengths or competencies. Objectives provide direction and control. Neither the strategic plan nor the marketing plan can be fully developed or evaluated without them.

Marketing objectives for long-term health care operations must be consistent with overall organizational objectives. Marketing-related objectives might be established with regard to market share, growth, room or bed occupancy, new product or service development, awareness among specific market segments, or image improvement, to name but a few areas. For example, a nursing home might pursue the goal of lowering its resident base, adding an Alzheimer's disease treatment service, or increasing recognition of its name by 3 percentage points among 46- to 60-year-olds, who are often involved in making nursing home decisions for their parents. Specific and measurable objectives guide the long-term care provider's strategic plan and marketing program.

The strategic plan is developed to answer the question of how to reach the objectives or how to compete more effectively. The plan may call for such strategies as market penetration, product and service development, market development, and diversification. For instance, product development focuses on new services offered to the health care provider's present clientele; market development concentrates on attracting previously untapped patient segments.

The marketing plan is the heart of strategy implementation. It specifies actions for carrying out marketing objectives. A marketing plan identifies target markets and the appropriate marketing mix. The remainder of the chapter is devoted to development of the marketing plan. Information gathering provides a solid foundation for marketing planning.

MARKETING RESEARCH FOR HEALTH CARE SERVICES

Marketing research provides information to allow effective marketing decisions. Common methods of information gathering include informal methods, such as experience surveys, secondary research (e.g., scanning published information), and focus groups, and more formal ones, such as observation and survey research.

In an experience survey, experts in the industry are interviewed. Discussions with effective administrators of long-term health care facilities or those with expertise in a related field provide useful insights about common marketing problems. For example, interviews with leading diabetes researchers could offer valuable information and advice to a health care provider exploring the possibility of adding a diabetes treatment program.

Secondary research uses information previously gathered inside and outside the organization. Periodic in-house reports are helpful for pinpointing trends, indicating gaps in the market or in the marketing program, or monitoring changes in the competitive environment requiring a response. For example, one long-term care provider found internal records showed a lack of patients from a nearby suburb. This resulted in a focused advertising campaign to this geographic segment to increase utilization. Reference books, journals, and government documents available in libraries also provide useful data for long-term health care organizations. The *U.S Census of Population* or the local City and County Data Book, for instance, can be used to estimate the size of any geographic or demographic market area for long-term patients. The *Journal of Health Care Marketing, Modern Healthcare's Eldercare Business,* and *Healthcare Marketing Abstracts* are among the publications reporting research in the health care field.

A focus group consisting of a small number of patients, potential patients, or sponsors meeting in a relaxed, informal atmosphere can be used to discuss topics related to extended care. A session may address the issue of fear about nursing homes or perceptions of area facilities. Although focus groups are exploratory in nature, they are easy to arrange, relatively inexpensive, and generally provide abundant information.

The most useful formal research tool for long-term care is the survey. Surveys can be conducted using personal interviews, over the telephone, or through the mail. The most common type in the health care industry is the patient satisfaction survey. Satisfaction levels of current patients can be monitored by asking them to rate the facility along a number of dimensions. Ratings for physicians and staff, administrative procedures, physical surroundings, and additional services reveal the likes and dislikes of patients. The Hanover Healthcare nursing home chain recently added a stock of toys for visiting children in response to suggestions in one of its quarterly surveys of residents and their families. In addition to patient satisfaction surveys, questionnaires can be used to evaluate promotional strategies, determine the best location for a new facility, or estimate the demand for a particular service.

Marketing research is an integral part of planning and is applicable to all phases of marketing strategy development. For effective target market development, attention must be given to the way consumers select health care services and the influences bearing on their decisions.

THE CONSUMER DECISION PROCESS

Who makes the decisions about long-term care—the decision to obtain treatment, the selection of the physician, and the choice of the health care facility? Is the decision maker different from the recipient of these services? What criteria are used in the decision process? Who and what influences these decisions? Answers to these questions are critical.

A general model of the consumer decision process includes five sequential steps:

1. problem recognition
2. information search
3. evaluation of alternatives
4. choice
5. postdecision evaluation

Problem recognition for long-term care most often occurs when an individual is no longer able to care for him- or herself or when the family and friends are no longer able to provide adequate care. It may occur when a disease such as Alzheimer's is initially diagnosed or when the disease reaches a certain point in its progression. Determining the common situations that lead to recognition of the need for long-term care is essential, since they are indicators of when information will be needed and can suggest ways of communicating with potential patients and other key decision makers.

Consumers (potential patients or their sponsors) seek information about extended care from personal sources such as friends, relatives, doctors, and even pharmacists. They can also obtain useful information during on-site visits with a long-term care facility's admissions personnel. Other marketer-dominated sources of information include listings in the yellow pages, brochures, newspaper and magazine advertisements, and television and radio commercials. Finally, some public information sources are available. Two frequently used sources are listings and descriptions of nursing facilities in local senior centers and newspaper articles profiling long-term health care organizations. Providing information to neutral and personal sources will enhance marketplace awareness and improve a health care organization's probability of being considered for selection. To reach elderly consumers in a small suburb of New Orleans, East Jefferson Hospital launched a program to circumvent referring doctors. Its Elder Advantage Program, a membership club, provides elderly consumers with a number of benefits, including physical exams, counseling services to help with health care-related paperwork, and interest-free financing for hospital charges above the insurance coverage amount. The members, over 13,000 of them, pay only $25 for a lifetime membership.

An information search typically results in defining a set of options to consider. The evaluation stage ultimately results in a choice. During this phase, consumers evaluate the options by comparing them against a particular set of criteria. The importance of the criteria varies according to the type of medical care sought.[7] In one study, nursing home resident sponsors indicated that cleanliness, safety, personnel skill, and services available to residents were the primary factors in their selection of a nursing home.[8] Financial aspects and costs, general appearance, and proximity to the sponsor's home were identified as the least important. Interestingly, though, the sponsors reported living within ten miles of the care facility, with the majority located within a five-mile radius. Each institution must determine the key criteria used by its target segments and properly manage the market's perception of how it meets those criteria. This may involve improving the facility, adding new services, or simply communicating better about what already exists.

Once the criteria are weighed and unwanted alternatives are eliminated, a decision is made. The decision to consider long-term care and the search for information is often carried out by the sponsor; however, the final choice decision still primarily rests with the elderly person. Failure by the long-term care provider to resolve the concerns of both parties may result in rejection.

The decision stage is followed by a postdecision evaluation. In this phase, the new resident of the long-term care facility measures perceived quality of service against expectations. If the quality exceeds expectations, the resident is satisfied; if quality fails to meet expectations, dissatisfaction results. This suggests the futility of making promises that cannot be lived up to. Follow ups with residents and sponsors are useful for monitoring expectation and satisfaction levels. Understanding consumer perceptions is also critical in establishing or changing a positioning strategy.

POSITIONING THE LONG-TERM CARE ORGANIZATION

The "position" of a long-term care organization is determined by how customers perceive the organization and how they differentiate it from other providers. Consumers rely on their image of health care organizations to evaluate health care options. It is important for the organization, then, to create a clear, distinct, unambiguous position that is consistent with the preferences of target consumers. Several positioning approaches are appropriate for the health care business: positioning by attribute, by user group, by usage occasion or type of care, and by dissociation. The following are some examples of these positioning strategies.

Positioning by Attribute or Benefit

The most direct method of positioning is to focus on one or two key attributes or benefits considered most important by potential residents or their sponsors. Communicating an image with slogans such as "Our home is your home" or "Give us the white glove test" keys in on the attributes of a homelike atmosphere and cleanliness that consumers look for in a nursing home.

Positioning by User Group

The American Hospital Association reported that women visit doctors 25 percent more often than men do and account for 63 percent of all surgery. Furthermore, of the 20 most common surgical procedures, 11 of them are performed on women only. In response, Women's Health Centers of America has created a "one-stop body shop" where women can receive total basic care. Each of the dozens of clinics across the country provide everything from mammograms and treatment for osteoporosis to advice on weight control and psychological counseling.

Positioning by Usage Occasion or Type of Care

Doctors' Hospital of Detroit is becoming known as "the place to go for emergency care." An advertisement shown on cable television promised that patients seeking emergency treatment would be seen within 20 minutes or receive free care. Baylor University Medical Center opened the Tom Landry Sports Medicine and Research Center focusing on rehabilitation, research, and fitness.

Positioning by Dissociation

People generally perceive nursing homes as undesirable, "last resort" options. Placement is often accompanied by other traumatic role changes such as widowhood, loss of independence, and loss of control over seemingly trivial matters. It is important, therefore, to develop a position for such an institution that defies those negative images. Emphasizing living with dignity, enjoying some comforts of home, and easing the financial burden all serve to dissociate an extended care facility from its undesirable perception.

Product positions are strengthened through promotion, pricing, and distribution strategies. The particular position an organization chooses to establish is dependent on the consumer segment it targets.

IDENTIFYING HEALTH SERVICES SEGMENTS

Consumers have varying needs; satisfying all potential consumer needs and wants with a single marketing program is virtually impossible. The case for long-term care is no exception. A marketing plan designed to please everyone rarely satisfies anyone. Instead, consumers can be divided into more homogenous sub-groups, along such dimensions as ability to pay, type of illness, or religious preference and a marketing plan developed to meet and satisfy the needs of one or some of these groups. The more well defined the target segments, the more precise and effective will be the marketing plan to reach those consumers.

Potential users of long-term care can be grouped by similarities in demographic characteristics, by physical condition or health need, by psychographic characteristics, or by benefits sought, to name a few. Generally, the most effective and most recommended method for identifying health care market segments is by benefits sought, or "benefit segmentation."[9] Benefit segmentation applied in the health care industry classifies individuals according to their needs and preferences for medical care. In this procedure, consumers provide importance ratings for a list of health care provision characteristics and are then grouped according to which characteristics they rate similarly. One study produced four distinct segments. The first was coined the "take care of me" segment. This group is most concerned about physical comfort during a hospital stay. The "cure me" segment consists of those who count on privacy and a quiet environment. The third was the "pamper me" segment that wants to be cared for, but doesn't want to be bothered by anything else. It also strives for psychological comfort. A fourth group is concerned with medical and administrative proficiency.[10]

Once possible segments are described, specific product, place, price, and promotion decisions can be directed toward meeting their desires. From the previously described segments, for instance, the pamper me group would be most appreciative of decorative bedding, fresh flowers in the room, and a body massage. The fourth segment described, however, is concerned about physician credentials and would prefer convenient parking and itemized billing statements. Advertising one of these sets of services would create a position for the care provider and attract a specific market segment.

THE LONG-TERM CARE "PRODUCT"

While health care is viewed as a service industry, many traditional product concepts in marketing can provide insights useful for effective marketing. Of particular relevance to the long-term health care market are the concept of the total product, branding issues, and product extensions.

The term "total" product refers to a bundle of tangible and intangible attributes providing satisfaction of consumer wants and needs during the entire stay "experience." A long-term health care product is the perception of the tangible (for example, the physical facilities and equipment, the perceived skills of individual doctors and nurses, the food, and opportunity for social interaction) and intangible features (such as the reputation of the provider and the perceived attitudes of personnel). Among the factors rated as extremely important in the selection of a health care provider are (aside from the formal qualifications of a doctor), how well the doctor listens, the willingness to discuss stress issues, and the willingness to discuss treatment alternatives.[11] Furthermore, since most health care consumers believe they lack the competence necessary to evaluate a physician's performance, they rely instead on personality, quality of interaction, and "art-of-care" to judge the quality of treatment.[12]

Any "brand" or name associated with a long-term care center serves to establish or strengthen an organization's position and improve name recognition. Some facilities have adopted brand names denoting specific types of surgery. Dallas-based Republic Health Corporation's hospitals, for instance, use "You're Becoming" (cosmetic surgery), "Gift of Sight" (cataract surgery), and "Step Lively" (podiatric surgery).

Research has shown that the words used to describe the long-term care institution convey meaning to potential residents and their sponsors. In a study where sponsors rated nine different institution titles in terms of desirability and how accurately they describe the function of the nursing home, none of them ranked high on both variables.[13] The name ranked highest in desirability was "extended health care facility." However, it was ranked only fifth in accuracy. The name ranked highest in accuracy was "extended care for the elderly." It was, however, ranked as one of the least desirable titles. "Nursing home" was ranked seventh of the nine in desirability, but second in accuracy. There clearly is considerable potential for improvement in long-term care institution titles.

Creating product line extensions, or expanded services, is another strategy used by health care organizations to distinguish themselves from competitors. For example, United Hospital in St. Paul and the Metropolitan Medical Center in Minneapolis market Nutritious Cuisine, a line of frozen dinners for the elderly. Mt. Sinai Medical Center sells soup under its own name. This, it believes, creates the image of a "warm and soothing" place. The center, located on 5th Avenue in New York, also employs a concierge to greet patients and assist in any special arrangements (such as preparing a conference room for a business meeting) during the patient's stay.

CREATIVE PRICING

Innovative pricing strategies are an effective tool for increasing health care demand and ultimately market share. Health care administrators tend to rely too heavily on cost-oriented pricing. Demand-oriented pricing offers more flexibility and opportunities to attract new customers. This approach recognizes that the value of a product or service is determined by patients' willingness and ability to pay. Although costs are rarely mentioned as the most important consideration in long-term care selection, price incentives can make the difference when choosing among options perceived as otherwise similar.

Several discount and allowance options are available to attract both private-pay and public-assisted patients. Some hospitals are waiving the Medicare deductible for inpatient care of senior citizens. Others are providing interest-free financing for charges not covered by Medicare or other insurance.

Off-peak pricing offsets costly overhead during slow occupancy periods. Sunset Hospital in Las Vegas offers a unique program to increase off-peak use of its services. If patients check in on Friday or Saturday, they are automatically entered in that week's prize drawing for a round-trip "recuperative cruise" to the destination of their choice. In another incentive program, Sunrise Center offered $5^1/4$ percent rebates on charges for patients checking in on Friday or Saturday. Long-term care occupancy may not fluctuate weekly, but facilities do experience occupancy lulls that could benefit from an off-peak pricing strategy.

Bundling services into packages and offering them at varying prices may be perceived as an attractive alternative to consumers of long-term care. They often feel they are getting a better value by selecting the services and extras important to them and not having to pay for those that are either inappropriate or unwanted. Furthermore, certain packages can be offered to appeal to different clienteles, such as "no frills" and "deluxe" versions of similar services.[14]

Other appropriate pricing strategies include offering cash discounts to private-pay patients who pay in advance or quantity discounts to those who stay for a certain length of time. Finally, for elderly individuals or their families reluctant to make a long-term commitment, the first month's stay could be offered free as a trial period.

APPLYING DISTRIBUTION CONCEPTS TO LONG-TERM CARE

The distribution component of the marketing mix comprises the physical environment (atmospherics) and the distribution or location of services.

Atmospherics

The physical environment plays an important role in the health care selection process. Just as consumers use the retail store atmosphere to judge the quality of its products, research has shown that patients use the quality of the physical surroundings to judge the quality of treatment.[15] To this end, "designer" decorated delivery rooms have been created for the upwardly mobile maternity patient. Pacific Presbyterian Medical Center in San Francisco offers rooms with Jacuzzi baths and a view of the Golden Gate Bridge. The Women's Hospital of Texas provides a limousine service and hors d'oeuvres for its maternity patients. St. Mary's Hospital in West Palm Beach supplies video equipment for taping birthing events. Patients claim some of these fashionable clinics look and feel more like a Ritz Carlton Hotel than a hospital.

In the case of nursing homes specifically, residents want the look and feel of a real domicile; they wish for some similarities to their former homes. A homelike appearance might include increased emphasis on residential as opposed to institutional furniture, wallpapered walls, a pleasant view from the window, and a place to display personal mementos.[16]

A sense of independence and control can also be maintained through thoughtful physical design. For instance, rooms can be designed to facilitate mobility and enhance independence for residents in wheelchairs by lowering closet rods and keeping other items easily accessible.[17]

Residents who are able to exercise some control by making choices on their own will experience greater satisfaction than those feeling completely dependent. Providing space for sitting, allowing room temperature control, accommodating eating preferences (including dining times), and respecting privacy will give residents a sense of autonomy.

Distribution of Services

The location of an institution is an important factor in long-term care. Given the knowledge that sponsors place elders in extended care facilities located near their homes, competition is kept primarily at the local level.

Other location options include bringing the care to the elders or establishing branch facilities for special services. The "Doc in a Box" concept was developed with this in mind. A "Doc in a Box" is a neighborhood center set up by a hospital for cash customers who need quick advice on cuts, colds, and other minor problems that are not viewed as serious enough for an emergency room visit.

Some institutions provide extended care service in elders' homes through the use of visiting nurses until it becomes necessary to transfer them to a permanent facility. The trend toward bringing the "place" to the patient is further evidenced by Meals on Wheels, mobile units for diagnostic testing, and even the return of physician house calls.

COMMUNICATING WITH TARGET MARKETS

The final element of the marketing mix is promotion. The purpose of the promotional strategy is to inform, persuade, and remind consumers of the benefits offered by the organization. The major components of promotion are advertising, publicity, personal selling, and sales promotion. Advertising refers to any paid form of nonpersonal communication from the identified marketer to the customer. Not long ago, advertising in the health industry was perceived as unethical; now it is generally accepted as a legitimate competitive activity. Advertising in the health care industry increased tenfold between 1983 and 1986 (expenditures went from $50 million to $500 million), and it continues to soar. More recent estimates put expenditures as high as $1 billion a year. Television and magazine advertising are useful for reaching large numbers of potential consumers over a wide geographic area, whereas radio and newspaper advertising generally have greater local penetration. Each of these media is heavily used in the health care industry.

The University of Chicago Hospital discovered through marketing research that its staff was not perceived as warm and approachable. Its solution: The hospital's ad agency produced a series of 20-second testimonials from several staff physicians for a television ad campaign. Faith Family Hospital in St. Louis ran profiles of its doctors in newspaper ads. Instead of using staff physicians, the Women's HealthCare and Wellness Center in Oak Park, Illinois, signed up Dorothy Hamill, Ann Jillian, and Rita Moreno as spokespersons to promote its opening.

Publicity, usually in the form of press releases, is the most common type of promotion in the health care industry. Publicity is not paid for by the organization; however, the press releases are not always published and the information is not always positive. One recommended strategy for developing media relations is to write an information column in the local newspaper. Administrators or staff could offer advice on such topics as identifying chronic illnesses or financial preparations for extended care. Information columns increase visibility, are less expensive than advertising, are more likely to be published than a press release, demonstrate social responsibility, and create a positive image.

Exercising another publicity option, the Franciscan Health System of New Jersey created House Calls, a cable television program. Viewers in 1.5 million homes are informed about health matters and the hospital's services. St. Agnes Hospital in Baltimore found another way of building community goodwill and promoting its services. It operates an in-house print shop for use by community organizations who publish newsletters. The service is offered without cost, and the hospital uses the excess space in the newsletters to promote its programs.

Personal selling involves face-to-face communication with the target customer. St. Elizabeth Medical Center in Dayton, Ohio, employs an unusual personal selling technique. It uses the "tupperware party" approach, complete with games, prizes, and refreshments, to inform potential patients of its services. Doctors and nurses conduct the parties in people's homes, providing answers to medical questions in a relaxed, informal atmosphere. This technique seems most appropriate for long-term care; potential residents and sponsors have much to learn.

Personal selling in the extended care facility occurs primarily during the on-site interview. In a study of first impressions in the nursing home interview, sponsors of prospective residents expressed clear preferences for a rather formal look of dress (sport coats rather than suits or sweaters) for facility personnel. The interview should be viewed as a selling opportunity; however, the soft-sell approach is likely to be most successful in this situation.

Sales promotion makes use of a wide array of tools, such as displays, coupons, event sponsorship, price specials, samples, and contests. Long-term care sales promotion opportunities are plentiful. Open houses for the community, special educational events for residents and their families, and sponsorship of local events are all appropriate and useful means of communicating with current and potential residents. Masonic Home and Hospital in Wallingford, Connecticut, caters to its residents' families (a primary referral group) through various programs that bring the residents and family members together. Its Masonic Railroad Club, for example, uses an elaborate model railroad displayed in one of the old wards to appeal to both residents and their grandchildren. The Greenhouse Club offers gardening activities and operates solely on donated plants and flowers. Residents, their families, and members of the community may join to learn more about gardening or just enjoy the attractive displays.

Each of these promotion methods has the potential to create community awareness of a long-term care facility, to communicate benefits and services offered, and to strengthen the facility's position.

CONCLUSION

Creating a marketing plan involves identifying potential consumers and developing a marketing action program. The effectiveness of the marketing plan depends largely on the extent and accuracy of the planning phase. Analyzing the organization's strengths and weaknesses, identifying marketing opportunities, and understanding the uncontrollable environmental factors provide the basis for a sound marketing program. A thorough knowledge of consumers' needs and wants will provide essential assistance in targeting market segments, designing a positioning strategy, developing health service offerings, specifying pricing and distribution strategies, and communicating to consumers the quality of care they can expect.

This chapter presented the basics for establishing a long-term care marketing program. Much more can be done, however, to fine-tune marketing decisions. The long-term care marketer must set up internal controls to monitor the environment, must institute market surveys to gauge resident satisfaction, and must continually evaluate and modify its product, price, place, and promotion strategies. Marketing must be viewed as a process and a philosophy; it is not just something to do but "a way to be."

NOTES

1. R.C. Atchley, *Aging: Continuity and Change* (Belmont, Calif.: Wadsworth Publishing, 1987).

2. For these facts and more, see U.S. Senate Committee on Aging, *Aging in America: Trends and Projections,* 1987–88 ed. (Washington, D.C.: U.S. Government Printing Office, 1988), 96–124.

3. J.A. Miller, Marketing Basics for Hospital Managers, *Hospital Forum* (July-August 1980):7–12.

4. R.C. Coile, Long-Term Care: Top Ten Trends for the 1990s, *Hospital Strategy Report* 3, no. 9 (July 1991):1–5.

5. J. Greene, Hospitals Can Boost Profits by Going According to Plan, *Modern Healthcare* 21, no. 31 (1992):36.

6. S. Majaro, Market Share: Deception or Diagnosis, *Marketing* (March 1977):43–47.

7. J. Boscarino and S.R. Steiber, Hospital Shopping and Consumer Choice, *Journal of Health Care Marketing* 2, no. 2 (1982):15–23.

8. M. Rogers et al., First Impressions: Preferences of Sponsors of Nursing Home Patients in the Search and Interviewing Processes, *Journal of Health Care Marketing* 8, no. 3 (1988):33–41.

9. D.W. Finn and C.W. Lamb, Jr., Hospital Benefit Segmentation, *Journal of Health Care Marketing* 6, no. 4 (1986):26–33.

10. Ibid.

11. D.W. Stewart et al., Information Search and Decision Making in the Selection of Family Health Care, *Journal of Health Care Marketing* 9, no. 2 (1989):29–39.

12. A. Cartwright, *Patients and Their Doctors* (New York: Atherton Press, 1967).

13. M. Rogers et al., First Impressions.

14. J.A. Miller, Marketing Basics for Hospital Managers.

15. P. Kotler and R.N. Clarke, *Marketing for Health Care Organizations* (Englewood Cliffs, N.J.: Prentice-Hall, 1987).

16. W.J. Brown, Tips on How To Plan for the Resident-Oriented Environment, *Provider* (1988):25–28.

17. J. Baker and C.W. Lamb, Jr., The Roles of Physical Environments in Health Care Marketing, paper presented at the Advances in Health Care Research Conference, Jackson Hole, Wyoming, March 1991.

Case Study 9-1

Marketing Admissions

Seth B. Goldsmith

Frank Fleet, Associate Director of the Grant Geriatrics Center, has just received the following confidential memo from the Center's director.

Grant Geriatric Center

From:	Ms. Wendy Field
To:	Mr. Frank Fleet
Subject:	OBRA regulations and our admissions agreement

As you are aware, our one-page admissions agreement is hopelessly out of date and fails to include a number of important points brought out in the OBRA regulations. Would you please review the section of the regulations on patients' rights and let me know how we could incorporate these rights into our admissions agreement and use them to our marketing advantage?

See Exhibit 9-1-1 for the relevant regulations.

Exhibit 9-1-1 OBRA Regulations: Resident Rights and Quality of Life

> **PART 483—REQUIREMENTS FOR STATES AND LONG TERM CARE FACILITIES**
>
> **Subpart B—Requirements for Long Term Care Facilities**
>
> **§ 483.1 Basis and scope.**
>
> (a) *Basis in legislation.* (1) Sections 1819 (a), (b), (c), and (d) of the Act provide that—
> (i) Skilled nursing facilities participating in Medicare must meet certain specified requirements; and

continues

Exhibit 9-1-1 continued

(ii) The Secretary may impose additional requirements (see section 1819(d)(4)(B)) if they are necessary for the health and safety of individuals to whom services are furnished in the facilities.

(2) Sections 1919(a), (b), (c), and (d) of the Act provide that nursing facilities participating in Medicaid must meet certain requirements.

(b) *Scope.* The provisions of this part contain the requirements than an institution must meet in order to qualify to participate as a SNF in the Medicare program, and as a nursing facility in the Medicaid program. They serve as the basis for survey activities for the purpose of determining whether a facility meets the requirements for participation in Medicare and Medicaid.

§ 483.5 Definitions.

For purposes of this subpart—

Facility means, a skilled nursing facility (SNF) or a nursing facility (NF) which meets the requirements of sections 1819 or 1919 (a), (b), (c), and (d) of the Act. "Facility" may include a distinct part of an institution specified in § 440.40 of this chapter, but does not include an institution for the mentally retarded or persons with related conditions described in § 440.150 of this chapter. For Medicare and Medicaid purposes (including eligibility, coverage, certification, and payment), the "facility" is always the entity which participates in the program, whether that entity is comprised of all of, or a distinct part of a larger institution. For Medicare, a SNF (see section 1819(a)(1)), and for Medicaid, a NF (see section 1919(a)(1)) may not be an institution for mental diseases as defined in § 435.1009.

§ 483.10 Resident rights.

The resident has a right to a dignified existence, self-determination, and communication with and access to persons and services inside and outside the facility. A facility must protect and promote the rights of each resident, including each of the following rights:

(a) *Exercise of rights.*

(1) The resident has the right to exercise his or her rights as a resident of the facility and as a citizen or resident of the United States.

(2) The resident has the right to be free of interference, coercion, discrimination, and reprisal from the facility in exercising his or her rights.

(3) In the case of a resident adjudged incompetent under the laws of a State by a court of competent jurisdiction, the rights of the resident are exercised by the person appointed under State law to act on the resident's behalf.

(4) In the case of a resident who has not been adjudged incompetent by the State court, any legal-surrogate designated in accordance with State law may exercise the resident's rights to the extent provided by State law.

(b) *Notice of rights and services.*

(1) The facility must inform the resident both orally and in writing in a language that the resident understands of his or her rights and all rules and regulations governing resident conduct and responsibilities during the stay in the facility. The facility must also provide the resident with the notice (if any) of the State developed under section 1919(e)(6) of the Act. Such notification must be made prior to or upon admission and during the resident's stay. Receipt of such information, and any amendments to it, must be acknowledged in writing;

(2) The resident or his or her legal representative has the right—

continues

Exhibit 9-1-1 continued

(i) Upon an oral or written request, to access all records pertaining to himself or herself including current clinical records within 24 hours (excluding weekends and holidays); and

(ii) After receipt of his or her records for inspection, to purchase at a cost not to exceed the community standard photocopies of the records or any portions of them upon request and 2 working days advance notice to the facility.

(3) The resident has the right to be fully informed in language that he or she can understand of his or her total health status, including but not limited to, his or her medical condition;

(4) The resident has the right to refuse treatment, to refuse to participate in experimental research, and to formulate an advance directive as specified in paragraph (8) of this section; and

(5) The facility must—

(i) Inform each resident who is entitled to Medicaid benefits, in writing, at the time of admission to the nursing facility or, when the resident becomes eligible for Medicaid of—

(A) The items and services that are included in nursing facility services under the State plan and for which the resident may not be charged;

(B) Those other items and services that the facility offers and for which the resident may be charged, and the amount of charges for those services; and

(ii) Inform each resident when changes are made to the items and services specified in paragraphs (5)(i) (A) and (B) of this section.

(6) The facility must inform each resident before, or at the time of admission, and periodically during the resident's stay, of services available in the facility and of charges for those services, including any charges for services not covered under Medicare or by the facility's per diem rate.

(7) The facility must furnish a written description of legal rights which includes—

(i) A description of the manner of protecting personal funds, under paragraph (c) of this section;

(ii) A description of the requirements and procedures for establishing eligibility for Medicaid, including the right to request an assessment under section 1924(c) which determines the extent of a couple's non-exempt resources at the time of institutionalization and attributes to the community spouse an equitable share of resources which cannot be considered available for payment toward the cost of the institutionalized spouse's medical care in his or her process of spending down to Medicaid eligibility levels;

(iii) A posting of names, addresses, and telephone numbers of all pertinent State client advocacy groups such as the State survey and certification agency, the State licensure office, the State ombudsman program, the protection and advocacy network, and the Medicaid fraud control unit; and

(iv) A statement that the resident may file a complaint with the State survey and certification agency concerning resident abuse, neglect, and misappropriation of resident property in the facility.

(8) The facility must comply with the requirements specified in subpart I of part 489 of this chapter relating to maintaining written policies and procedures regarding advance directives. These requirements include provisions to inform and provide written information to all adult residents concerning the right to accept or refuse medical or surgical treatment and, at the individual's option, formulate an advance directive. This includes a written description of the facility's policies to implement advance directives and applicable State law.

(9) The facility must inform each resident of the name, specialty, and way of contacting the physician responsible for his or her care.

continues

Exhibit 9-1-1 continued

(10) The facility must prominently display in the facility written information, and provide to residents and applicants for admission oral and written information about how to apply for and use Medicare and Medicaid benefits, and how to receive refunds for previous payments covered by such benefits.

(11) *Notification of changes.* (i) A facility must immediately inform the resident; consult with the resident's physician; and if known, notify the resident's legal representative or an interested family member when there is—

(A) An accident involving the resident which results in injury and has the potential for requiring physician intervention;

(B) A significant change in the resident's physical, mental, or psychosocial status (i.e., a deterioration in health, mental, or psychosocial status in either life-threatening conditions or clinical complications);

(C) A need to alter treatment significantly (i.e., a need to discontinue an existing form of treatment due to adverse consequences, or to commence a new form of treatment); or

(D) A decision to transfer or discharge the resident from the facility as specified in § 483.12(a).

(ii) The facility must also promptly notify the resident and, if known, the resident's legal representative or interested family member when there is—

(A) A change in room or roommate assignment as specified in § 483.15(e)(2); or

(B) A change in resident rights under Federal or State law or regulations as specified in paragraph (b)(1) of this section.

(iii) The facility must record and periodically update the address and phone number of the resident's legal representative or interested family member.

(c) *Protection of Resident Funds.* (1) The resident has the right to manage his or her financial affairs, and the facility may not require residents to deposit their personal funds with the facility.

(2) *Management of personal funds.* Upon written authorization of a resident, the facility must hold, safeguard, manage, and account for the personal funds of the resident deposited with the facility, as specified in paragraphs (c)(3)–(8) of this section.

(3) *Deposit of funds.* (i) *Funds in excess of $50.* The facility must deposit any residents' personal funds in excess of $50 in an interest bearing account (or accounts) that is separate from any of the facility's operating accounts, and that credits all interest earned on resident's funds to that account. (In pooled accounts, there must be a separate accounting for each resident's share.)

(ii) *Funds less than $50.* The facility must maintain a resident's personal funds that do not exceed $50 in a noninterest bearing account, interest bearing account, or petty cash fund.

(4) *Accounting and records.* The facility must establish and maintain a system that assures a full and complete and separate accounting, according to generally accepted accounting principles, of each resident's personal funds entrusted to the facility on the resident's behalf.

(i) The system must preclude any commingling of resident funds with facility funds or with the funds of any person other than another resident.

(ii) The individual financial record must be available through quarterly statements and on request to the resident or his or her legal representative.

(5) *Notice of certain balances.* The facility must notify each resident that receives Medicaid benefits—

(i) When the amount in the resident's account reaches $200 less than the SSI resource limit for one person, specified in section 1611(a)(3)(B) of the Act; and

continues

Exhibit 9-1-1 continued

(ii) That, if the amount in the account, in addition to the value of the resident's other nonexempt resources, reaches the SSI resource limit for one person, the resident may lose eligibility for Medicaid or SSI.

(6) *Conveyance upon death.* Upon the death of a resident with a personal fund deposited with the facility, the facility must convey within 30 days the resident's funds, and a final accounting of those funds, to the individual or probate jurisdiction administering the resident's estate.

(7) *Assurance of financial security.* The facility must purchase a surety bond, or otherwise provide assurance satisfactory to the Secretary, to assure the security of all personal funds of residents deposited with the facility.

(8) *Limitation on charges to personal funds.* The facility may not impose a charge against the personal funds of a resident for any item or service for which payment is made under Medicaid or Medicare (except for applicable deductible and coinsurance amounts). The facility may charge the resident for requested services that are more expensive than or in excess of covered services in accordance with § 489.32 of this chapter. (This does not affect the prohibition on facility charges for items and services for which Medicaid has paid. See § 447.15, which limits participation in the Medicaid program to providers who accept, as payment in full, Medicaid payment plus any deductible, coinsurance, or copayment required by the plan to be paid by the individual.)

(i) *Services included in Medicare or Medicaid payment.* During the course of a covered Medicare or Medicaid stay, facilities may not charge a resident for the following categories of items and services:

(A) Nursing services as required at § 483.30 of this subpart.

(B) Dietary services as required at § 483.35 of this subpart.

(C) An activities program as required at § 483.15(f) of this subpart.

(D) Room/bed maintenance services.

(E) Routine personal hygiene items and services as required to meet the needs of residents, including, but not limited to, hair hygiene supplies, comb, brush, bath soap, disinfecting soaps or specialized cleansing agents when indicated to treat special skin problems or to fight infection, razor, shaving cream, toothbrush, toothpaste, denture adhesive, denture cleaner, dental floss, moisturizing lotion, tissues, cotton balls, cotton swabs, deodorant, incontinence care and supplies, sanitary napkins and related supplies, towels, washcloths, hospital gowns, over the counter drugs, hair and nail hygiene services, bathing, and basic personal laundry.

(F) Medically-related social services as required at § 483.15(g) of this subpart.

(ii) *Items and services that may be charged to residents' funds.* Listed below are general categories and examples of items and services that the facility may charge to the residents' funds if they are requested by the resident, if the facility informs the resident that there will be a charge, and if payment is not made by Medicare and Medicaid:

(A) Telephone.

(B) Television/radio for personal use.

(C) Personal comfort items, including smoking materials, notions and novelties, and confections.

(D) Cosmetic and grooming items and services in excess of those for which payment is made under Medicaid or Medicare.

(E) Personal clothing.

(F) Personal reading matter.

(G) Gifts purchased on behalf of a resident.

(H) Flowers and plants.

continues

Exhibit 9-1-1 continued

(I) Social events and entertainment offered outside the scope of the activities program, provided under § 483.15(f) of this subpart.

(J) Noncovered special care services such as privately hired nurses or aides.

(K) Private room, except when therapeutically required (for example, isolation for infection control).

(L) Specially prepared or alternative food requested instead of the food generally prepared by the facility, as required by § 483.35 of this subpart.

(iii) *Requests for items and services.*

(A) The facility must not charge a resident (or his or her representative) for any item or service not requested by the resident.

(B)The facility must not require a resident (or his or her representative) to request any item or service as a condition of admission or continued stay.

(C) The facility must inform the resident (or his or her representative) requesting an item or service for which charge will be made that there will be a charge for the item or service and what the charge will be.

(d) *Free choice.* The resident has the right to—

(1) Choose a personal attending physician;

(2) Be fully informed in advance about care and treatment and of any changes in that care or treatment that may affect the resident's well-being, and

(3) Unless adjudged incompetent or otherwise found to be incapacitated under the laws of the State, participate in planning care and treatment or changes in care and treatment.

(e) *Privacy and confidentiality.* The resident has the right to personal privacy and confidentiality of his or her personal and clinical records.

(1) Personal privacy includes accommodations, medical treatment, written and telephone communications, personal care, visits, and meetings of family and resident groups, but this does not require the facility to provide a private room for each resident;

(2) Except as provided in paragraph (e)(3) of this section, the resident may approve or refuse the release of personal and clinical records to any individual outside the facility;

(3) The resident's right to refuse release of personal and clinical records does not apply when—

(i) The resident is transferred to another health care institution; or

(ii) Record release is required by law.

(f) *Grievances.* A resident has the right to—

(1) Voice grievances without discrimination or reprisal. Such grievances include those with respect to treatment which has been furnished as well as that which has not been furnished; and

(2) Prompt efforts by the facility to resolve grievances the resident may have, including those with respect to the behavior of other residents.

(g) *Examination of survey results.* A resident has the right to—

(1) Examine the results of the most recent survey of the facility conducted by Federal or State surveyors and any plan of correction in effect with respect to the facility. The facility must make the results available for examination in a place readily accessible to residents, and must post a notice of their availability; and

(2) Receive information from agencies acting as client advocates, and be afforded the opportunity to contact these agencies.

(h) *Work.* The resident has the right to—

(1) Refuse to perform services for the facility;

(2) Perform services for the facility if he or she chooses, when—

continues

Exhibit 9-1-1 continued

(i) The facility has documented the need or desire for work in the plan of care;

(ii) The plan specifies the nature of the services performed and whether the services are voluntary or paid;

(iii) Compensation for paid service is at or above prevailing rates; and

(iv) The resident agrees to the work arrangement described in the plan of care.

(i) *Mail.* The resident has the right to privacy in written communication, including the right to—

(1) Send and promptly receive mail that is unopened; and

(2) Have access to stationery, postage, and writing implements at the resident's own expense.

(j) *Access and visitation rights.* (1) The resident has the right and the facility must provide immediate access to any resident by the following:

(i) Any representative of the Secretary;

(ii) Any representative of the State;

(iii) The resident's individual physician;

(iv) The State long term care ombudsman (established under section 307(a)(12) of the Older Americans Act of 1965);

(v) The agency responsible for the protection and advocacy system for developmentally disabled individuals (established under part C of the Developmental Disabilities Assistance and Bill of Rights Act);

(vi) The agency responsible for the protection and advocacy system for mentally ill individuals (established under the Protection and Advocacy for Mentally Ill Individuals Act);

(vii) Subject to the resident's right to deny or withdraw consent at any time, immediate family or other relatives of the resident; and

(viii) Subject to reasonable restrictions and the resident's right to deny or withdraw consent at any time, others who are visiting with the consent of the resident.

(2) The facility must provide reasonable access to any resident by any entity or individual that provides health, social, legal, or other services to the resident, subject to the resident's right to deny or withdraw consent at any time.

(3) The facility must allow representatives of the State Ombudsman, described in paragraph (j)(1)(iv) of this section, to examine a resident's clinical records with the permission of the resident or the resident's legal representative, and consistent with State law.

(k) *Telephone.* The resident has the right to have reasonable access to the use of a telephone where calls can be made without being overheard.

(l) *Personal property.* The resident has the right to retain and use personal possessions, including some furnishings, and appropriate clothing, as space permits, unless to do so would infringe upon the rights or health and safety of other residents.

(m) *Married couples.* The resident has the right to share a room with his or her spouse when married residents live in the same facility and both spouses consent to the arrangement.

(n) *Self-Administration of Drugs.* An individual resident may self-administer drugs if the interdisciplinary team as defined by § 483.20(d)(2)(ii), has determined that this practice is safe.

(o) *Refusal of certain transfers.* (1) An individual has the right to refuse a transfer to another room within the institution, if the purpose of the transfer is to relocate—

(i) A resident of a SNF from the distinct part of the institution that is a SNF to a part of the institution that is not a SNF, or

(ii) A resident of a NF from the distinct part of the institution that is a NF to a distinct part of the institution that is a SNF.

continues

Exhibit 9-1-1 continued

(2) A resident's exercise of the right to refuse transfer under paragraph (o)(1) of this section does not affect the individual's eligibility or entitlement to Medicare or Medicaid benefits.

[56 FR 48867, Sept. 26, 1991, as amended at 57 FR 8202, Mar. 6,1992; 57 FR 43924, Sept. 23, 1992]

§ 483.12 Admission, transfer and discharge rights.

(a) Transfer and discharge—

(1) *Definition:* Transfer and discharge includes movement of a resident to a bed outside of the certified facility whether that bed is in the same physical plant or not. Transfer and discharge does not refer to movement of a resident to a bed within the same certified facility.

(2) *Transfer and discharge requirements.* The facility must permit each resident to remain in the facility, and not transfer or discharge the resident from the facility unless—

(i) The transfer or discharge is necessary for the resident's welfare and the resident's needs cannot be met in the facility;

(ii) The transfer or discharge is appropriate because the resident's health has improved sufficiently so the resident no longer needs the services provided by the facility;

(iii) The safety of individuals in the facility is endangered;

(iv) The health of individuals in the facility would otherwise be endangered;

(v) The resident has failed, after reasonable and appropriate notice, to pay for (or to have paid under Medicare or Medicaid) a stay at the facility. For a resident who becomes eligible for Medicaid after admission to a facility, the facility may charge a resident only allowable charges under Medicaid; or

(vi) The facility ceases to operate.

(3) *Documentation.* When the facility transfers or discharges a resident under any of the circumstances specified in paragraphs (a)(2)(i) through (v) of this section, the resident's clinical record must be documented. The documentation must be made by—

(i) The resident's physician when transfer or discharge is necessary under paragraph (a)(2)(i) or paragraph (a)(2)(ii) of this section; and

(ii) A physician when transfer or discharge is necessary under paragraph (a)(2)(iv) of this section.

(4) *Notice before transfer.* Before a facility transfers or discharges a resident, the facility must—

(i) Notify the resident and, if known, a family member or legal representative of the resident of the transfer or discharge and the reasons for the move in writing and in a language and manner they understand.

(ii) Record the reasons in the resident's clinical record; and

(iii) Include in the notice the items described in paragraph (a)(6) of this section.

(5) *Timing of the notice.* (i) Except when specified in paragraph (a)(5)(ii) of this section, the notice of transfer or discharge required under paragraph (a)(4) of this section must be made by the facility at least 30 days before the resident is transferred or discharged.

(ii) Notice may be made as soon as practicable before transfer or discharge when—

(A) the safety of individuals in the facility would be endangered under paragraph (a)(2)(iii) of this section;

(B) The health of individuals in the facility would be endangered, under paragraph (a)(2)(iv) of this section;

continues

Exhibit 9-1-1 continued

(C) The resident's health improves sufficiently to allow a more immediate transfer or discharge, under paragraph (a)(2)(ii) of this section;

(D) An immediate transfer or discharge is required by the resident's urgent medical needs, under paragraph (a)(2)(i) of this section; or

(E) A resident has not resided in the facility for 30 days.

(6) *Contents of the notice.* The written notice specified in paragraph (a)(4) of this section must include the following:

(i) The reason for transfer or discharge;

(ii) The effective date of transfer or discharge;

(iii) The location to which the resident is transferred or discharged;

(iv) A statement that the resident has the right to appeal the action to the State;

(v) The name, address and telephone number of the State long term care ombudsman;

(vi) For nursing facility residents with developmental disabilities, the mailing address and telephone number of the agency responsible for the protection and advocacy of developmentally disabled individuals established under Part C of the Developmental Disabilities Assistance and Bill of Rights Act; and

(vii) For nursing facility residents who are mentally ill, the mailing address and telephone number of the agency responsible for the protection and advocacy of mentally ill individuals established under the Protection and Advocacy for Mentally Ill Individuals Act.

(7) *Orientation for transfer or discharge.* A facility must provide sufficient preparation and orientation to residents to ensure safe and orderly transfer or discharge from the facility.

(b) *Notice of bed-hold policy and readmission*—(1) *Notice before transfer.* Before a nursing facility transfers a resident to a hospital or allows a resident to go on therapeutic leave, the nursing facility must provide written information to the resident and a family member or legal representative that specifies—

(i) The duration of the bed-hold policy under the State plan, if any, during which the resident is permitted to return and resume residence in the nursing facility; and

(ii) The nursing facility's policies regarding bed-hold periods, which must be consistent with paragraph (b)(3) of this section, permitting a resident to return.

(2) *Bed-hold notice upon transfer.* At the time of transfer of a resident for hospitalization or therapeutic leave, a nursing facility must provide to the resident and a family member or legal representative written notice which specifies the duration of the bed-hold policy described in paragraph (b)(1) of this section.

(3) *Permitting resident to return to facility.* A nursing facility must establish and follow a written policy under which a resident, whose hospitalization or therapeutic leave exceeds the bed-hold period under the State plan, is readmitted to the facility immediately upon the first availability of a bed in a semi-private room if the resident—

(i) Requires the services provided by the facility; and

(ii) Is eligible for Medicaid nursing facility services.

(c) *Equal access to quality care.*

(1) A facility must establish and maintain identical policies and practices regarding transfer, discharge, and the provision of services under the State plan for all individuals regardless of source of payment;

(2) The facility may charge any amount for services furnished to nonMedicaid residents consistent with the notice requirement in § 483.10(b)(5)(i) and (b)(6) describing the charges; and

(3) The State is not required to offer additional services on behalf of a resident other than services provided in the State plan.

continues

Exhibit 9-1-1 continued

(d) *Admissions policy.*

(1) The facility must—

(i) Not require residents or potential residents to waive their rights to Medicare or Medicaid; and

(ii) Not require oral or written assurance that residents or potential residents are not eligible for, or will not apply for, Medicare or Medicaid benefits.

(2) The facility must not require a third party guarantee of payment to the facility as a condition of admission or expedited admission, or continued stay in the facility. However, the facility may require an individual who has legal access to a resident's income or resources available to pay for facility care to sign a contract, without incurring personal financial liability, to provide facility payment from the resident's income or resources.

(3) In the case of a person eligible for Medicaid, a nursing facility must not charge, solicit, accept, or receive, in addition to any amount otherwise required to be paid under the State plan, any gift, money, donation, or other consideration as a precondition of admission, expedited admission or continued stay in the facility. However,—

(i) A nursing facility may charge a resident who is eligible for Medicaid for items and services the resident has requested and received, and that are not specified in the State plan as included in the term "nursing facility services" so long as the facility gives proper notice of the availability and cost of these services to residents and does not condition the resident's admission or continued stay on the request for and receipt of such additional services; and

(ii) A nursing facility may solicit, accept, or receive a charitable, religious, or philanthropic contribution from an organization or from a person unrelated to a Medicaid eligible resident or potential resident, but only to the extent that the contribution is not a condition of admission, expedited admission, or continued stay in the facility for a Medicaid eligible resident.

(4) States or political subdivisions may apply stricter admissions standards under State or local laws than are specified in this section, to prohibit discrimination against individuals entitled to Medicaid.

[56 FR 48869, Sept. 26, 1991, as amended at 57 FR 43924, Sept. 23,1992]

§ 483.13 Resident behavior and facility practices.

(a) *Restraints.* The resident has the right to be free from any physical or chemical restraints imposed for purposes of discipline or convenience, and not required to treat the resident's medical symptoms.

(b) *Abuse.* The resident has the right to be free from verbal, sexual, physical, and mental abuse, corporal punishment, and involuntary seclusion.

(c) *Staff treatment of residents.* The facility must develop and implement written policies and procedures that prohibit mistreatment, neglect, and abuse of residents and misappropriation of resident property.

(1) The facility must—

(i) Not use verbal, mental, sexual, or physical abuse, corporal punishment, or involuntary seclusion;

(ii) Not employ individuals who have been—

(A) Found guilty of abusing, neglecting, or mistreating residents by a court of law; or

(B) Have had a finding entered into the State nurse aide registry concerning abuse, neglect, mistreatment of residents or misappropriation of their property; and

continues

Exhibit 9-1-1 continued

(iii) Report any knowledge it has of actions by a court of law against an employee, which would indicate unfitness for service as a nurse aide or other facility staff to the State nurse aide registry or licensing authorities.

(2) The facility must ensure that all alleged violations involving mistreatment, neglect, or abuse, including injuries of unknown source, and misappropriation of resident property are reported immediately to the administrator of the facility and to other officials in accordance with State law through established procedures (including to the State survey and certification agency).

(3) The facility must have evidence that all alleged violations are thoroughly investigated, and must prevent further potential abuse while the investigation is in progress.

(4) The results of all investigations must be reported to the administrator or his designated representative and to other officials in accordance with State law (including to the State survey and certification agency) within 5 working days of the incident, and if the alleged violation is verified appropriate corrective action must be taken.

[56 FR 48870, Sept. 26, 1991, as amended at 57 FR 43924, Sept. 23,1992]

§ 483.15 Quality of life.

A facility must care for its residents in a manner and in an environment that promotes maintenance or enhancement of each resident's quality of life.

(a) *Dignity.* The facility must promote care for residents in a manner and in an environment that maintains or enhances each resident's dignity and respect in full recognition of his or her individuality.

(b) *Self-determination and participation.* The resident has the right to—

(1) Choose activities, schedules, and health care consistent with his or her interests, assessments, and plans of care;

(2) Interact with members of the community both inside and outside the facility; and

(3) Make choices about aspects of his or her life in the facility that are significant to the resident.

(c) *Participation in resident and family groups.*

(1) A resident has the right to organize and participate in resident groups in the facility;

(2) A resident's family has the right to meet in the facility with the families of other residents in the facility;

(3) The facility must provide a resident or family group, if one exists, with private space;

(4) Staff or visitors may attend meetings at the group's invitation;

(5) The facility must provide a designated staff person responsible for providing assistance and responding to written requests that result from group meetings;

(6) When a resident or family group exists, the facility must listen to the views and act upon the grievances and recommendations of residents and families concerning proposed policy and operational decisions affecting resident care and life in the facility.

(d) *Participation in other activities.* A resident has the right to participate in social, religious, and community activities that do not interfere with the rights of other residents in the facility.

(e) *Accommodation of needs.* A resident has the right to—

continues

Exhibit 9-1-2 continued

(1) Reside and receive services in the facility with reasonable accommodation of individual needs and preferences, except when the health or safety of the individual or other residents would be endangered; and

(2) Receive notice before the resident's room or roommate in the facility is changed.

(f) *Activities.*

(1) The facility must provide for an ongoing program of activities designed to meet, in accordance with the comprehensive assessment, the interests and the physical, mental, and psychosocial well-being of each resident.

(2) The activities program must be directed by a qualified professional who—

(i) Is a qualified therapeutic recreation specialist or an activities professional who—

(A) Is licensed or registered, if applicable, by the State in which practicing; and

(B) Is eligible for certification as a therapeutic recreation specialist or as an activities professional by a recognized accrediting body on or after October 1, 1990; or

(ii) Has 2 years of experience in a social or recreational program within the last 5 years, 1 of which was full-time in a patient activities program in a health care setting; or

(iii) Is a qualified occupational therapist or occupational therapy assistant; or

(iv) Has completed a training course approved by the State.

(g) *Social Services.* (1)—The facility must provide medically-related social services to attain or maintain the highest practicable physical, mental, and psychosocial well-being of each resident.

(2) A facility with more than 120 beds must employ a qualified social worker on a full-time basis.

(3) *Qualifications of social worker.* A qualified social worker is an individual with—

(i) A bachelor's degree in social work or a bachelor's degree in a human services field including but not limited to sociology, special education, rehabilitation counseling, and psychology; and

(ii) One year of supervised social work experience in a health care setting working directly with individuals.

(h) *Environment.*

The facility must provide—

(1) A safe, clean, comfortable, and homelike environment, allowing the resident to use his or her personal belongings to the extent possible;

(2) Housekeeping and maintenance services necessary to maintain a sanitary, orderly, and comfortable interior;

(3) Clean bed and bath linens that are in good condition;

(4) Private closet space in each resident room, as specified in § 483.70(d)(2)(iv) of this part;

(5) Adequate and comfortable lighting levels in all areas;

(6) Comfortable and safe temperature levels. Facilities initially certified after October 1, 1990, must maintain a temperature range of 71–81°F; and

(7) For the maintenance of comfortable sound levels.

[56 FR 48871, Sept. 26, 1991, as amended at 57 FR 43924. Sept. 23, 1992]

The Unwanted Resident

Seth B. Goldsmith

Mr. and Mrs. Jack Ross investigated nursing homes for their elderly and impoverished aunt, Ms. Janet Horner, who was living with them. On their visit to California's College Valley Home, they met with its administrator, Mr. Albert Press, who explained to them that even though Ms. Horner would be on Medi-Cal, prior to and as a condition of admission Mr. Ross (who was known as a wealthy man in the community) would have to make a donation of $10,000.00 to the home. Mr. Ross made the donation, and Ms. Horner was admitted. A few weeks after her admission, Mr. Ross called the home to tell Mr. Press that he was quite dissatisfied with the care at the home, particularly the quality of nursing care, which he found disrespectful and unresponsive to Ms. Horner's needs. Mr. Press then wrote Mr. Ross the following letter.

College Valley Home
Prentice Hill
Southern, California

November 1, 19____

Dear Mr. Ross:

I am sorry to hear that you are unhappy with the care that we are providing to your aunt, who actually seems perfectly happy, particularly with our food. However, in light of your dissatisfaction we have decided to discharge her on November 10, 19____. Please make the appropriate arrangements to pick her up on that date.

Finally, because of your negative attitude toward the home, I hereby bar you from visiting Ms. Horner at any time prior to her discharge.

Sincerely,

Albert Press, Administrator

* * *

Discussion Question

1. What OBRA compliance issues are raised by this case?

Chapter 10

Total Quality Management

Marianne Raimondo

Quality has become one of the most prevalent business topics of the decade. Quality of products, quality of service, quality in management. The health care industry has not been immune to this quality revolution. Increasing attention is being paid to the problem of appraising and improving the quality of health care and health services. The complexities of defining quality, finding valid measurements of quality, and ensuring quality in health care organizations continue to be debated by providers, payers, regulators, policy makers, and researchers in the industry, not to mention patients.

In the search of how to best ensure quality in health care organizations, the latest entry is total quality management (TQM). Since the late 1980s, hospitals, health centers, managed care organizations, and physician clinics have begun to implement TQM. Very recently, long-term care organizations have also begun to recognize that TQM holds potential for them as well. TQM has grown naturally out of the steady progression in quality assurance from implicit peer review to medical audits to systematic quality assurance. It is the next step in the evolution of quality assurance and provides solutions to many of the weaknesses that characterize traditional quality assurance methods. Many contend that TQM will result in major advances in the quality and effectiveness of health care.[1]

TQM represents a much broader approach to quality than traditional quality assurance, which can be viewed mainly as a method of evaluation. Quality assurance is a function, lodged in the quality assurance or nursing department, and its basic purpose is to monitor the quality of products or services produced and delivered by an organization in order to identify poor quality outcomes and the persons responsible for the problems or errors. It has been referred to as a "search for bad apples."[2]

TQM is a much more encompassing management approach to organization-wide quality improvement. Also referred to as continuous quality improvement, TQM is a management philosophy and practice that establishes quality as an organization's highest priority—as a fundamental determinant of an organization's viability and growth. It is based on the premise that a focus on quality will ultimately manage costs in an organization and offer improved value. As an organization attempts to provide quality products and services, it will focus on "doing the right things right the first time," thereby reducing duplicative effort, rework, and waste and consequently improving efficiency and productivity and reducing costs. An organization that differentiates itself on the basis of quality will enhance its reputation, which will lead to increased market share and organizational growth.

TQM has been formally defined as an approach to management that focuses on giving top value to customers by building excellence into every aspect of the organization and by creating an environment that encourages everyone to contribute to the organization. It also encourages the development of skills that enable people to scientifically study and constantly improve every process by which work is accomplished.[3]

Simply put, TQM puts quality as the top priority in an organization—quality that is defined by the customers, that is achieved, not by inspection, but by the improvement of work processes, and that requires the total cooperation of everyone in the organization.

Not to be viewed as a short-term program or project, TQM is a long-range strategy or process intended to mold organizational culture so that it is driven by a relentless search for quality, and to implement management practices and systems that ensure the delivery of quality products and services. TQM is often referred to as a way of running a business, a structured, systematic process for creating organizationwide planning and for implementing continuous improvements in quality.

THE ESSENTIALS OF TOTAL QUALITY MANAGEMENT

Customer Focus

At the core of the total quality management principle is a focus on the customer. According to TQM, quality begins with delighting customers. In fact, TQM defines quality as meeting or exceeding the needs and expectations of customers. Customers can be internal or external to an organization. External customers of a nursing facility comprise those who receive and use the products and services of the facility, including residents, families, physicians, payers, hospitals, and the community. Regulatory agencies such as HCFA and the state department of health and accreditation bodies such as the Joint Commission on Accreditation of Healthcare Organizations (Joint Commission) are also customers. Individuals within organizations, however, receive from other individuals products and services that are necessary for performing their job. That is, within an organization there exists a chain or network of internal customer–supplier relationships. Employees are customers when they receive a product or service from fellow employees and are suppliers when they provide a product or service to someone else who relies on that product or service.

Examples of internal customer–supplier relationships in long-term care facilities include the interaction between housekeeping and nursing, dietary and nursing, pharmacy and nursing, and admissions and billing. The expectations, requirements, and needs of the final or ultimate external customer, the resident or resident's family, can only be met when the requirements and needs of all internal customers are met.

To gain knowledge of customer needs, requirements, expectations, and satisfaction, TQM long-term care facilities use proactive methods such as focus groups, surveys, and interviews, recognizing that annual or quarterly resident satisfaction surveys are often biased and insufficient to gain insights about customers.

These insights are then translated into the provision of quality services through the improvement of the systems and processes by which work is accomplished. Unlike traditional quality assurance, which is essentially an evaluation or monitoring process to detect errors, adverse outcomes, or problems, TQM is directed toward building quality into work processes and systems. Monitoring outcomes such as patient falls, medication errors, complications, and infections may identify isolated problems but often fails to identify the causes of those problems. Furthermore, quality problems are most often due, not to human errors, but to system or process failures. Quality by inspection is costly and is provided too late—the quality problem has already occurred, resulting in waste, rework, duplicative efforts, and perhaps dissatisfied customers.

Contrary to this approach of monitoring final outcomes, TQM is based on the premise that quality is improved by understanding how processes work. Sorting through failures does little to guarantee that a process will do the right things, the right way, the first time, and every time. Systems that focus on identifying bad outputs and that fail to associate output failures with variations in the process do not improve quality as effectively as systems that prevent quality failures before they happen. In TQM, quality is built in during the process, not inspected at the end. Examples of work processes in a long-term care organization include admissions, administering medications, feeding patients, billing, and purchasing.

Quality Improvement Tools

Process improvement is accomplished though systematic problem solving and decision making based on data and factual information rather than anecdotes, innuendo, or guesswork. According to W. Edward Deming (whose theories contributed most to TQM as we know it today), the first step in quality control is to judge and act on the basis of fact supported by quality improvement tools, including flow charts, histograms, Pareto charts, check sheets, control charts, run charts, and scatter diagrams. These tools, briefly described below, facilitate the problem-solving process, enabling data to be collected and analyzed so that process operations can be understood and the root causes of problems can be identified and eliminated. The quality improvement tools described are also useful in identifying and measuring variations in systems and processes. Uncontrolled variations in processes prevent managers and staff working in the processes from ensuring desirable outcomes. Once sources of variation in a process are identified, they can be removed, increasing the consistency and predictability of output.

Flow Chart. A flow chart (Figure 10-1) is a pictorial representation showing all of the steps of a process. Flow charts provide excellent documentation of a process or project and can be useful for examining how various steps in a process are related to each other.

Pareto Chart. A Pareto chart (Figure 10-2) is a special kind of vertical bar graph that helps in determining which problems to solve in what order. It is based on the Pareto principle, which suggests that most effects come from relatively few causes.

Histogram. A histogram (Figure 10-3) displays the distribution of measurement data. It reveals the amount of variation that any process has within it.

Cause and Effect (Fishbone) Diagram. A cause and effect diagram (Figure 10-4) is a special type of chart that is used to organize all the causes of a problem. It helps to identify the root causes of a problem and how the causes relate to each other.

Control Chart. A control chart (Figure 10-5) shows how much variability in a process is due to random variation and how much is due to unique events or individual actions in order to determine whether a process is in statistical control.

Run Chart. A run chart (Figure 10-6) is used to monitor a process to see whether or not the long-range average is changing.

Employee Involvement

Statistical thinking is certainly a key component of a total system. TQM is based on the principle that the quality of services cannot be realized unless processes are understood and controlled. Another fundamental principle is that quality cannot be improved without involving employees in the improvement process.

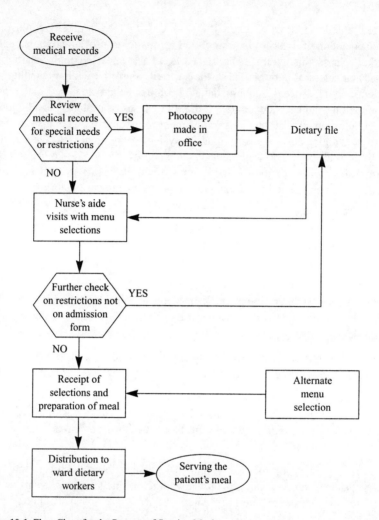

Figure 10-1 Flow Chart for the Process of Serving Meals

The underlying idea is that most employees in an organization want to do a good job and do seek to participate in and contribute to efforts to improve quality in their organization. Deming proposes that management should accept that employees want to do their best and are not willfully lazy or incompetent. It then becomes management's responsibility to provide employees with the necessary training and education as well as clear descriptions of expectations, systems that work, and assistance removing whatever obstacles prevent them from doing a good job.

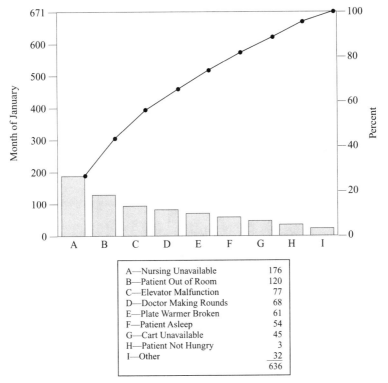

Figure 10-2 Pareto Chart of Reasons for Patient Receiving Cold Food. *Source:* Reprinted from *Total Quality Management Concepts and Methods,* p. 30, with permission of Applied Management Systems, Inc., © 1992.

It is management's job not simply to delegate responsibility of fixing problems to employees but to help employees do their jobs better and to involve them in decisions that affect their work. Believing that employees want to contribute to organizational improvements, TQM embraces an approach to management that empowers employees by involving them in problem solving and decision making and providing opportunities for them to contribute to the achievement of quality goals. Specifically, TQM requires teamwork in an organization, since employees offer different experiences, talents, skills, and knowledge that must be tapped for maximum gain. If an organization is to be truly excellent in every function, activity, work process, and provided service, everyone in the organization must work together to improve processes.

Teamwork means two things: first, a spirit of loyalty and collegiality throughout the organization, and second, extensive use of team and participative processes in the conduct of business. Teamwork of both kinds results from a common under-

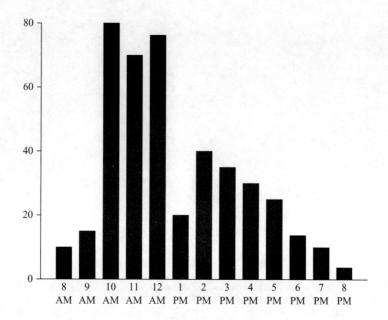

Figure 10-3 Distribution by Time of Discharge

standing of the organization's vision and values, a dedication to pleasing customers, an understanding of the organization's systems and processes, and a shared commitment to the ongoing improvement of those systems and processes. All employees in a quality organization understand where their work fits into the larger systems and processes and know how their work relates to the final products or ultimate users or customers. Optimizing individual or departmental quality does not necessarily result in organizational excellence. TQM requires emphasizing cooperation and collaboration across functions and departments that are working in concert for organizational goals.

Quality improvement teams represent one way employees are involved in quality improvement efforts. Quality improvement teams are composed of employees from all organizational levels who are responsible for performing the work in a particular process. Teams follow a systematic problem-solving approach, using the quality improvement tools previously described.

Finally, from the perspective of TQM, quality is the result of a never-ending cycle of continuous improvement. Unlike quality assurance, which establishes standards as the tool for quality, TQM treats standards as minimum requirements. Quality leaders are dissatisfied with the status quo; their goal is not getting by but getting better.

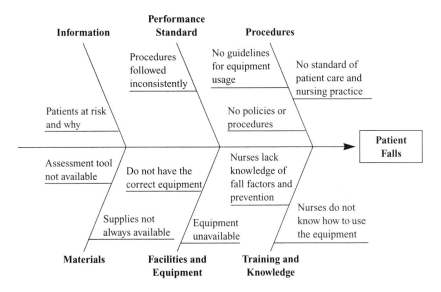

Figure 10-4 Cause and Effect Diagram for Patient Falls. *Source:* Reprinted from *Journal for Healthcare Quality,* Volume 14, Issue 5, with permission of the National Association for Healthcare Quality, 5700 Old Orchard Road, First Floor, Skokie, IL 60077-1057. Copyright © 1992. National Association for Healthcare Quality.

HISTORY

The concepts and principles of TQM are mainly credited to W. Edward Deming, an American statistician who developed, taught, and wrote about management practices and statistical techniques required to design, produce, deliver, and market quality products and services. Deming's ideas and methods were employed by American manufacturers during the 1940s for wartime production, but after the war his teachings on quality were ignored as American companies focused on quantity, production, and short-term profits. Deming's teachings, however, were heeded by the Japanese, who became familiar with his work while he was in Japan assisting the U.S. Secretary of War conduct a population census after World War II. Deming spent over 30 years in Japan, lecturing, consulting, and writing about his statistical techniques and his method of management. Many attribute the rebirth of Japanese industry and Japan's rise as a worldwide economic force to Deming. Joseph M. Juran, an engineer who followed Deming to Japan, is also credited with some of TQM's concepts. He is noted for his ideas on planning for quality.

Total quality management was introduced to the health care industry in the middle to late 1980s. The impetus came from several fronts. The Hospital Corpo-

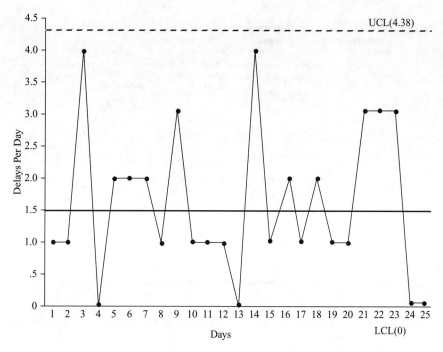

Figure 10-5 Control Chart for Operating Room Delays

ration of America (HCA), a for-profit company that owned and managed over 390 hospitals throughout the United States and abroad, made a corporate-level decision to implement an adapted version of the Deming method of TQM entitled Hospitalwide Quality Improvement Process (HQIP). By 1990, HCA had 75 of their hospitals voluntarily involved in this program.

In 1987, Dr. Donald Berwick, Vice President for Quality of Care Measurement at the Harvard Community Health Plan, initiated with Dr. Blandan Godfrey, then an executive with AT&T Bell Laboratories, the National Demonstration Project (NDP) on Industrial Quality Control in Health Care Quality. Twenty-one health care organizations, including Beth Israel in Boston; the University of Michigan Medical Center, Ann Arbor; Ferry Hospital in Atlanta; and Strong Memorial in Rochester, New York, were trained by professionals from 21 manufacturers, including Xerox, AT&T, and Ford Motor Company, to apply TQM methods to health care processes. The project, funded by the Hartford Foundation, was intended to assess whether quality management theory and techniques could be successfully applied to health care. Given the success of the initial project, the NDP was refunded and expanded. It included more health care organizations, provided training seminars and conferences on TQM,

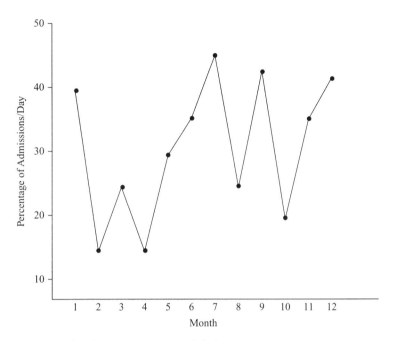

Figure 10-6 Run Chart for Emergency Room Admissions

and sponsored networking opportunities for organizations involved in TQM to share information and experiences.

Hospitals throughout the country have since announced their commitment to TQM implementation. The initial group included the Alliant Health System, Louisville, Kentucky; the University of Michigan Medical Center, Ann Arbor; Henry Ford Health System, Detroit; and Rush Presbyterian St. Luke's, Chicago. In the fall of 1991, the NDP became the Institute for Health Care Improvement (IHI). Headed by Dr. Berwick, the institute was formed to offer educational programs on TQM for hospitals and other health care entities.

Long-term care facilities are beginning to adopt TQM as well. Examples include the Sherrill House, Boston; the Evanswood Center for Older Adults, Kingston, Massachusetts; Villa Clement Manor, Greenfield, Wisconsin; and the Jewish Home for the Aged of Worcester County, Worcester, Massachusetts.

The Joint Commission has also begun to embrace TQM. Changes in the *1992 Accreditation Manual for Hospitals* reflect the beginning of a transition from quality assurance to quality improvement. The chapter called "Quality Assurance" has been changed to "Quality Assessment and Improvement," and new standards are intended to promote (1) more interdepartmental and interdisciplinary quality improvement activities, (2) a focus on processes and systems and not just individual performance, (3) increased efforts to improve the performance of the entire organization rather than focusing only on outliers, and (4) increased communication and collaboration. The manual also contains new leadership standards that require the leadership of hospitals to set priorities for organizationwide quality improvement activities, provide training and education in quality improvement for staff, foster communication and collaboration within the organization, and become personally involved in quality improvement. Some speculate the Joint Commission will eventually change its standards for nursing facilities to reflect TQM.

IMPLEMENTATION

The implementation of a total quality process begins with management's intense commitment to quality and its belief that TQM is the means to achieve not only improved quality but increased market share, improved customer satisfaction, improved productivity, and reduced costs. Although there is no roadmap or instruction manual for becoming a total quality organization, there are some key components of the TQM implementation process, which are described below.

Assessing Readiness

The total quality process can only be initiated after an organization's senior management group is educated in TQM concepts and methods. This can be accomplished through attending conferences, seminars, and courses and making site visits to long-term care and other organizations already using TQM. This awareness-building effort is critical to getting off to the right start. Once senior managers are knowledgeable about TQM and what the approach will involve, they can begin to explore its applicability to their organization.

Before implementing a total quality process, administrators in a long-term care facility should assess whether TQM is compatible with the values, goals, and management practices in their organization. The long-term success of TQM will require intense commitment and dedication of management to the values of quality, customer focus, teamwork, employee involvement, and continuous improvement. Managers should answer several key questions:

• Why implement TQM in the organization?
• What are the potential benefits?
• What obstacles might be encountered in the implementation process?

Administrators should only decide to implement TQM if it makes sense for them based on their leadership style and the organization's goals. Further, the CEO must remain personally involved in the implementation process to ensure a long-term strategic commitment to change and must be willing from the start to maintain that involvement and leadership.

Managers should also articulate a vision of their organization. This vision answers these questions:

- What kind of organization do we want to be?
- How will we look as a total quality organization?

For example, the Evanswood Center for Older Adults developed the following vision statement as part of its ongoing efforts to create a quality culture.

The Evanswood Vision

We pledge uncompromising dedication to excellence in helping older adults grow in spirit, live with a sense of fulfillment, experience dignity, and meet the challenges of their changing lives. We aspire to be consistent in our quality of care, distinctive in our approach, outstanding in performance, and to provide leadership in the field of service to older adults. We welcome others who will join us in pursuit of our vision.

Laying the Foundation

The implementation process begins with senior managers laying the foundation for the total quality process. During this initial phase of implementation, administrators revisit their organizational mission to assess its compatibility with total quality values. The mission statement should answer these questions: Why do we exist as an organization? What is our purpose? What business are we in? The statement should clearly articulate the key customers of the organization, the services provided, and the expected outcomes of such services.

In addition to establishing the organizational mission and vision, an organization implementing TQM should also identify and articulate the values and norms that guide and hold meaning for the employees. The values emphasized by TQM include quality, the primacy of the customers (especially the residents), internal teamwork, employee involvement, and continuous improvement. Finally, the organization may also establish a broad definition of how it defines quality.

Simply drafting mission, vision, quality, and value statements and posting them up throughout the organization is not sufficient to create a total quality organization. They must be communicated constantly to establish and maintain quality-mindedness among all employees.

This initial phase of the quality improvement process is often initiated at a one- to two-day retreat for the organization's senior managers and steering council. The objectives of this session are to explore the benefits of TQM for the organization, to begin to identify potential barriers and obstacles to the process, and to begin to lay out the strategic plans and goals.

Quality Planning

Once the foundation is laid for creating a total quality organization, a plan is developed that outlines the strategy for the implementation process and the expected outcomes of the process. The quality plan is not a static document but is revised throughout the implementation process.

The quality plan lays out the steps of the implementation process, including training managers and employees, forming quality improvement teams, recognizing and rewarding teams for quality improvement, building employee awareness of quality concepts and organizational values and goals, establishing strategies to empower employees, and introducing mechanisms to communicate the quality initiatives continuously. The plan should also include outcome objectives that define how the total quality process should improve quality. These objectives are usually measured in terms of patient satisfaction, employee satisfaction, clinical outcomes, productivity and efficiency, and market share. TQM implementation therefore requires ongoing evaluation to assess whether the process is progressing as planned and objectives are being met. The information gained as a result of this assessment guides the ongoing implementation of TQM.

Gaining Knowledge of Customers

The customer is clearly the focus of the total quality process; the quality improvement process is driven by customer needs, expectations, and requirements. This means that a TQM organization must remain close to its customers, whether they be residents, residents' families, payers, or community agencies. Knowledge of customers can be gained through surveys, focus groups, or interviews. Long-term care organizations implementing TQM need to identify their key customers and then organize efforts to determine customer needs, expectations, and requirements. Task forces are often convened to help in these efforts.

Senior managers should also encourage middle managers to undertake activities to understand internal customers better. Satisfying internal customers is the way to delight external customers. Departments that rely on each other for supplies, products, information, and other services should initiate strategies to learn more about each other's work processes, needs, and requirements. When customer–supplier relationships are strengthened, system improvements can be pursued to increase the quality of the organization's services and products.

Customer satisfaction (of internal and external customers) must be measured on an ongoing basis. Meetings, focus groups, and interviews with residents, employees, hospitals, physicians, and other customers are more effective ways to learn of customer satisfaction than annual, often abbreviated, close-ended surveys.

Making Process Improvements

Knowledge about customers is translated into quality products and services through systems design and process improvement. The emphasis in TQM is prevention, not inspection.

Process improvements are pursued not only by managers of those processes but also through the involvement of employees who perform the work. Quality improvement teams are composed of five to ten employees from all levels in an organization (e.g., nurses, housekeepers, clerks, supervisors, social workers, technicians, etc.) who have knowledge of how work processes operate. Teams are led by team leaders, who are individuals who have ownership of and responsibility for the processes being improved. Team leaders are often supervisors or managers, but they need not be. They are responsible for guiding and directing team efforts, and they are members of the teams and participate fully in the work of the teams. Teams are also guided by facilitators. Unlike team leaders, facilitators are not members of teams; they are outside consultants who remain neutral and objective in providing technical assistance to teams, helping them stay on track and reach consensus.

Quality improvement teams utilize a systematic approach to problem solving to enable them to understand how processes operate, identify and quantify problems in current processes, identify the root causes of the problems, and implement improvements in the performance of the processes.

Much of a quality improvement team's activities involve data collection and analysis supported by the quality improvement tools described previously. These tools enable teams to base decisions on data rather than anecdote, innuendo, or guesswork. The motto adopted by many organizations engaged in quality improvement is: In God We Trust; All Others Bring Your Data.

Use of all quality improvement tools and techniques is not required for every improvement process. Combined they represent a toolbox of available instruments that can be utilized as needed.

Team leaders and facilitators receive extensive training to help them develop the interpersonal and analytical skills required for effective teamwork. Training courses for team leaders and facilitators cover problem solving, how to conduct effective meetings, the use of quality improvement tools, data collection and analysis, team building, and group dynamics.

Quality improvement is a long-term process; teams often meet routinely (usually weekly) for six months or more to improve processes or design new systems. In addition to actual team meetings, team members often work in data gathering, flow charting, and other activities between meetings.

In addition to the actual improvement of work processes, there are many positive outcomes from teamwork in organizations. Teamwork builds respect and understanding among team members from different departments, which leads to greater cooperation and collaboration. As team members gain greater understanding of each other's work and their needs as internal customers and suppliers, they are more likely to work together to improve quality.

Involving employees in resolving problems and improving the processes that affect their everyday work also fosters increased pride of workmanship and an increased sense of ownership. Teamwork also provides an opportunity for employees to learn new tools, develop new skills, and gain new knowledge that will enable them to continue pursuing improvements in their work.

Communication

Communication is critical to the quality improvement process. What should be communicated? First, the basics: The organization's mission, vision, plans, and objectives should be communicated, not in a brochure that is provided at employee orientation or formally recited at an annual staff get-together, but constantly during staff meetings and management meetings and in daily conversations. Communication of the big picture builds teamwork in an organization; employees feel that their work is not menial or trivial but makes an important contribution to the organization.

Second, the values of the organization: Quality, customer focus, continuous improvement, and teamwork must be communicated. This begins during the hiring process, is emphasized in employee orientation, and is continuously re-emphasized daily by all managers.

Third, achievements and progress of the quality improvement process must be communicated, including an announcement of the teams formed, the progress of the teams' work, and team successes. It is crucial that feedback from customer surveys, interviews, or focus groups be communicated, whether it be positive or suggest opportunities for improvement.

Celebrating quality initiatives, besides communicating progress and success, recognizes and rewards employee efforts. Many TQM organizations hold events for teams such as luncheons with the board, recognition dinners, or "team days," which are special days set aside to allow quality improvement teams to present their work at a poster session open to all employees or through formal presentations open to the entire organization. Existing communication mechanisms such as newsletters, bulletin boards, and staff meetings should also be utilized to incorporate quality improvement initiatives and successes.

Quality Deployment

Quality improvement teams, being mostly cross-functional in nature, provide a mechanism to horizontally integrate quality values and initiatives in an organization. However, to infiltrate an entire organization with quality thinking and action also requires vertical alignment. That is, TQM thinking, methods, and practices must be filtered from the top to all departments in a long-term care facility (see Figure 10-7).

Eventually, all managers (i.e., department heads and supervisors) must be educated in TQM concepts and methods and encouraged to pursue quality improvement in their functional areas. This requires that all managers clearly articulate their mission and vision for their departments, establish means to better meet customer requirements and improve customer satisfaction, develop the problem-solving skills of their employees, and build teamwork not only intradepartmentally but interdepartmentally. Most important, it requires that all managers promote the philosophy of continuous quality improvement and be role models for quality improvement practices by constantly seeking ways to get close to customers, pursuing improvement rather than being content with the status quo, being impatient with guesswork, and fostering teamwork.

Systems Integration

If TQM is meant to be a way of life in an organization, then it must mean more than scattered customer surveys or a few isolated teams in the entire organization. It must be integrated into existing organizational rituals, events, activities, and systems, such as planning, budgeting, marketing, information systems, quality assurance, and human resource systems. Systems integration is necessary to ensure constancy of purpose in an organization, consistency in values, and compatibility of organizational objectives. For example, if an organization's priority truly is quality, then performance appraisal systems may need to be revised to recognize an employee's contributions to quality. If an organization truly values

The total quality management model has three major focuses:

1. Vertical alignment through leadership and planning
2. Horizontal integration through teams and customer-driven improvement of processes
3. Daily control through systems, statistical methods, and employee involvement

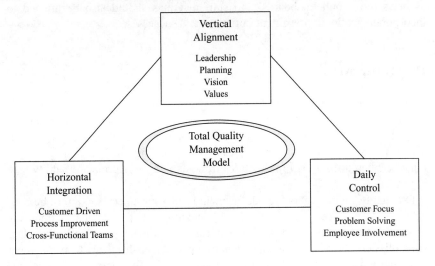

Figure 10-7 Organizationwide Integration of Quality Improvement

teamwork, then performance appraisals should recognize and reward team efforts rather than individual accomplishments, which may have been realized at the expense of collaborative relationships. Likewise, if managers are serious about quality, then management objectives, discussions, strategies, and plans should focus on ways to improve quality rather than contain cost or increase productivity. Managers committed to the concepts of TQM recognize that if processes are improved, duplicative effort, waste, and rework are reduced, thereby decreasing operating costs. Again, if an organization improves the quality of its products and services, it will improve its reputation for quality, thereby increasing market share.

Assessment and Evaluation

The implementation of TQM requires evaluation or assessment to ensure that expected outcomes are attained and that the process that guides those outcomes is continuously improved. A successful total quality process is measured in terms of improved patient satisfaction, improved employee satisfaction, reduced costs, improved productivity, increased market share, and improved performance.

An infrastructure for total quality management must be developed. It should include a leadership body or group, an implementation coordinator, and teams of employees to pursue quality improvements. The leadership body, typically referred to as the quality steering council or committee, energizes the efforts by developing the TQM implementation plan, establishing expectations and objectives for the total quality process, providing resources for training and education, supporting and assisting quality improvement teams, establishing priorities for process improvement, and integrating TQM with other management systems. The steering council is typically composed of senior managers or a combination of senior managers and middle managers. Some steering councils also include a board member. Steering council meetings are scheduled on a weekly or biweekly basis and are held in addition to routinely scheduled management meetings.

The TQM coordinator is responsible for facilitating teams; providing some of the training for the organization; providing assistance and guidance to teams; maintaining a library of information resources and training materials; communicating quality efforts organizationwide; organizing events to recognize and celebrate QI efforts; arranging for seminars, workshops, courses, and other educational opportunities; and working with managers in Human Resources, Finance, Information Systems, and QA to integrate such management systems with TQM. Often the TQM coordinator facilitates the steering council and has direct responsibility for developing the TQM implementation plan. The background of the TQM coordinator can vary. In long-term care organizations, the coordinator could be an administrator, department director, nurse manager, quality assurance professional, staff development coordinator, or human resources manager. The TQM coordinator should report directly to the administrator.

THE ROLE OF MANAGEMENT IN TQM

For some managers, TQM may represent a transformation of their management practices. Rather than a directive, controlling style of management, TQM requires a more participative approach, including open communication with employees and the involvement of employees in decision making. It requires that managers be leaders, exemplars, and teachers of quality. To translate these objectives into action managers must

- be advocates for quality
- see themselves as suppliers to a variety of customers

- seek ways to determine customers' needs, expectations, and requirements and initiate improvements to meet those needs
- seek to improve systems instead of seeking someone to blame
- listen to employees at every level to learn of employees' concerns, problems, or ideas
- help remove obstacles preventing employees from providing quality services and products
- understand how to manage processes and that unless variation is removed from processes, optimal outcomes may be unrealistic for employees to achieve
- become impatient with guesswork and require that data be collected to ascertain the facts
- continuously communicate organizational plans, strategies, problems, goals, issues, concerns, and successes
- provide resources for education and training for employees to improve job skills, understand TQM concepts, and develop the skills necessary for pursuing quality improvement
- find out what stands in the way of teamwork in their organization
- find out what would make employees feel more a part of their organization
- continuously seek ways to integrate quality thinking into existing management systems, such as planning, marketing, quality assurance, and management information systems
- commit to providing jobs for employees instead of creating the fear of job loss
- promote ways to bring employees closer to their customers
- commit to continuous improvement instead of being content with the status quo
- support the work of quality improvement teams by becoming knowledgeable about their activities, providing assistance as needed, and working with them to implement improvements
- seek ways to find out what customers need or expect and initiate improvements to meet those needs or expectations

BARRIERS TO TQM IMPLEMENTATION

There are many barriers to implementing a total quality process. The first barrier is thinking that total quality is a program to be overlaid on traditional management practices rather than a way of life in an organization. TQM should not be equated with a guest relations program or quality circles. It is a comprehensive approach to managing an organization. Managers should not be seduced into thinking they are implementing TQM because they have launched quality improvement projects or teams. Quality improvement teams do achieve laudable results and are excellent vehicles for education, but in and of themselves they do not represent a transformation. TQM is not intended to be a haphazard, fragmented effort but rather an organizationwide, systematic effort. It requires planning, training, direct management involvement, intense commitment, and long-term vision. Managers who form quality improvement teams but fail to change their leadership style to involve employees in decision making, fail to remove obstacles facing employees, continue to focus first on budgets and the bottom line rather than quality, and continue to base performance appraisals solely on tasks performed or objectives met rather than on collaborative teamwork are not implementing TQM. Likewise, managers who, under the guise of improving quality, attempt to use TQM as a cost-cutting tool will probably not be able to rally the support and cooperation of employees, who will tend to view TQM as just another management trick to cut staff, cut budgets, and make them work harder.

Another barrier to implementing TQM in long-term care organizations, a barrier that may not be as significant in hospitals, is the relatively low educational level of employees. Although this problem does not preclude a successful quality improvement process, it needs to be recognized and addressed. Managers in long-term care organizations must be willing to invest in training and education for their staff. Trainers hired should also be sensitive to the fact that the learning process may be gradual and should be experienced in presenting material so that it is understandable and relevant to staff-level employees. Members of quality improvement teams who experience difficulty in data gathering and analysis will need to be assisted and coached by trainers, team leaders, facilitators, and their managers.

Viewing TQM as a quick fix, short-term project is also a way to sabotage quality improvement efforts. TQM is a strategy for long-term improvement; it requires patience. Although some improvements in process performance and employee morale will be experienced within the first year of implementation, increased customer satisfaction, cost reductions, and improved productivity will take longer.

A very real threat to TQM is pseudo-participation. Pseudo-participation occurs when managers form quality improvement teams, communicate to the teams that they are empowered to make changes and improvements, then ignore or reject the teams' recommendations or fail to help the teams implement their improvements. Telling teams they can meet to identify problems but then failing to involve them in the decision to implement improvements is a signal to employees that TQM means business as usual—decision making by management alone. Employees will soon view TQM as a facade and become discouraged and skeptical of management's motives.

Finally, the biggest mistake organizations make in trying to implement TQM is failing to provide education and training for managers and employees. Training and education should be viewed as an investment in human resources. For the total quality improvement process to be effective, employees need to be trained to focus on their customers, work as members of teams, and develop problem-solving skills.

CONCLUSION

Because TQM has only recently begun to be implemented in health care, there has been no formal evaluation of its effectiveness. Early reports of its application have provided some anecdotal evidence of cost reductions, improved customer satisfaction, improved process performance, and improved clinical outcomes, especially in the hospital area.

It is still too early to determine whether TQM is a fad or an approach to management that has significant potential for improving quality in health care. Yet the challenges administrators face in running long-term care facilities in an environment characterized by fragmented and shrinking reimbursement systems, older and sicker patients, higher costs, and intense regulation suggest that TQM is at least worth looking into.

NOTES

1. D.M. Berwick et al., *Curing Health Care: New Strategies for Quality Improvement* (San Francisco: Jossey-Bass, 1990).
2. D.M. Berwick, Sounding Board: Continuous Improvement as an Ideal in Health Care, *New England Journal of Medicine* 320 (1989):53–56.
3. B.L. Joiner, *Total Quality Leadership vs. MBO* (Madison, Wis.: Joiner Associates, 1985), 1–10.

The Salon

Lorrie A. Higgins

For 14 years the Century Nursing Home had an arrangement with Jenny Martin, a licensed beautician, whereby Ms. Martin would operate a salon at the nursing home. Over the years an informal pattern of communication existed whereby financial issues were discussed with the home's administrator and service issues were dealt with by the nursing department, usually the director or assistant director.

Recently, a number of incidents occurred that caused the administration and some members of the board to reconsider both the issue of the home delivering salon services as well as the relationship with Jenny Martin. The incidents included resident complaints that Jenny rushed them out of the salon, failed to keep appointments, and did not listen to resident's requests about style preferences.

Michelle Diamond, the home's administrator, also became rather concerned about the salon and its impact on the quality of life at the home. She decided to use the home's newly formed TQM initiative to deal with the problem.

* * *

Discussion Questions

1. What is the significance of the salon service to the residents of the nursing home?
2. How is the quality of life impacted for the residents by this service and the concerns raised?
3. Illustrate the customer expectations and confidence in light of the history of the situation and the concerns raised.
4. How have the customers been identified by the home and by the salon?
5. How can the service strategy between the home and salon be compared?

Communication at Hallie G.

Marvin A. Goldberg

The mission statement of the Hallie G. Geriatric Center, a 150-bed skilled facility, reads in part:

> The Hallie G. Geriatric Center is committed to providing quality services to needy older persons. These services may be institutional or noninstitutional and are offered to members of the community at large.

To accomplish this mission, Hallie G.:

> recognizes and supports the talent and dedication of our staff and encourages their continuous improvement.
>
> ... is committed to a continuous quality improvement philosophy that benefits both resident and staff.

For months, the nursing department, the largest department (105 staff members) has had recurring differences of opinion among the shifts. Each shift feels it is the responsibility of another shift for ongoing functions such as morning care, bathing, documentation, and record keeping. Shift change has been a tension point as some staff barely nod to each other in passing. Morale is low and there are some indications that more time is spent complaining than providing basic nursing care. In addition, some staff have language problems.

Aware of this pressing problem, the director of nursing and her supervisors met several times. The purpose of these meetings was to discover the cause or causes of the problem and to develop and implement a strategy that would enable staff members to better communicate with each other and to continue to provide quality services to the residents.

The plan was unveiled to the nursing staff at a series of meetings with the director of nursing and the supervisors. The plan was very specific and staff were requested to cooperate in order to continue to provide good service. It was also announced that the plan would be evaluated within 30 days and then every 90 days thereafter for one year to ensure compliance. At the one-month evaluation it was discovered that the problem was as serious as ever. In fact, three staff members had resigned, including a supervisor.

* * *

Discussion Questions

1. Was continuous quality improvement used appropriately in this case? What could be done to change the organizational climate? Who should be involved in such a change process and why should those people be involved? What improvement measures could be utilized?
2. After rereading the mission statement consider the following: How does the mission statement relate to the current situation?
3. How does management get "buy-in" when trying to solve a problem? What happens when staff members choose not to "buy-in" and continue their current behaviors?

Chapter 11

Financial Management of Long-Term Care Organizations

Seth B. Goldsmith and Solomon Goldner

A central premise of this book is that long-term care facilities are increasingly complex organizations functioning in an extremely demanding and often hostile regulatory environment. The complexity of organization results from the demands being placed on homes to provide a broad array of services to residents needing basic custodial care up to what could be classified as subacute hospital care. Regulatory demands range from those that have a broad application, such as the Americans with Disabilities Act, to those that are more targeted at nursing home reform, such as certain sections of the Omnibus Budget Reconciliation Act of 1987. Unfortunately the problem with many of these well-meaning legislative initiatives is that they cost the long-term care facility money that is simply not fully reimbursed. To deal with this situation requires a strong and informed management that can read and understand financial statements, deal with reimbursement issues, and work with the financial team on developing creative and effective mechanisms to collect all revenues due the institution, generate new sources of revenue, and control expenses without compromising the quality of care provided to the residents.

To meet these challenges, managers in long-term care institutions need a basic understanding of three major topics: (1) the financial organization of long-term care institutions and programs; (2) the elements of health finance, including the revenue cycle; and (3) the budgeting process.

THE FINANCIAL ORGANIZATION OF LONG-TERM CARE INSTITUTIONS

Managers of long-term care organizations are most often in the situation of having major financial decisions made by a top level of owners, corporate officers or, in the case of nonprofit homes, a governing board. This top level of decision making is usually not involved in the day-to-day financial management of the organization but rather exerts its control by allocating funds through annual capital and operating budgets, approving new jobs, and establishing approval levels for spending, such as requiring owner, corporate, or board approval for any expenditure in excess of $2,000. To a large extent, the size of the home may dictate the expectations owners or trustees have of management as well as the resources management has available for financial management. For example, in a 50-bed home it is unlikely that a manager will be able to afford much more support than a bookkeeper, with the result that owners or trustees may themselves try to direct the fiscal management of the home or alternatively may expect that the manager is in fact primarily a finance person. Additionally, the nature of services provided in a home, as well as a state's Medicaid reimbursement system, may dictate either a higher or lower level of financial involvement by the licensed administrator than the owners or trustees expect.

Quite often when there is a board of directors at the top, it will delegate responsibility for the finance function to a subordinate committee. This committee may have limited direct authority or may be just a fact-finding group for the entire board. There is, of course, no simple formula for how all this should work. The key point is that in many organizations the board of directors or owners are ultimately responsible and do indeed exercise that responsibility. This responsibility includes a critical role in ensuring that the home's assets are properly utilized and that all major decisions are financially sound. Although the board and the owners are most often involved in the kind of financial policy making that establishes the parameters of decision making for management, they must also continually oversee the fiscal health of the organization. This is simply not a responsibility that can be delegated to management.

It should be noted that these overseers of the organization's financial health are under no obligation to select only "financial wizards" to serve on the finance committee or to be their guiding light on financial matters. In some instances, a board's finance committee is composed of lawyers or businesspeople who have no particular expertise in finance, much less long-term care finance, and have learned what they need to know by years of experience. For example, in one nursing home, the long-time board treasurer was a stockbroker who had no knowledge of the intricacies of long-term care finance. On one hand, such a situation may be helpful, in that the staff must make its case understandable to those who have only a general knowledge of finance. On the other hand, the board is almost entirely dependent on the staff for its information and is in a sense a captive of its own employees.

Within the long-term care organization or program, the focus of financial activities is the comptroller or vice-president for finance. The nomenclature is so unstandardized that the same position may have scores of different titles. Most comptrollers are trained in accounting. Sometimes they are certified public accountants, and occasionally they have special training in finance. The comptroller is the chief financial officer of the organization and plays a major part in developing and policing the systems that gather, analyze, and interpret financial and related operational data. In some organizations, the comptroller and his or her staff play a key role in all managerial decisions, since they most often have the clearest understanding of the financial implications of any decision.

The major problem with such an accounting and finance staff (and, some might say, their major value) is that they often lack experience in and a perspective on long-term care operations. For example, most of the training programs in accounting and finance focus on the for-profit sector of the economy. Working in long-term care, particularly for the government or nonprofit sector, requires an understanding of slightly different accounting systems, new nomenclature, and different objectives—some of which present problems to a person trained on Exxon financial statements. To compensate for these differences, many organizations send promising individuals to special training programs and encourage them to enroll in the various health-related professional societies. Such educational and professional involvement serves two major purposes: It acquaints these people with the nature of long-term care organizations and their concerns, and it assists them in utilizing their professional skills to maximum effectiveness in the organization. It is also essential that financial officers attend professional meetings, such as the annual meetings of the American Health Care Association or the American Association of Homes for the Aging.

The administrator, whether called president or executive director, is the person who is most accountable for the financial management of the organization. Usually, administrators are not formally trained in finance or accounting but have a general management education background, which typically includes some minimal coursework in accounting and finance. The result of this situation is that administrators utilize the input of their finance staff in making crucial institutional decisions that involve weighing the broad range of quantifiable costs against unquantifiable benefits. So, for example, one administrator pushed ahead on a money-losing day-care program because she felt it was important to the relationship between her nursing home and the community. From a purely financial perspective, it might have been a bad decision; from a political perspective, it was certainly a reasonable choice.

Others in long-term care organizations are also important to the financial management of the organization. Among these are business office staff, who are involved in the credit and collection systems of the organization; data processing staff, who are involved in the systems that set up and record transactions; purchasing staff, whose decisions affect the cash flow and hence the financial health of the organization; and the personnel department, which through its policies affects turnover, vacation substitutions, and a range of other activities that can be translated into dollars and cents. Also, of increasing importance are the medical staff, who should play a role in educating staff, owners, and board members on the implications of new technology for the institution and its residents.

Essentially then, any long-term care organization operates with a series of cash registers that, if properly utilized, take in or ensure the receipt of revenues and disburse money in an organized and objective-related way. For example, the nurse on the resident care floor of a nursing home must ensure that the proper form is filled out when physical therapy is ordered; otherwise, the business office will not bill the resident, Medicare, or Medicaid for the service. If a service is not billed, then the organization has expended resources, such as the nurses' and therapist's time, the machinery and supplies to perform the test, and all the over-head systems necessary to support the physical therapy, without even the opportunity to be reimbursed. Thus, everyone in an organization is part of the revenue-generating function.

ELEMENTS OF LONG-TERM CARE FINANCE

Taxes

Most long-term care organizations are incorporated as for-profit organizations and are taxed as any other organization is taxed. Approximately 25 percent of nursing homes are incorporated as nonprofit organizations and are typically exempt from a range of federal, state, and local taxes. These exemptions do not preclude nonprofit nursing homes from making a profit or force them to operate at the break-even point or at a loss; rather, it requires that any profit made by such organizations must not directly benefit any single person or group of stockholders. In general, the tax laws differentiate between related and unrelated income. Income from activities that are related to the operation and objectives of the organization, such as a profit-making cafeteria run for the convenience of the staff and residents, is tax-exempt. Clearly unrelated income would be taxable. For example, if a nonprofit organization owned a spaghetti factory, the profits from the spaghetti factory would have to be taxed before they could be transferred to the nonprofit organization. Farfetched example? Not really, since the Mueller Spaghetti Company was for many years owned by New York University's law school. Perhaps of greater importance is the increasing vigilance by the Internal Revenue Service regarding the activities of tax-exempt organizations and the increasing pressure by local taxing authorities to collect real estate taxes from nonprofit organizations.

Philanthropy

Occasionally, a wealthy benefactor wills a nursing home or university millions of dollars. While that type of philanthropy is becoming rare, philanthropy on a smaller scale has continued to play a role in financing institutions. However, as a percentage of total revenue, philanthropic giving has declined. Philanthropy is important to an organization for spiritual as well as financial reasons. Spiritually, it tells the organization that it has friends and supporters, and in today's often hostile climate of management and regulation, such statements of support are comforting. From a financial perspective, philanthropy provides funds. Many of the philanthropic gifts that long-term care organizations receive, however, are specially targeted funds, that is, given for a single purpose, such as funds for a building or a program endowment. When money is put into an endowment, the use of the principal is restricted and the interest is available for the purposes of the endowment. Typical problems regarding philanthropic gifts include the source of the money, the restrictions placed on the money, and the cost of getting the money. When money is given, it appears to be less often transferred to the recipient in an unrestricted fashion than it was in the past. The problem with conditions on the money is that operational costs are rarely endowed; thus, for example, money may be provided for a new wing at a nursing home but not for maintenance, heat, or cleaning, and it is the cost of these items that is sometimes too high for an organization to bear. Finally, it should be noted that it takes considerable time and money to raise funds for any organization. Long-term care organizations must compete for limited charitable dollars with a range of other health care programs, particularly hospitals, as well as a broad range of important social programs.

Revenues and Reimbursement

Revenues of long-term care organizations can be broken down into two categories: operating and nonoperating. The operating revenues are generated by the clients or residents who request the services that the organization is in business to offer. The nonoperating income is generated independently of the residents in the organization, although it is directly related to the organization's existence and mission. Operating income from residents may be financed by one of a variety of sources, including the government (through Medicare and Medicaid), private insurers, and the residents themselves. Each of these different payers operates with a different set of reimbursement rules for services, and this translates into different billing and often different collection services. To further complicate matters, each state has different rules affecting nursing home rates. For example, Massachusetts allows nursing homes to charge private-pay residents whatever the home wishes, whereas Minnesota sets the private rate in concert with the Medicaid rate. The income itself is generated by the resident who uses the nursing or professional services. In nursing homes, because of differing agreements with the various payers, residents who have similar limitations, diagnoses, and treatment regimens and are being treated by the same physicians in similar accommodations may in fact generate different revenues for the nursing home. This is analogous to the airline business: Despite the fact that all the passengers on a plane are flying between the same two cities, they are not all paying the same fare. Some are paying first class fare, others are paying full economy fare, others are paying excursion fares (and staying over Saturday night), others are traveling on half-fare coupons, and so forth.

Managing Medicaid and Medicare reimbursement is perhaps the core of financial management for most institutions. State variability in Medicaid methodology and reimbursement is significant. For example, several years ago I visited three comparable nonprofit homes in Dallas, Texas; Kansas City, Missouri; and Fairfield, Connecticut. The Dallas home was reimbursed under a flat rate system at $34.60 per day, the Missouri home received $51.60 per day, and the Connecticut home received $93.84 per day. Yet the Texas home was able to operate with the least restrictions regarding numbers of private-pay residents, whereas the Connecticut home had to respect a tough access law that required it to admit residents on a first-come basis. Finally, if there is an immutable law in Medicaid reimbursement, it is probably that nothing is certain. For example, in 1991 Connecticut relaxed its tough access law in order to allow homes to build their private-pay census and thus cross-subsidize the Medicaid recipients.

Medicare is a program that some homes have been reluctant to develop for a variety of reasons, including a fear of not making money on this program, which is one of the last of the cost-reimbursement programs. This fear may be exaggerated for several reasons. For example, Medicare "cost" includes overhead expenses from every department, including administrative salaries. Thus, every dollar of overhead that is legitimately shifted to a Medicare cost center removes a dollar of overhead from the flat-rate residents, who are usually private-pay residents and in some states Medicaid recipients. In addition, Medicare Part B services, such as physical, occupational, and speech therapy, are often overlooked as sources of revenue. Many nursing homes, while providing space and equipment for these services (as well as the clients), literally give way to outside vendors, who direct bill for the services and leave the nursing home with no fiscal benefit but some real expenses.

Obviously in the world of reimbursement there are numerous tricks of the trade, most of which are based on careful and thoughtful cost accounting, proper recordkeeping, and capturing of all charges. Attention to these details may mean the difference between fiscal viability and insolvency.

Nonoperating revenue comes from grants for projects or development, philanthropy, and other activities, such as parking lots, cafeterias, and gift shops. This income is important, particularly when operating revenues are tight, since funds generated from these sources can often provide the seed money for future development and thus help the organization maintain a competitive edge in its area.

This competitive edge is equally dependent on the effective management of the revenue cycle.

The Revenue Cycle

Effective management of the revenue and accounts receivable cycle is key to the survival of a long-term facility. No matter how good the service is, if the facility does not bill for the service and collect accounts receivable, it cannot stay in business for long. It sounds too simple, but in many organizations there is a significant loss due to unbilled charges through preventable omissions and errors, resulting in the ultimate noncollectibility of accounts. Long-term collection results will depend on effective systems and controls—every step of the way.

Intake and Admissions

A key element of the entire process is the presence of proper intake and admitting procedures. This starts with the building of an accurate and complete database from the time an inquiry for service is received by facility personnel. The persons taking inquiries should be well trained in the financial aspects of the admission process as well as the marketing aspects. They must be capable of developing a preliminary assessment of a prospective resident's condition, needs, and financial resources while simultaneously marketing the facility to the prospective resident. The data gathered is evaluated and a determination is made as to the appropriateness of the admission.

Verification of the prospective resident's third-party coverage should be an integral part of the admissions process. Additionally, because of the debilitated health status of most applicants, a visit to the hospital to meet with and evaluate the prospective resident may help avoid inappropriate placements. The need for and extent of these measures will depend on the relationship with the referral source. Ideally, the nursing home will build relationships of trust with referral sources over time, and they will be able to work with each other effectively to meet the needs of all parties involved.

If the applicant is admitted to the nursing home, the next step in the admission process is a review and execution of the admission agreement. Such agreements have become complex legal documents in their own right, with new requirements added every day. It is imperative that the new resident and his or her representative understand the obligations they are undertaking as well as their rights as health care consumers. If the resident is deemed incompetent, a duly authorized representative who can legally act on behalf of the resident must be identified and assume the role of "responsible party."

When discussing payment, it is important that the resident or responsible party know what is included in the facility's base rate and what is extra and that it is a possibility that, after proper notice, rates and payment arrangements will change. Likewise, care must be taken that they understand what third-party coverage might be available, as well as the limitations of any such coverage. In some states, such as California, Medicaid requires that a "liability" be met by the resident before Medicaid coverage commences, a concept very much akin to a deductible in private insurance policies. Similarly, Medicare has certain deductibles and coinsurance that must be met by the resident or responsible party. If the resident is private pay, it is recommended that the facility collect a deposit equivalent to several months' charges at the time of admission, and the ground rules as to when payment is expected on an ongoing basis should be discussed. Generally, private-pay residents should pay in advance for the month upcoming.

One dilemma often facing the facility is how to deal with residents who have applied for Medicaid but have not yet been approved. These residents are commonly referred to as Medicaid pending and present a risk to the facility inasmuch as it remains questionable whether it will be paid for its services. Where applicable, a deposit covering at least the first 30 days of care should be requested and a thorough evaluation of the resident's Medicaid application performed. Here, too, the extent to which the family cooperates in the process and the known experience and accuracy of the referral source are factors that can minimize the facility's exposure.

Medicare admissions are among the most complex, since a number of additional steps must be performed. In addition to verifying the resident's Medicare coverage, a determination must be made as to whether the resident's condition meets Medicare's strict eligibility criteria from a level-of-care standpoint. This determination is based on a combination of the resident's diagnosis and the nature and extent of "skilled care" required. For this reason it is important to have the input of a qualified nurse who is well versed in the Medicare program. If it is determined that Medicare coverage is not applicable, the facility is required to issue to the resident or responsible party a "Medicare denial letter." The resident may challenge the facility's determination and request that an independent review be performed by the facility's Medicare intermediary. This can be done by requiring the facility to submit a "demand billing" to the intermediary and await its decision. The facility cannot request payment for services until a decision is made by the intermediary, which could have a negative impact on cash flow. However, in most cases effective communication between the facility and the resident or responsible party will obviate many of these problems.

Medicare admissions also require screening other coverage such as HMO membership, since Medicare regulations mandate payment to be sought first from any other existing coverage. This screening is required under the regulations commonly known as the "Medicare secondary payer" rules. In fact, with the accelerating growth of HMO senior plans, in which Medicare participants sign over their benefits to the HMO in return for full medical coverage by the HMO, the facility should routinely check out other coverage for all admissions. Besides the fact that Medicare will generally not pay for the stay of residents enrolled in an HMO, most HMOs require the facility to have a contract with their plan before authorizing services or to contact them, at least, for prior authorization.

Clearly, the best protection for avoiding problems in collection down the road is to have good policies and procedures up front during the admission process as well as well trained staff performing the intake and admission functions. It is the job of the staff to be sure that these policies are well explained to the resident, the family members, or the responsible party. A possible approach that provides additional protection to the facility against costly mistakes in this area is to have all admissions signed off by a committee consisting of the administrator, director of nursing, and business office manager.

Billing for Services

Once again, having proper systems and procedures throughout the billing cycle is of paramount importance. Controls must exist that ensure that charges are generated and posted for all services and supplies that are considered chargeable. A complete "chargemaster," that is, a facility-specific comprehensive price list identifying these items and reflecting appropriate mark-ups over cost, is essential, as is the frequent monitoring of the nursing staff. In this regard, a central supply person who has the full backing and support of management is key to the program's success. Equally important is having proper documentation in the residents' records, such as physician orders and nursing notes detailing usage. One of the most effective ways of achieving control in this area is by utilizing a bar code system, such as the one described later in this chapter.

The three major categories of revenue that we are concerned with are the following:

1. *Basic care.* This is also referred to as room and board. The key here is maintaining an accurate census at all times. It must be balanced daily and reflect all admissions, discharges, and transfers virtually immediately. This type of up-to-the-minute accuracy is essential for the efficient operation of the intake and placement activities as well as for controlling billing.

2. *Ancillary review.* This type of revenue includes physical, speech, and occupational therapy, laboratory and x-ray services, pharmaceuticals, and billable supplies. It represents an increasingly significant source of revenues, since patients are being transferred to nursing homes with higher acuity than ever before. A major portion of this revenue is covered by Medicare Part B, which has the advantage that it is not subject to a specific cap, as is the "routine cost" associated with room and board under Part A.

3. *Personal items.* Revenue can be generated through such items as personal laundry, television rental, beauty shop, and so on. Policies vary from facility to facility as to how these items are charged for, if at all. Given the cost of these items, they should not be overlooked as a potential source of revenue.

The key to maximizing revenue is to avoid lost charges that disappear through cracks in the system, often through staff indifference and lack of controls. A tight, fully integrated order entry and charging system is essential, as discussed earlier. Another significant control step with regard to ancillary charges is to tie the processing of the vendor invoices for contracted services or supplies to the billing cycle. Evidence that a charge has been posted to the revenue system should accompany the invoice sent to accounts payable for processing.

The information generated from the census and the charging systems is then posted to the resident's account, along with any cash receipts and adjustments, and the facility is ready to bill. The concepts are the same whether the facility uses a computer for billing or a manual system. The key here from a cash flow perspective is to condense the cycle as much as possible so as to get the bills out as quickly as possible. In addition, the following suggestions are offered as ways to speed up cash flow:

- Prebill private residents for the next month's room and board charges, mailing statements between the 20th and 25th of the month. Cut off charges for ancillary services and personal items on the 20th of the month, billing the charges from the 21st through the end of the month on the following month's statement.
- Consider "split-billing" Medicaid accounts, sending out two semimonthly invoices instead of one monthly invoice (in those states that allow this). This will have the effect of evening out cash flow over the month.
- Process ancillary charges soon after month's end so that Medicare bills can be mailed early in the month. Securing cooperation from outside vendors in furnishing their invoices soon after month's end is a very important step.

Follow-up and Control

The administrator should, as an integral part of his or her job, monitor the billing process on an ongoing basis, being alert to identify possible bottlenecks or snags in the system. It is ultimately the administrator's responsibility to ensure that a bona fide source of payment exists for every resident who is admitted to the facility and that the systems for billing and collecting for services are in place and functioning properly. The administrator can be aided in this task by receiving at a minimum the following key reports:

- *Monthly revenue and billing report.* This report would indicate revenue by resident type (e.g., Medicare, Medicaid, private, etc.) and category (e.g., room and board, ancillary, personal items) *actually billed.* By comparing these data to the census and other indicators, the administrator would be able to identify and research any variances.
- *Monthly unbilled report.* Complementing the first report is a detailed listing of those accounts *not billed,* along with an explanation as to why each could not be billed, such as "awaiting Medicaid approval." It is critical that the administrator periodically follow up on these unbilled accounts and use this report as a control document.

In addition, the administrator should receive a monthly aging of accounts receivable report, review it, and initiate appropriate follow-up billing and collection activity. Left unattended by the administrator, follow-up activities tend to take a back seat to current, ongoing activities in the business office. The result is that unresolved accounts get older and become progressively more difficult to collect. The simple fact is that the earlier a problem with an account is detected, the greater the likelihood collection will be successful. Therefore, the facility should have a comprehensive collection policy that outlines the various actions to be taken at different times (e.g., a telephone call on fifth of month if no payment is received, followed by letter on the tenth, etc.). Letters and calls should become progressively stronger, with the ultimate action being eviction or the filing of a lawsuit. The point is that the facility should pursue real collection efforts and should not be inhibited in asking for money it is entitled to for services rendered and for which the client has undertaken to pay.

Expenses

The other side of the financial equation is expenses. In most long-term care organizations, the major expense is labor. Depending on the organization, anywhere between 55 and 60 percent of the budget is devoted to salaries and wages, with an additional 10–15 percent going toward taxes and fringe benefits. One 210-bed nonprofit facility in Connecticut offering a range of community services issued an annual report in 1991 that broke down its expenses as follows: wages, salaries, 55.1 percent; employee benefits, 15.9 percent; interest expenses, 4.4 percent; fuel utility and depreciation expenses, 9.3 percent; and supplies and expenses, 15.3 percent.

Cost

The trick for most long-term care organizations, in particular nursing homes, is to maximize their revenue or reimbursements for the services they offer. As previously noted, residents, like airline passengers, each pay a different amount for the same service. While Medicare is a federal system using a cost-based methodology, Medicaid, a joint federal-state program, is the major source of income and headaches. States take differing approaches to Medicaid, ranging from cost caps to paying on the basis of intensity of care provided. Regardless of the system utilized, it is imperative that the nursing home examine the methodology so that it can capture all potential costs. To do this, the home must first have in place a cost-accounting system that can accurately identify costs, and then these costs must be converted into billable charges, which must be followed by timely collection.

Further, it should be recognized that within the commonly accepted principles of accounting and finance, there is considerable discretion for cost allocation to maximize reimbursement. In some instances, institutions have reorganized to take advantage of the reimbursement formulas. Caution should be used, however, because reimbursement strategy is one of the most complex and technical areas long-term care organizations have to deal with. For that reason, expenditures for specialized consultants are often worthwhile.

Cost Containment, Avoidance, and Reduction

Much of the regulatory activity that has occurred over the past few years in the health field has been intended to prevent further escalation in the costs of health care. In general, several strategies can be followed by organizations wishing to contain, avoid, and reduce costs. These strategies include paper work improvements, productivity improvements, scheduling, and training. Typical problems faced by many long-term care organizations include cash shortages, overstaffing, poor utilization of present staff, low productivity, and equipment breakdown. With regard to cash shortages, an organization can establish a budgeting system that contains mechanisms for more accurate forecasting. In order to ensure appropriate cash flow billing and collection, systems must be developed and maintained. The key word is *systems*. It is always amazing to find out how poorly many long-term care organizations handle billing. Even a day's delay in sending out bills or asking for reimbursement is costly to an organization. In one horrendous example, a nursing home failed to collect from a private-pay resident who eventually was $40,000 in arrears.

Rare is the organization that does not have too many staff in certain departments and poorly utilized staff in others. Both under- and overutilization are costly and can be alleviated by better planning and coordination of personnel actions. It cannot be emphasized too strongly that, in a labor-intensive industry such as long-term care, all steps must be taken to ensure the most efficient and effective utilization of staff. This, unfortunately, is not often done.

The related problem of low productivity could be a function of numerous factors. For example, low productivity may result from recruiting inappropriate staff (i.e., people with poor skills or the wrong kind of skills). Productivity problems are often the result of poorly developed expectations for workers, a problem that can be solved by analysis of the jobs in question and related activities. Sometimes low productivity is related neither to production standards nor to the caliber of staff but rather to the basic systems for getting the job completed. The potential for this kind of problem occurs in any process that requires input or material from any other component of the organization before it can proceed. On the Ford assembly line, each of the various functions must be carefully articulated with the previous ones, and materials must be readily available. Without the wheel assembly, the tires cannot be put on, and so forth. Even within nursing homes there is a considerable amount of integration required: The work flow on a nursing unit can bog down because of a breakdown in the laundry, or the business office can be slowed down because information has not arrived from the ancillary service areas or other revenue-generating parts of the facility. All of these breakdowns are expensive simply because they result in unproductive staff time that must be paid for.

Management of Working Capital

Because most nursing homes are dependent on receiving funds from Medicaid, they are increasingly being held hostage to the fiscal machinations of state governments. Whether it is the use of IOUs (as in California) or delayed payments (as in Massachusetts), the problem presented to nursing homes is to pay bills and meet payrolls. To avoid having to borrow money, a home must carefully manage its working capital. Working capital can be thought of as those assets of the organization that are essentially current, such as cash, accounts receivable, and inventory, as opposed to its fixed assets, which might include land and buildings. The basic idea of working capital management is to utilize the current assets to keep the organization in the strongest financial position. Regarding the management of working capital, there are three especially important areas of concern: inventory, accounts receivable, and accounts payable.

Inventory

The basic concern in inventory control is to balance the cost of not having enough with the cost of having too much. Inventory costs money to purchase, and this money is essentially out of circulation until the inventory is used and then converted back to cash. In addition, inventory costs money to store. A final problem is that some items have a limited shelf life; if not used during their shelf life, they must be destroyed. A typical question facing a long-term care manager is how many disposable underpads to buy: a day's supply at a time, a week's supply, a month's supply? It is not so very different from the question the consumer faces when the supermarket has a special on tuna fish. How many cans should the consumer buy? If the consumer uses the entire grocery budget for tuna, then no money is left over for other needs. The consumer also deals with limitations of storage space and shelf life. So it is with the disposable underpads. All the money in central supply cannot be allocated to this item, even if it is bargain priced and the cost is going up in the future, since central supply needs other items that are equally important.

An additional factor in the inventory equation may be the likely availability of the product from suppliers. The reason most people do not maintain large inventories of groceries is that large inventories are readily available in neighborhood stores. An interesting example in the acute care field occurred several years ago when a hospital in Brooklyn, New York, took this approach with its oxygen systems. Since oxygen tank supplies were readily available, why should the hospital install a more expensive (capitalwise) central system that required a large storage tank? Rather, the administration reasoned, it would be better to buy tanks in small amounts and bring in new supplies a few times weekly. This worked well until a strike occurred and the oxygen tanks could not be found. Finally, an imminent disaster was averted when oxygen was located some 50 miles away in New Jersey. When things settled down, the hospital began work on its new central oxygen system, having changed its attitude toward the cost-benefit ratios.

One emerging method for maintaining inventories is the bar code scanning systems typically seen in grocery stores. One of the many systems that presently exist was explained by Michael Barrett of the Minneapolis-based Red Line Corporation, who noted that Red Line's ORBITS system uses bar codes and portable scanners to "track the use of products and services to specific residents and bill it to the appropriate financial class." He went on to note that, when inventory is dispensed, the system automatically records usage and produces reports identifying reorder points based on predetermined levels. As with other automated systems, ORBITS has the capacity to generate budgeting and Medicare reports, case-mix data, and specific usage patterns by individual resident, groups of residents, or units.

Accounts Receivable

Accounts receivable constitute an integral component of cash management, since they are the monies owed the organization for services rendered. Most long-term care organizations operate on a noncash basis; residents or third parties are billed for services, and these bills take some period of time to collect. On the other hand, the organization has obligations to pay the staff who have rendered the services that generate the bills. A nurse is not told that she will be paid as soon as Medicaid pays Mrs. Smith's bill. Rather, the nurse and the rest of the staff are paid periodically, even though a good deal of receivables do not come in on such a regular basis.

The key in accounts receivable is to set up an efficient billing and collection system so that bills are sent expeditiously and contain all the proper information (this is particularly important when dealing with the third-party reimbursers) and that follow-up takes place. As noted earlier, receivables can deteriorate to such a point that it becomes progressively more difficult to collect on them, particularly from private-pay residents. There are no easy solutions to accounts receivable problems, but the importance of organized systems must be emphasized. Organizations should carefully evaluate what have in the past been unacceptable alternatives, such as the use of credit cards or the development of time payment schemes for residents. Finally, it must be recognized that a dollar collected today is worth more than a dollar collected in two months and that investment in a good system therefore can have clear financial benefits.

Accounts Payable

To some extent, accounts payable are the other side of the equation. They are monies the organization is paying out for services and supplies that it has acquired or is planning to acquire. The major account payable for most long-term organizations is the payroll. From an organization's financial perspective, it is best to pay over the longest stretch possible. For example, a monthly payment of staff means 12 processings a year, which saves the organization considerably more cash on hand each month than under a weekly system, where 52 processings a year are required (and higher costs are involved). In business, suppliers often offer incentives for rapid payment, such as 1 percent off the bill if it is paid within ten days. In one nursing home, the working capital was so poorly managed that the home was months and months behind in its payments (some argued that this was actually good management). In some instances, suppliers had cut off deliveries to the home until old bills were cleared up, and thereafter they would supply the home only if cash was paid for the supplies. Again, the key is having an organized system for paying obligations, but this system must be integrated into the total working capital system, which is designed to ensure that money owed the organization is received as rapidly as possible and that funds are properly expended in purchasing inventory.

THE BUDGETARY PROCESS

A budget is essentially a statement of expected expenses and expected revenues over a certain period of time. Most organizations have some sort of budget and a budgetary process. Some organizations, such as nursing homes, must meet federal and sometimes state requirements for budgets of varying lengths. Indeed, some states (e.g., Connecticut) use the budget as a key regulatory device. Also, virtually every government-run or government-financed program is required at the least to prepare a budget at its outset. In theory, then, a budget is a financial timetable, a plan for the organization that has been translated into dollars and cents. Such an approach means that a budget can serve as a guide, a target, and a yardstick for measuring results. A different way of viewing the budget is as a political document that often involves a complicated bargaining process within the organization. Thus, forecasting (or in some cases educated guessing) becomes a key element in the entire budgeting process. Because of the political nature of budgeting and the control that management has when it makes decisions affecting department budgetary levels, the budget and the process can become very significant management tools.

For practical purposes, there are three types of budgets many organizations use: cash, capital, and expense. The cash budget is concerned with cash receipts and disbursements; it is developed to ensure that the business of the organization proceeds at a smooth pace. The capital budget is concerned with capital acquisitions, such as buildings, land, or equipment. Finally, the major budget is the expense budget, which is essentially a statement of the planned operation for a subsequent period of time. The budgetary document, at least superficially, does not vary much from organization to organization, but the process to get to that document does vary substantially. In the end, though, a financial document is prepared. Some documents are program-based, whereas others itemize each expense individually (line item budgets), but with minor effort each type can be translated into the other.

Traditional Budgetary Process

The typical budgetary process has four stages: (1) dissemination of instructions, (2) preparation of initial budget, (3) review and adjustment, and (4) appeal. Dissemination of instructions is exactly that. The instructions to be followed in the preparation of next year's budget are sent to those people who have been designated as responsible for their section of the budget. This is in reality the beginning of management's political statement about the budget and its seriousness about the budget. The first question is, Who prepares the instructions? Is budget preparation by fiat from the management or finance department, or is the instruction rule-making process itself open to question and negotiation? The instructions must also contain some parameters and forecasts, which again provides an opportunity for management to use its control. For example, in the instructions, it might say, "Because of our tight fiscal situation, do not budget any new positions in your department or plan expense for consumable supplies at a level of 2.25 percent higher than last year."

Effectively, management has sent a stark message to the department through the process itself. Another way management makes an important statement about the budget is by its choice of staff to prepare the budget. In one large organization, the department secretaries were responsible for budget preparation, while in another it was the department heads. Different message?

Having read through and digested the mechanics of the instruction, someone within the department is now ready to prepare the initial budget. Within a given department, the budgetary process may reflect the entire organization's approach or the management style of that department's manager. For example, the department may have an open process in which members of the department discuss their plans for the coming year and the money needed to translate those plans into action, or the manager may decide what should happen next year and plan accordingly. Sometimes there is no room in the budget for more than incremental financial plans for the future.

Review and adjustment occurs at the next higher management level (perhaps the second level of management). Here requests are pruned and coordinated. Since the final budget must be adopted at the highest management level (in many organizations, the board or corporate level), it is in everyone's interest to make sure that the document, when finally presented, is as defensible as possible. A strong defense of requests is possible when the forecasts are good and the requests are reasonable. In the review stage, it is important to see that each department has interpreted the forecasting data properly and is using assumptions similar to those of other departments. The review stage also provides an opportunity to ensure that there is no duplication.

The budget is then returned to the originating department. Depending on management's approach, a final appeal to top management is possible. If the department secretary has prepared the budget, there will be few appeals, since the secretary is not likely to be in a power position. Also, by asking the secretary to prepare the budget, management has said that it really considers the process just an academic exercise. On the other hand, if the process is serious and has consumed much energy of "powerful" department-level personnel, an appeal process to override decisions of the coordinating-level managers may be necessary. Here, the case for an increase or change is again made and the budget may be adjusted. It should be remembered that the budget may be reviewed by the board's finance committee before it goes to the full board.

At every one of these stages of review and negotiation, questions are asked. If clarifications are not forthcoming, the budget may not be adopted. Negotiation is the key to this type of process. In many senses, top management and lower-level management are negotiating. The two groups are, to a degree, adversaries, and if each is operating at a high level of competence, the organization stands to benefit from the competition. For example, different groups may have different forecasts based on different interpretations of trends; it behooves the organization to analyze these interpretations before making a decision on the budget. In a closed and managerially dominant system, the opportunity for interaction and negotiation is limited, which is probably not in the best interests of the organization.

Even the timetable of the budgetary process is a statement of how serious and open management is about the process. Too short a timetable gives management total control of the process and the input data for decisions, whereas a reasonable timetable gives the individual departments the opportunity to analyze their own experiences and plans.

The final budget should be an important and weighty document that presents management with a tool to evaluate department heads regarding their ability to meet expectations. Additionally, since the budget sets up the targets, variances from the budget act as flags alerting management of the need to investigate financial problems in a timely manner. Without timely intervention, financial problems simply get out of hand.

CONCLUSION

In sum, money is the fuel of long-term care organizations. A wisely managed institution will use its economic resources well and plan for the future. A poorly run institution not only endangers its own fiscal viability but compromises the health of its residents.

Case Study 11-1

Asset Shifting at Lenoxville

Seth B. Goldsmith

Several years ago, the Lenoxville Nursing Home, a nonprofit community nursing home, revised its admission agreement to include the following paragraphs for private-pay residents:

> The resident or the resident's responsible party agrees to pay the Home a deposit equal to one month's charges, with said deposit being applied to any final charges due upon the discharge of the resident. No interest will accrue to this deposit.
>
> All monthly bills are payable within five days of receipt. Residents or their responsible parties will be billed for monthly bed and board charges on the first of each month. All late payments are subject to a $100.00 late payment fee. It is further understood that failure to pay all charges will subject residents to discharge from the Home.

Mrs. Wilma Jefferson was admitted to the home 20 months ago as a private-pay resident. Because of her frail condition, her son and sole heir William Jefferson III, MD, was designated as the responsible party, that is, the person responsible for paying her bills with her funds. Shortly after her admission to the home, her son began to transfer Mrs. Jefferson's assets to his name with the idea of transferring enough of her assets out of her accounts that she would be eligible for Medicaid.

At present, there is an outstanding balance due the home of $27,000.00. Dr. Jefferson now claims that his mother is financially destitute and that she must go on Medicaid. The home's administrator has also learned that as of last month Dr. Jefferson had shifted all of his mother's assets to his own accounts.

At the most recent board of trustees meeting, the administrator brought the situation to the attention of the board and asked for guidance. Several board members were horrified to learn that the home had been carrying the account for almost a year and they were only now being informed. A second group of trustees was anxious to start litigation against Dr. Jefferson and proceed to discharge Mrs. Jefferson. A third group, composed primarily of members with the longest tenure, suggested that the home attempt to negotiate a compromise with Dr. Jefferson. One member of this last group also stated, "Jefferson is an important man in this community, president of the hospital medical staff, and probably the town's wealthiest surgeon, and we don't want to antagonize him."

Finally, the following motion was made, seconded, and passed with a slight majority:

> It is moved that the administration develop a plan and strategy to get Dr. Jefferson to pay the bill and present this plan and strategy to the board at next month's regular meeting.

* * *

Discussion Questions

1. Assuming you are the administrator, what would be your plan and strategy for dealing with the Jefferson situation? What impediments do you expect?
2. How could you avoid a similar situation in the future?

Finances at Lotta Rest Nursing Home

Howard L. Braverman and Robert R. Merry

Lotta Rest Nursing Home
Lotta, Massachusetts

To: I. Getknow, President
From: Ed Debenture, Director of Finance
Date: April 26, 1993
Subject: 1993 Financial situation

Attached is the final income statement for our 1992 fiscal year (Table 11-2-1). As you can see, we did much better than expected. My concern arises in that the Commonwealth has indicated that it will be cutting back substantially on our reimbursement for 1994. These cutbacks could be in excess of one million dollars.

We should start looking at ways of cutting back on our operating costs before the situation becomes critical.

I would like to arrange a meeting with you to further discuss this situation.

Table 11-2-1 Comparative Income Statement (Year Ended 12/31/___)

	1991 Actual	1992 Actual	1992 Budget	Budget Variance
Revenue				
Patient Care Revenue				
Private	$1,688,850	$1,897,873	$1,870,500	$27,373
Medicaid	5,531,434	5,481,482	5,382,955	$98,527
Medicare	190,152	263,783	143,847	$119,936
Veteran	43,139	43,033	43,802	($769)
Blind	251,269	198,466	270,864	($72,398)
Total Patient Revenue	$7,704,844	$7,884,637	$7,711,968	$172,669
Other Revenue	$427,953	$453,177	$408,882	$44,295
Total Revenue	$8,132,797	$8,337,814	$8,120,850	$216,964
Expenses				
Nursing	$3,909,852	$3,997,575	$4,107,888	($110,313)
Physical therapy	85,516	98,175	76,529	$21,646
Occupational therapy	87,225	94,434	89,201	$5,233
Medical services	98,498	117,831	110,237	$7,594
Social services	83,644	88,298	79,643	$8,655
Activities	81,962	83,942	82,552	$1,390
Education	56,507	54,078	53,825	$253
Food service	1,198,080	1,248,673	1,271,580	($22,907)
Housekeeping	441,103	451,470	467,956	($16,486)
Laundry	204,630	212,533	217,422	($4,889)
Maintenance	551,794	542,676	559,825	($17,149)
Day care	164,060	163,466	160,878	$2,588
Business office	272,012	300,612	280,538	$20,074
Administration and general	649,825	605,890	548,322	$57,568
Volunteers	47,925	46,081	44,949	$1,132
Property and related	365,071	331,015	372,300	($41,285)
Total Expenses	8,297,704	8,436,749	8,523,645	($86,896)
Operating Profit (Loss)	($164,907)	($98,935)	($402,795)	$303,860

	1991 Actual	1992 Actual	1992 Budget	Budget Variance
Private	12,809	12,181	12,470	(289)
Medicaid	54,714	54,954	54,616	338
Medicare	1,693	2,938	1,453	1,485
Veteran	365	335	362	(27)
Blind	2,566	1,784	2,639	(855)
Total	72,147	72,192	71,540	652

Lotta Rest Nursing Home
Lotta, Massachusetts

To: Ed Debenture, Director of Finance
From: I. Getknow, President
Date: April 27, 1993
Subject: Your Memo of April 26, 1993

I have reviewed the financial statement you provided me. Before we meet there is some important information that I would like you to prepare. This information is imperative so that we can appropriately plan for any reimbursement adjustments.

Let me also commend you on the successful financial operation of last year. However, I am concerned as to how we achieved this success. To what do you attribute the increases in revenues and decreases in expenses? Did we overcharge our residents for services? Did we cut expenses and compromise our services? Please explain!

Most notably, why are we so underbudget in our nursing costs? Did Ms. Nightingale cut staffing in any way? Was resident care jeopardized in any way?

I am also interested in the details of all departments that were either over or under their budget by more than 3 percent.

On the revenue side, I am very interested in knowing how our Medicare revenues are double what was projected. Was it all attributed to Part A or did we receive additional Part B income? Also, why is Medicaid so much higher? I believe that with case-mix reimbursement in place and with the freeze of rates, Medicaid income was to be flat.

Looking toward the future, please provide me some projections with regard to income and expenses if the new reimbursement methodology goes into effect. You need to prepare a series of contingencies for reducing costs and increasing revenues. Can our foundation provide us with the additional income to help offset these cost reductions?

If there are any other areas you feel we need to address, please bring them to my attention.

Chapter 12

Principles of a Successful Capital Campaign

Donna G. Michaels and Charles S. Wolfe

PHILANTHROPY: OUR ROOTS, OUR STRENGTH

Peter F. Drucker, management guru wrote,

> America needs a new social priority to triple the productivity of the non-profits and to double the share of gross personal income—now just below 3% they collect as donations.
>
> Federal, state and local governments will have to retrench sharply, no matter who is in office. Moreover government has proven incompetent at solving social problems. Virtually every success we have scored has been achieved by the non-profits.[1]

Drucker sees the nonprofits as constituting the social sector of society, which could become as significant as the public sector (government) or the private sector (business).

Drucker's formula for success in the social sector is as follows: "The average non-profit must manage itself as well as the best managed do. . . we need a change in the attitude of government and government bureaucracies. . . and finally non-profits have to learn how to raise money."[2]

Nonprofit nursing homes serving older people have played and continue to play an exceptionally important role in our society. As the public sector continues to withdraw support from these homes, the gap between what is minimally required and what is responsibly desirable will continue to grow.

Philanthropy has often been the means of providing the physical plant, equipment, special services, and desirable levels of staff and of fulfilling our social contract with the elderly of our communities. Today perhaps more than anytime in our past, the need for increased philanthropy is clear.

Although appropriate fund raising is a complex and carefully developed activity that must be based on individual circumstances, we will attempt in this chapter to provide a framework for understanding how the fund-raising process flows. We believe this chapter should be viewed as a springboard to further inquiry and as an aid in assessing any particular environment's potential for sustaining a capital campaign.

The United States has a history of encouraging its citizens to concern themselves with social problems and to underwrite constructive change privately. This unique facet of American society is described in de Tocqueville's familiar quote:

> These Americans are the most peculiar people in the world. You'll not believe it when I tell you how they behave. A citizen may conceive of some need which is not being met. What does he do? He goes across the street and discusses it with his neighbor. A committee comes into existence, and then the committee begins functioning on behalf of that need, and you won't believe this, but it's true: All of this is done without reference to any bureaucrat. All of this is done by private citizens on their own initiative.[3]

The word *philanthropy* derives from the Greek words *phil,* meaning love, and *anthropos,* meaning man. The term *philanthropie* first appeared in the English language in 1628, but philanthropy can trace its earliest roots back thousands of years to the Greeks, Romans, Hebrews, Egyptians, and ancient Chinese. Philanthropy has funded wars, erected temples, built universities, established monuments, transformed the image of tyrants into benevolent statesmen, preserved the arts, and changed the course of world history.

Although the first U.S. charitable foundations appeared after the Civil War, they are considered a phenomenon of the 20th century. By 1915, only 27 foundations had been set up, including those of Andrew Carnegie (1911) and Rockefeller (1913). By 1985, over 32,000 foundations had been formed. The Foundation Center estimates over 95 percent have been established since World War II.[4]

A FRAMEWORK FOR DEVELOPMENT

Development, in its broadest sense, includes the destiny of an institution and can be realized only by an effort on the part of the institution to analyze its philosophy and activities, to crystallize its objectives, and then to project them into the future.

A development program has three major objectives:

1. building acceptance for the organization

2. providing the kind and quality of membership that the institution wants and can best serve
3. obtaining financial support for current operation, special projects, and capital growth

A comprehensive program for financial support will include:

- the annual fund
- ongoing efforts to fund specific projects
- a planned giving program
- major capital funds

Such a program is best managed by a development department responsible for a range of functions. These functions include marketing research, development of marketing strategies, and development of a long-range plan. The department also prepares brochures and newsletters to inform constituents. It has a primary responsibility for developing and directing the several separate giving programs, such as annual giving, deferred giving, and capital giving, as well as requests for foundation funding and government funding. Additionally, the department provides leadership for a speakers bureau, handles gift acknowledgments, and maintains accurate and effective gift-reporting systems.

Ideally, the development department should be managed by a senior development officer, whose responsibilities include the direction and overall supervision of the staff and volunteers who are part of the development effort. The senior development officer has the main responsibility for designing the development program and recommending appropriate goals to the CEO and the board of directors, including specifying the programs and activities necessary to meet funding priorities. The senior development officer also serves in special situations as the spokesperson for the organization and bears the responsibility for organizing support services and materials for development volunteers. The senior development officer plays the role of chief of staff in identifying and cultivating major gift prospects. In this role, the senior development officer will be involved in motivating and training the CEO, the board, and the staff to become an effective fundraising team.

MANAGING A CAPITAL CAMPAIGN

A capital campaign is basically an intensive and concentrated program to raise an agreed-upon amount of money for specific needs. Such a campaign is usually launched and carried out in a limited time period. This means that the institution's leadership (staff and volunteers) will need to devote significant amounts of time and energy to this endeavor. The involvement of a large number of people working together will be required. There should be a clearly defined financial goal. The target amount is essential if the institution's organizational goals are to be accomplished. Setting a financial goal suggests that the institution has engaged in long-range planning. From this planning, specific organizational plans have emerged to address well-defined needs.

The campaign should set datelines. There is some urgency to raise money within those datelines so that the organizational goals can be accomplished. Capital gifts are usually received for specific projects over and above the annual giving budget. Often, the projects are construction-related, such as a new building or an addition to or renovation of an existing building. However, capital gifts may also be used to build an endowment or for specific endowed projects, such as endowed chairs or endowed scholarship programs.

Launching a fund-raising campaign requires a major institutional commitment. Time, energy, financial resources, and willingness to take risks are all necessary in the planning and implementation of the campaign. The commitment to fund raising does not develop all at once. This type of commitment evolves over time, especially if fostered by success. Achieving success requires the implementation of a systematic program to create the conditions under which people will want to contribute. Ultimately, the board and administration control the creation of the conditions necessary for success. According to Crawford,[5] the requirements are

- public awareness of how donations will impact the institution's ability to fulfill its mission
- the direct involvement of persons of affluence and influence (people give when they are involved)
- public awareness that the institution seeks and receives financial support (people give if they are asked and if they know that others are giving too)
- acknowledgment that the institution appreciates the support (people continue to give when they feel appreciated)

The Benefits of a Capital Campaign

A well-conceived capital campaign will raise the dollars immediately needed for the project in question and will increase interest in and good will toward the institution. There are multiple positive campaign outcomes that the CEO and the board of directors need to consider, such as rearticulating the mission of the organization and reviewing and possibly realigning priorities. A capital campaign helps the organization to develop a new leadership base, enhance the loyalty of its constituency, and create a better understanding among its friends and potential supporters. It also helps to provide a more in-depth information base about constituents and potential donors for future fund-raising efforts.

Requirements for Success

For capital campaigns to be successful, several criteria must be met. The sponsoring organization needs an identifiable and relevant constituency that has the potential to meet the fund-raising objective and is also prepared to give the project a reasonably high priority. In addition, the constituency must understand the need and accept the plan. The organization must be prepared to follow sound standards based on time-tested fund-raising principles. There must be a visible plan and a timetable that is experientially based. The plan must be undergirded by an organization built on informed, influential, and effective leadership and a sufficient corps of volunteer solicitors. The campaign must have adequate staff to support the technical work and the volunteers. Above all, the senior leadership group must be unified and possess a sense of common purpose.

BASIC PRINCIPLES OF CAPITAL CAMPAIGNING

Implementation of important fund-raising principles is essential for success. Capital campaign fund raising is unique in several important ways:

1. It is usually done for purposes of an urgent nature.
2. It seeks much larger amounts than normal giving to annual causes.
3. It schedules payments of installments over a period of time.
4. It invests its returns in permanent property or programs.
5. It takes place only when absolutely necessary.
6. It requires planned effort and often involves giving of securities or property.

THE BIG GIFT

The generalization that 80 percent of the funds in a successful capital program come from 20 percent of the donors is a useful guide for most programs. No matter how sophisticated and experienced the organization leadership may be in fund-raising matters, the importance of major gifts cannot be stressed enough. Energy and attention must be focused on obtaining the top 15 to 20 gifts that will be needed in order to establish the pace and pattern of support essential to accomplish the objective of the campaign.

What Leads a Donor To Make a Major Gift?

Dunlop suggests that the specific experiences of each major gift giver are bound to be different.[6] Nonetheless, there are some stages of the process of deciding to give that are common to all. Understanding these common steps can provide insight into how to help others go through the same steps, which will increase the likelihood of their making a major gift. Dunlop outlines the five steps as follows:

1. *Awareness* is critical and can be brought about by a wide range of stimuli: the printed word, comments by a friend, a speech, a broadcast, a public event, or a private experience.
2. *Knowledge* and understanding do not always follow awareness. Knowledge of an institution or a project can only be developed from the information that is made available and that the prospect chooses to assimilate.
3. *Caring* for an institution or a project does not necessarily follow knowledge. Some of the factors that make a person care about a project are personality, values, experience, interests, proximity, relevance, timing, and friendships.
4. *Involvement* develops from caring. Some gifts are made by people who simply care and are not involved. Substantial giving usually results from caring that has turned into involvement. Without involvement, even caring people give only token gifts. Involvement is the key to shifting a person's perspective of an institution or a project from the third person to the first person. When that shift occurs, the process of giving is a matter, not of giving resources away, but of giving to a purpose the giver has become invested in.
5. *Commitment* occurs when the elements of relationship between a person and an institution create in that person a feeling of being a part of a community. The prospective giver will seek out means to express his or her commitment most effectively. The term *commitment* is often used as synonymous with *gift* or *pledge*.

THE PRECAMPAIGN PHASE

In his seminal work, Seymour states that precampaign procedures are paramount.[7] What one does ahead of time usually decides a success or failure. If the services of a professional could be had for only one period, before or during the campaign, the preference would clearly be before the campaign. A capital fund-raising campaign usually involves the conduct of a feasibility or planning study to find out how much can be raised, who will contribute, who will help raise the money, and who will provide campaign leadership. This process begins with a needs assessment aimed at achieving agreement between the administration and trustees concerning essential programs and projects. The needs are concisely described in a prospectus or case statement, which is then shared with those who will be interviewed as part of the needs assessment. Interviews with people who can make or implement the largest gifts to a campaign are critical elements of feasibility studies. Of equal importance are interviews with those who might offer effective leadership. About 50 interviews are usually sufficient to get an overview of the situation. The number will depend on the size of the institution and the number of different constituencies that support it. For smaller institutions, as few as 25 interviews may suffice, but for larger institutions, 100 may be needed. After a list of candidates for interviewing has been developed (the list should be about one-third longer than the number of interviews planned), a letter from the chairperson of the board and the CEO should be sent to the candidates. The letter should explain the nature of the proposed interview and be mailed along with the prospectus.

The Feasibility Study

A feasibility study is essential to the development of a campaign plan because it provides necessary information. Properly carried out, such a study can test the general attitudes of donors and community leaders toward the goals of the campaign. It can reveal unseen problems that may affect the conduct of the campaign. The study will probe reactions, determine the potential level of support, and measure the relative willingness and enthusiasm of the organization's constituencies regarding support and participation in the campaign. It will help to discover appropriate promotional themes and to build early support. The organization should not underestimate the potential of the study for identifying the key leaders and organizations that will be necessary to ensure success.

For public relations purposes and to bring more people into the planning process or to cultivate them as donors in advance of the campaign, it is helpful to add several consultation or focus groups to the individual interviews. Focus group meetings require the attendance of an institution's CEO. They are intended to bring together potential campaign leaders and donors for a presentation of plans and future needs. The guests are invited to question the various proposals and to offer comments and suggestions. When the interviews are completed and the focus groups have met, the feasibility study report is compiled. It should contain suggestions and recommendations regarding every facet of the proposed campaign, including points of emphasis to be made in the promotional case statement and the campaign goal. The report may contain anonymous interviewee quotes. These are often the most carefully read portions of the report.

A feasibility study may require as much as two or three months from start to finish. Ample time is required to arrange and conduct interviews. Depending on the size of the study, it can cost from several thousand dollars to many tens of thousands. The majority of studies range between ten and twenty-five thousand dollars. The investment is usually justified, since the feasibility study is the foundation on which the capital campaign is built. One direct result of the study is the central campaign case statement.

The Case Statement

According to Seymour, the case statement is the definitive document of the campaign.[8] It tells all that needs to be told, including answering all the important questions and explaining the proposed plan for raising the money. With the development of a solid case statement, half of the fund-raising communications task is already completed. The case statement becomes the database. From the case statement, all other materials will flow.

Researching and planning for the case statement should involve directors, key executives, and volunteers who are large gift donors. The case statement should be clear, concise, and compelling; is usually 10–20 typewritten, double-spaced pages; and should be aimed at convincing prospective donors why they should invest their resources in the institution or project. The basic ingredients of a good case statement are as follows:

1. A statement of the need to be addressed by the project. Clear documentation is essential.
2. A clear description of the project the institution has designed to respond to the need. Be specific. For example, describe the

   - program objectives
   - operating procedures
   - expected results (or options)
   - professional staffing
   - timetable
   - costs
   - evaluation and reporting methods

3. Evidence that the institution is capable of carrying out the program. Include the institution's

- history
- achievements and recognition
- professional capabilities
- capacity to serve

4. Dollar requirements for the project and where the institution intends to seek support. List gifts and contributions to date and names of major donors.
5. The project's operating timetable and cash flow requirements and the timetable for fund raising.
6. An explanation of how success in this effort will benefit the project's clientele, society at large, and the donors.
7. A request for a specific gift. Be sure to indicate how a gift can be made.

Selecting a Model for the Campaign

Three kinds of campaigns dominate the philanthropic marketplace: (1) traditional or building fund campaigns, (2) campaigns to build endowment, and (3) combined campaigns that merge capital, endowment, and annual fund objectives.

The selection of the appropriate campaign model will be influenced by a number of factors. The key factors include the experience and abilities of the campaign leadership, the potential for cultivating major prospects, the range and scope of the campaign effort, and the experience and abilities of the development staff. The selection will also depend on the level of sophistication and maturity of the development program and the organization's commitment to strategic planning. It is important to understand that there is no one correct campaign model. What is crucial to remember is that the goal must be reasonable, credible, attainable, and challenging. In the development of the goal, the key actors must be aware of the organization's fund-raising history and the quality of the data in the feasibility study. In addition, the abilities of the campaign leadership and the potential size of the top ten gifts are crucial factors. Finally, the experience of similar institutions in such campaigns and the nature of local experience are important to consider. The development team that ignores these factors risks failure.

The campaign plan delineates organizational requirements, timetables, deadlines, job descriptions, prospect review procedures, the publicity plan, the record-keeping system, and campaign policies. The plan must fix the responsibilities of the staff, leadership, volunteers, and board. And of course it must be approved by the campaign steering committee.

THE ROLE OF LEADERSHIP IN A CAPITAL CAMPAIGN

Nothing is more fundamental to a successful campaign than committed leadership from the top volunteers. The leadership must be the first ones to give, and they must give at a level appropriate to their means, or beyond. They must be among the largest donors. They bear witness that the campaign is personally important, and their donation commits them to the success of the project. It is these leaders who must be depended upon to raise campaign funds from others. Potential donors often prefer to be asked by their peers for support. They do not like to be hit for money by fund-raising professionals and may suspect such professionals of being self-serving, less than candid, or the recipients of unacknowledged benefits. The volunteer leader who has already shown commitment by giving is able to motivate prospects to positive action.

In a good campaign, the fund-raising professional focuses on planning, acts as a resource, and deals with the nuts and bolts. It is the enthusiastic volunteer armed with the plan who goes out and wins the hearts and minds of the donors.

The integration of fund-raising responsibility and values into the thinking of the board of directors is essential for creating the proper climate for the development program's efforts. It is the board's responsibility to establish the fund-raising goal and to be prepared to commit an appropriate portion of the organization's resources, including board member time, to the achievement of the goal. Every board meeting should have time devoted to the progress of the fund-raising effort. The board and key staff should understand that they are expected to participate in training programs that hone their fund-raising skills and enhance their effectiveness in the recruitment of campaign volunteers. The organization and the board should be prepared to show appreciation to the volunteers and to organize appropriate events to honor them.

THE CAMPAIGN CHAIR: THE KEY TO SUCCESS

The campaign chair is the key leader of the campaign. No individual is too important for this post. The best that the community has to offer is just barely good enough. The chair must be a person who can command respect without demanding it, who has the determination to overcome all obstacles. Problems will arise in every campaign. To someone with the right abilities, they are but a signal to go to work. There is an axiom in fund raising: People give and work for people, not for causes. There are many good causes that lack support until a person of influence and ability assumes command. Such a person should have power and influence and be willing to use it. It is also axiomatic that it is impossible to do a first-team job with second and third teams. In fund raising, this means that the chair must have access to the top business structure of the community and must be a person of proven capabilities, dedicated to seeing that the job gets done on schedule.

Duties of the Campaign Chair

1. To serve as chair of the campaign cabinet and hold regular meetings.
2. To follow the campaign plan and schedule and the procedures outlined.
3. To recruit the division chair.
4. To exercise influence on behalf of the campaign, be willing to make a pace-setting personal investment, and be willing to secure dramatic pacesetting investments.
5. To be accessible to the campaign director and other key leaders of the campaign for consultation.
6. To inspire the division chair and ensure that he or she is meeting his or her assigned campaign responsibilities on schedule.
7. To attend meetings and special functions when necessary for the success of the campaign.

CULTIVATING DONORS

Prospect Identification

This is what Benjamin Franklin had to say about getting people committed to a cause:

> My practice, is to go first to those who may be counted upon to be favorable, who know the cause and believe in it, and ask them to give as generously as possible. When they have done so, I go next to those who may be presumed to have a favorable opinion and to be disposed to listening, and secure their adherence. Lastly, I go to those who know little of the matter or have no known predilection for it and influence them by presentation of the names of those who have already given.[9]

Evaluation and prospect review is the process of identifying potential sources of large gifts and determining what would be a reasonable request. Evaluation should answer the question, "How much can this prospect give if interested and seen by the right person?" It is a painstaking process and must involve key volunteer leaders who are knowledgeable about potential donors. The evaluation must be in relation to the required standards for giving—the top gift, the top ten, and top hundred according to the plan. Amounts must be both realistic and challenging. The acceptance of the evaluation by the key campaign leaders and the advance gift prospects will add credibility to the campaign plan.

Helping Donors Make the Right Gift

The key to obtaining the best gift possible is matching the gift opportunity that most interests the donor with the donor's assets and the most suitable gift method. The assets can include cash, securities (marketable or closely held), life insurance, real estate (a residence or vacation property), and tangible personal property (art, antiques, yachts, etc.). Additionally, the general methods of giving include an outright gift; a bequest; a trust providing income to the organization for a period of years, after which it reverts to the family of the donor or the beneficiaries; and a trust providing income to the donor and beneficiaries until the donor's death, after which the assets are transferred to the organization.

Acknowledging Donors

The responsibility for acknowledging gifts in an accurate and timely fashion is a development office responsibility that cannot be underestimated or overlooked. The senior development officer must ensure that appropriate systems are in place for this to be done. Dedications, memorials, and appropriate signs and symbols are just some of the ways to recognize major gifts and principal donors. Additionally, it is essential to ensure compliance with federal, state, and local rules applicable to exempt organizations.

CAMPAIGN COSTS

You cannot raise money without spending money. Within reasonable limits, the return is likely to be commensurate with the investment. In all campaigns, the cost will vary with scope, time, and size of goal. Annual campaigns run for less than 10 or 15 percent of return have all the cost respectability anyone has a right to expect—and in some communities perhaps a touch of uniqueness. Capital campaigns might go as high as that when the goals are low, but the ambitious ones often keep their costs well below 5 percent.

With good management and planning, the expenses will be minimal. Every campaign should have a budget. The following is a guide to preparing a sound campaign budget:

1. salaries and fees

   - professional staff, clerical staff, consultants
   - federal deductions and fringe benefits
   - fees for professional firms, auditors, etc.

2. organization expenses

   - luncheons, dinners, and meetings
   - local and long-distance travel

3. promotion and publicity

   - printed materials
   - artwork
   - models and visualizations
   - direct mail
   - stills and motion pictures
   - special presentations
   - radio and TV

4. general operating expenses

   - rent
   - furniture and fixtures
   - business machines
   - office supplies
   - telephone
   - postage
   - freight and express
   - messenger service
   - electricity and water
   - service and repairs
   - insurance
   - bank charges and interest

5. contingencies

FUND-RAISING CONSULTANTS

A good consultant can provide the expertise and management of detail and technical requirements that are so necessary to a successful campaign. The consultant can maintain momentum during slow periods by keeping on schedule and maintaining the enthusiasm. The consultant's experience and professional objectivity can facilitate problem solving. The professional consultant can bring a critical perspective to both failures and successes. The consultant can also generate excitement and creativity by understanding what is unique and by suggesting remedies. Comradeship is essential in a campaign, and the consultant can help spread the spirit of comradeship among the staff and lay leadership. Most important, hiring a consultant means there is someone who assumes accountability for the problems that can occur.

The following list enumerates the tasks that a campaign consultant will typically be assigned:

1. performing a feasibility or planning study and making recommendations
2. developing and drafting the case statement
3. creating a detailed campaign plan and a timetable
4. setting realistic financial goals based on study results
5. helping with the hiring of appropriate staff
6. helping with the recruiting of the volunteer leadership
7. assisting with office systems, such as the computerization of donor records
8. drafting a fund-raising letter and special proposals for foundation and major gift prospects
9. helping to set up the public relations and communications programs
10. training volunteers
11. providing volunteer support or engaging in donor solicitation
12. performing prospect research
13. determining the campaign budget and maintaining cost controls
14. assisting with postcampaign planning

A fund-raising consultant can do many things and help the organization with many others, but he or she cannot do it all. Particularly, a consultant cannot raise money. The campaign leadership and volunteers have to do that. Of course, a consultant can help. But a consultant cannot replace the keys to good capital fund raising, such as a good case for support, strong and committed leadership, a potential donor base, and sufficient volunteers. A consultant will not relieve the organization staff and board of their campaign responsibilities. In fact, their responsibilities and workload will most likely increase.

Selecting the Right Consultant

The first thing to consider is who should research and short-list the potential consultants and who should sit on the selection committee. The committee should probably include the CEO, the development officer, and representatives of the organization board, the staff, and the volunteers.

After creating a list of consultants who appear to match the institution's needs and who have successful track records, those responsible should interview the candidates and prepare a short list of no more than three. They should then invite the chosen candidates to make formal presentations to the selection committee. The committee members should ask themselves the following questions:

- How well were the candidates prepared for their presentation?
- Did they answer all questions?
- What is their professional reputation?
- Have they had success with other campaigns?
- Do they have good references?
- Do they offer a campaign approach designed to meet the unique needs of the institution?
- Do they have experience in fund raising?
- What is their record on cost per dollar raised?
- Is their style compatible with the institution?

General guidelines can be the starting points for making the final decision, but they are no substitute for in-depth analysis. A good fund-raising consultant will have integrity, experience, commitment, and adaptability in addition to the characteristics required by the particular situation of the institution.

The Contracts

After making the decision on which consultant to hire, the organization will want to state the terms of the business arrangement in a written contract. Although a consultant can be brought in at any time during a capital campaign, many consultants prefer to enter as early as possible (i.e., as soon as the organization begins to consider a campaign seriously). By entering early, a consultant can help develop the strategic fund-raising plan, can convince volunteers that fund raising is crucial to an institution's long-range finances, and can act as the catalyst in making the decision to proceed.

SOLICITOR TRAINING

A good development department places substantial emphasis on the effective training of solicitors. The following model of an ideal solicitor should form the basis of the solicitor training program.

John D. Rockefeller, Jr., said, "Never think you need to apologize for asking someone to give to a worthy objective, any more than as though you were giving him an opportunity to participate in a high-grade investment. The duty of giving is as much his as the duty of asking is yours."[10] Solid commitments from prospects are not obtained by browbeating. They will give if the solicitor

- believes in the mission of the organization
- understands the needs for building projects and endowment programs
- understands something of the background, interests, and capabilities of the prospect
- brings personality to the solicitation
- is not afraid to ask
- knows how to ask open-ended questions, listen, overcome objections, and adapt
- proves by example that the project is worthy of the prospects' support

HOW MUCH TO ASK FOR

Staff and committee evaluation will result in a general range of gift amounts for consideration. It is advisable to aim high enough to challenge and flatter the prospect. If the figure is too high, the prospect will reduce the request. However, very few prospects give more than the amount requested. Setting a solid, high figure in advance of the meeting is crucial to the success of sequential fund raising. Keep in mind the possibility of asking for a pledge for installment payments over a five- or ten-year period as well as the possibility that the prospect's company, family, or private foundation may wish to join together in a gift.

One of the objectives of aiming high and asking the prospect to make the largest possible commitment is that it raises his or her sights. Along with an amount, it is worthwhile to consider how the money will be used. There will be tangible results from receipt of the gift, and a special dedication of a space, floor, or building could be proposed. There are also many special endowment opportunities that provide the satisfaction of having given a perpetual gift.

Like many of the decisions that need to be made before a visit to the prospect, determining the right combination of opportunity and amount is based on the knowledge obtained about the prospect, especially his or her interests and financial situation.

SOLICITATION

A fund-raiser once said, "You don't get a good pickle by squirting brine on a cucumber, you have to let it soak awhile." A good gift will result after proper attention is given to the donor. A two-visit system has proven to have positive results. The first call is more for probing and cultivation. The fact that a solicitor is serious enough to persist will impress the people who are being called and will also begin to raise their sights. It is generally ineffective to mail a sample pledge card. The key to success is face-to-face solicitation.

The First Visit

There is no need to be concerned about closing a gift on the first visit. The first visit is just that—a first visit. A thoughtful gift is usually made on the second visit, after careful consideration of an earlier presentation. Accordingly, it is appropriate to just talk about the facility, its recent achievements, and its future needs. Ultimately, convincing the prospect of the worth and promise of the facility should be the only goal.

The solicitor should try to learn what interest the prospect may already have in the facility. One way to do this is by mentioning a gift opportunity at the appropriate financial level. Mention could be made of the possibility of a combination gift or a gift named to honor the donor, the donor's family, an individual, a corporation, a foundation, or another organization. It is important to use polite locutions like "We hope you will consider giving x dollars" or "We would like to suggest naming y project" rather than "We have you down for x dollars" or "Will you give x dollars?" The prospect should be informed that the suggested gift is proportionate with what others are being asked to consider and that a five- to ten-year pledge period is also an option.

Assessing the Prospect's Reaction

There is no need to worry about closing a gift on the first visit. An excuse may not mean no; it could just mean "not yet." A lower amount suggested by the donor may ultimately be acceptable, but it should not necessarily be either accepted or rejected out of hand. It is essential to listen without judging.

The Follow-up Visit Appointment

One way to make an appointment for a follow-up visit is to say, "I can appreciate that you will want to think this over before making a commitment. Why don't we meet next week at this same time?" Coming back also provides the opportunity to determine the right response to unanswered questions. If, for example, the prospect wants more information about a specific issue, an opportunity to return has been created.

The Pledge Card

Whatever happens, it is essential to keep control of the pledge card and not leave it with the prospect. Too often, leaving the unsigned card results in a much lower gift than anticipated or eventual loss of the prospect completely. It is common practice to leave behind the gift opportunity material or questions and answers and any specifically prepared proposal. The prospect should also be encouraged to discuss the matter with family, business associates, and financial advisors.

The Follow-up Visit

The follow-up visit should be used to review just how important the proposed gift is and to discuss the details of the gift. It is preferable to secure the pledge verbally and then use the card to record the pledge and the details of how it will be handled. The solicitor should review it with the donor and state that a confirming letter will be sent from the development office. To avoid misunderstandings, the solicitor needs to listen carefully and then restate to the prospect what has been heard. If there is any uncertainty about the donor's position, the solicitor can offer to return with a written proposal for the donor to consider and sign. It is often better to turn down a gift or postpone acceptance if a commitment is made that is considerably below expectations. Even if the gift is turned down, the prospect now has a greater understanding of the organization, and an opportunity for a future relationship has been established. Soliciting major gifts is not a science but an art. Usually, if there is one variable that determines success or failure, it is the degree of enthusiasm the solicitor conveys to the prospect. A solicitor must feel excited about the campaign and show it.

CONCLUSION

Philanthropy, despite its centuries' old history, is still an evolving and dynamic field. It is growing and changing to keep pace with the changes in human needs and the priorities of communities. This chapter has presented the basic principles and guidelines for capital campaigns that every professional development officer should know. However, it is important to keep in mind that, in this changing world, creativity, imagination, and the willingness to modify and innovate are the cornerstones of successful philanthropic campaigning.

NOTES

1. P.F. Drucker, *Wall Street Journal,* December 19, 1991, A 14.

2. Ibid.

3. A. de Tocqueville, *Democracy in America,* trans. H. Reeve, ed. R.D. Heffner (New York: New American Library, 1956).

4. E.F. Andrews, *Philanthropy in the United States* (New York: The Foundation Center, 1978).

5. J. Crawford, Perspectives on Consulting: Part I, *Journal of the National Association for Hospital Development* (Spring 1988):27–29.

6. D. Dunlop, *Concepts for Educational Fundraising,* Presentation. (Miami: University of Miami, 1984).

7. H.J. Seymour, *Designs for Fund Raising,* 2d ed. (Ambler, Pa.: Fund Raising Institute, 1984).

8. Ibid.

9. B. Franklin, *Familiar Quotations,* ed. John Bartlett (Boston: Little, Brown, 1980), 12.

10. J.D. Rockefeller, Ten Principles (Address on Behalf of United Service Organizations, New York, July 8, 1941), 8.

Case Study 12-1

The Cedars Fund-Raising Project

Charles S. Wolfe and James N. Broder

In 1929, moments before the Great Depression took hold of America, the Jewish community of the Portland, Maine, area opened a home for the Jewish aged. By the mid-1980s, and after three expansions, the 88-bed facility was in desperate need of rehabilitation or replacement. After careful analysis by the home's board leadership, it was decided that the best solution was to build an entirely new, 99-bed facility on a wooded site approximately two miles from the home's current downtown location.

The board anticipated that in order to make the project feasible, it would be necessary to raise at least $2,000,000 from the community. Complicating the fund raising were the following issues:

1. Although the nursing home was sponsored by the Jewish community and identified with that community, approximately half of the residents were not Jewish.
2. Only those people who were closely involved with the home thought the care was excellent. Most people in the community were unclear about their assessment of the home.
3. With the exception of a handful of people, the Jewish and non-Jewish community had no history of providing significant financial support to the home.
4. There was no history of major gifts to the home for new projects.

After some discussion the board decided that in order for the project to be successful, it was necessary to engage a fund-raising professional.

* * *

Discussion Questions

1. Does the Cedars project appear to be an appropriate circumstance for a fund-raising professional?
2. If a fund-raising professional is not engaged, how should the community organize itself to raise the money?
3. If a decision is made to utilize a fund-raising professional:
   - What experience and skills should the board look for in such a person?
   - How can such a consultant be investigated?
   - What issues should be clarified in a contract between the client and consultant?
4. What are the major factors that need to be in place in order for a successful fund-raising campaign to take place? Do those factors appear to be in place in the Cedars situation?

Chapter 13

Architecture for Long-Term Care Facilities

Ronald L. Skaggs and H. Ralph Hawkins

INTRODUCTION

Long-term care facilities design emerged as a result of changes in reimbursement mechanisms. The advent of Medicare and Medicaid in 1967 focused attention on the extended care setting as a means of reducing the cost of hospitalization and delivering more cost-effective care. This new emphasis reduced the then-current utilization of hospitals through shortening the length of stay. As the average American grew older and the benefits of extended care became available, many facilities were designed and built in the form of "nursing homes." However, the relevant government programs proved to be costly, and resources for funding began to dwindle. Eventually, reimbursement was reduced, which greatly impacted the fledgling long-term care industry.

Currently, the industry is facing new challenges. Hospitals, which were once a source of referrals, are getting into the market of providing long-term care as part of the continuum of care. This tactic has been relatively simple to implement, since hospitals could convert underutilized nursing units into long-term care, skilled, or intermediate nursing beds. In addition, other organizations, such as home health agencies, provided extended care to patients at home so that they would not have to be institutionalized at all. Day-care programs also allowed the elderly to be under supervision during the day, when family members were working, but at home in the evening and overnight, when family members were at home. All of these programs were aimed at keeping costs to a minimum while providing appropriate long-term care.

Long-term care may take place in a variety of facilities. The setting may be a hospital or a free-standing center. The facilities may provide individually or jointly a range of services, including skilled nursing, intermediate care, assisted living, and specialized services (e.g., services for those who are ventilator-dependent or have Alzheimer's). Other programs may augment these services, such as day care, respite, or independent living programs.

Initiating the design and construction of a long-term care project involves a variety of tasks. However, if the development is handled using experienced professionals, it can result in a well-designed, aesthetically pleasing, and functional facility. The following section is a brief overview of the development process and the main design considerations.

THE ARCHITECT'S ROLE

Architects are responsible for the design of buildings that accommodate the space requirements for the organizations' operational goals. When designing for a long-term care facility, an architect seeks to balance the functional requirements against the aesthetics (building appearance), cost (budget constraints), technology (how the building will be put together), and time (schedule for design and construction). The architect works with the long-term care facility administrator and others involved in the planning process to establish project requirements, design the appropriate facility to meet these requirements, and assist in administering the construction activities as they relate to the design documents.

Services provided by the architect can include feasibility consultation, facility development (master) planning, functional and space programming, site evaluation, basic architectural and engineering services, interior and graphic design services, facility management services, and other services that may be deemed appropriate. Various owner-architect contracts are available from the American Institute of Architects. The most common contract form is the AIA B-141, which outlines basic architectural and engineering services, along with methods of payment, and provides for the inclusion of additional services.[1] The planning and design process often is carried out by a multidisciplined team of planning consultants, architects, engineers, equipment planners, interior designers, graphic designers, landscape architects, and other specialists.

Feasibility Consulting Services

These services are often required at the beginning of a project to assess current market conditions, projected needs, and financial capacity. The resulting database provides the mechanism to determine the advisability of beginning a new long-term care facility project. Feasibility services are often provided by a health planning consultant, although many architectural firms offer such services. Also, individual institutions may have in-house planners capable of accomplishing required feasibility tasks.

Facility Development (Master) Planning Services

A facility development plan establishes a framework for existing building and site use that can accommodate future facility and program needs. Such a plan is based on current institutional considerations, including project goals, present site features, building size and capacity, and existing programs. After the investigation of current status, the information gathered is reviewed and evaluated for program compliance, functional performance, and establishment of space needs for immediate, intermediate, and long-range development. Subsequently, a final facility plan can be devised that identifies facility development strategies, proposed site development, future locations of departmental activities, and proposed growth options.

Functional and Space Programming Services

The functional and space program serves as the basis for the design of a long-term care facility. It describes how the building is to work and includes documentation describing appropriate relationships between various departments within the facility. Individual department operational considerations are outlined, and room-by-room space specifications are provided. Establishment of the functional and space program occurs after extensive data collection and reviews with operational entities. The program sizes each department and its component spaces based on operating concepts, staffing requirements, equipment needs, and patient accommodations.

Basic Architectural and Engineering Services

Typically, the basic architectural and engineering design process as defined in the AIA B-141 consists of five phases of activity, each subsequent phase characterized by more specificity and a greater level of detail. The first phase is the schematic design phase, in which the architect prepares preliminary sketches, models, drawings of room-by-room plans, preliminary specifications, and an early statement of probable construction cost for owner review and approval.

After approval of schematic design, the design development phase is initiated. In this phase, the size and character of the long-term care facility are described in greater detail. This includes indicating major materials, room finishes, and mechanical, electrical, and structural systems. Typically, a more detailed estimate of probable construction cost is presented, along with the design development documents, for owner review and approval prior to moving into the next phase.

During the construction documents phase, the architects and engineers prepare the detailed working drawings and specifications that the contractor will use to build the project after establishing final construction prices. These drawings and specifications will ultimately be made a part of the construction contract established between the owner and contractor.

The bidding or negotiation phase can vary substantially from one project to another. In certain cases, a contractor may become involved in the project prior to the completion of contract documents with the intent of arriving at a negotiated maximum construction price prior to the completion of plans. In other cases, a list of qualified contractors may bid completed plans and specifications. In either case, great care is required in evaluating the competence of the contractors under consideration as well as the mechanical, electrical, and plumbing subcontractors.

After the contractor is selected and a contract for construction is established, the construction phase begins. There should be a preconstruction conference between the owner, architect, and contractor prior to actual construction, which is the longest phase of the development process. The architect serves as the owner's agent, making periodic visits to the construction site to observe construction progress. Back in the office, the architect and engineers review shop drawings, process contractor pay requests, change orders, and perform other administrative functions in support of the construction activity.

Additional Services

Interior and graphic design services are often offered as an option in addition to basic services. Such services typically include space and furniture planning; selection of such building interior items as draperies, bedspreads, carpets, indoor plants, and special lighting; and color coordination of furniture and furnishings with the building materials and finishes. Graphic design typically includes the development of exterior signage, interior signage, and wall graphics.

Facility management services are of relatively recent development. They are in part an offspring of computer-aided design and drafting. Capital investment in facilities is an ever-increasing management burden. Following initial construction and occupancy of a building, computer-aided facilities management provides the resources to coordinate the ongoing necessary modifications of the internal configuration of the facility and the associated furnishings, equipment, and mechanical and electrical systems. Computer-aided facilities management provides the ability to rapidly produce the necessary drawings and related documents for ease of alteration while simultaneously maintaining a continuous record of the current state of the facility and its associated systems, furnishings, and equipment.

The best time during the development process to bring the architect on board is as early as possible, preferably at the feasibility study stage or during site selection. The organization may wish to institute an architect selection process. Architect selection should begin with the establishment of a select list of qualified architectural firms. Each firm on the list should be invited to submit its qualifications based on an established set of criteria. A sample application is included in *Selection of Architects for Health Facility Projects*, which is published by the American Hospital Association.[2]

After the receipt of the qualifications of the firms and the evaluation of their appropriateness for the proposed project, a smaller number of firms, possibly three to five, should be invited to be interviewed. In addition to interviewing each firm, the organization may wish to contact previous references as well as visit similar projects designed by each firm. Interviews can take place at the owner's place of business or at the architect's office. Visiting each firm's office can be an effective means of understanding the firm's internal operations.

TYPES OF LONG-TERM CARE FACILITIES

Long-term care facilities come in a wide variety of types. There are, in addition to facilities for the elderly, facilities for physical rehabilitation, psychiatric care, mental retardation, and head trauma. Detailed discussions on architecture for rehabilitation and psychiatric facilities are available in the *Encyclopedia of Architecture*.[3] Regarding facilities for the elderly, there is a full spectrum of facility types that differ primarily in terms of level of dependence. At the lower end of the spectrum are elderly housing units and senior centers.

Elderly Housing

Elderly housing comprises numerous housing types, ranging from single-family residences to multiunit apartments. Facilities also range from single-level to high-rise buildings and often include a variety of shared support functions, including social centers, meal service, housekeeping, and related services. The common denominator is that they contain dwelling units, which vary to meet different housing and life-style needs. Typically, an elderly housing complex has a mix of efficiency, one-bedroom, and two-bedroom accommodations.

Senior Centers

Senior centers provide day-care and community interaction services to the elderly in a nonresidential setting. Such centers can be free-standing, part of a church or school, or the focus of a continuing care retirement community. Most senior centers consist of a large group meeting lounge and activity rooms supported by meal service capabilities, administrative and counseling services, and outdoor recreation space.

In the middle of the long-term care facility spectrum are residential care facilities typically referred to as independent living and assisted living centers. The major difference between such facilities is the level of dependence or assistance required by facility residents.

Independent Living Centers

Independent living facilities are intended to support a variety of levels of independence. Facilities at one end of the continuum are similar to elderly housing or leisure retirement communities in that health care is not available. The other end of the continuum consists of housing where the average resident can maintain an independent life style while also having access to on-site health care services and often assisted living or nursing services.

Assisted Living Centers

Assisted living facilities offer personal services that support various daily activities including bathing, dressing, taking medications, and dining. Such facilities would typically include health care and often nursing services on site. The primary feature of an assisted living facility is that the residents are unable to function independently and require some level of personal services on a daily basis.

At the higher end of the long-term care facility spectrum are nursing-related facilities, including intermediate care, skilled nursing, and specialized care facilities. Such facilities are often free-standing, although there is a growing trend toward combining such facilities with independent and assisted living centers as a way of providing a full continuum of care.

Intermediate Care Facilities

Intermediate care facilities are designed to provide minimal nursing services to residents requiring limited medical care. Residents are often able to get around but require continuous supervision in regard to medication or activities of daily living and often require periodic physical, occupational, or recreational therapy. Nursing units in intermediate care facilities commonly contain semiprivate rooms and are supported by a central meal service as well as housekeeping and various therapeutic support functions.

Skilled Nursing Facilities

Residents of skilled nursing facilities are typically bedridden and often have multiple health problems requiring continuous nursing care and supervision.

Many residents are incontinent or have debilitating illnesses affecting their ability to function on their own. Skilled nursing facilities commonly consist of nursing units that contain 40–60 beds each and have a mixture of private and semiprivate rooms.

Special Care Facilities

Special care facilities provide special services for individuals with distinct medical needs. Alzheimer's facilities, which are increasing in number, have physical design characteristics that address the special needs of residents with Alzheimer's disease. Such facilities require special provisions for security because of the tendency of these residents to wander. Careful attention to lighting, color, and signage can assist in orienting facility residents while appropriate assignment of space and views to the outside or other areas can help staff maintain awareness. Other types of special care facilities include facilities for individuals who are ventilator-dependent, are comatose, or have suffered head trauma. Such facilities often include selected acute care-related diagnostic and treatment functions in order to satisfy resident treatment needs and state licensing requirements.

CODES AND STANDARDS

Long-term care facility design, depending on types of services provided, may be subject to a wide range of codes and standards as well as licensing requirements. When acquiring, renovating, or designing a new facility, it is prudent for an architect and engineer to perform an evaluation of all applicable design requirements. These requirements vary significantly from state to state. Even within a single state, application and interpretation may vary among the various local, state, and federal regulatory agencies. This multiplicity of review can be time consuming and ultimately costly to a long-term care facility operator seeking to respond to pressing facility needs. In the case of conflicting codes and standards, the most restrictive regulation usually applies.

The purpose of codes and standards is to assure the public that long-term care facilities are safe and that their design contains the functional components necessary to provide the appropriate services.

The codes that apply to long-term care facilities generally will include a model building code, such as the Uniform Building Code or Standard Building Code. In addition, model building codes may be amended by the government prior to being promulgated. These codes are generally used in conjunction with a compatible mechanical, electrical, plumbing, and fire code. Many times, these local codes are interpreted differently by the chief building official and the local fire department officials. Another code frequently used is the National Fire Protection Association 101–Life Safety Code.

All of these codes are intended to provide for the safety of occupants and ensure proper construction techniques. There are many sections addressing structural integrity, mechanical systems, and electrical systems, but the major concerns are occupant safety and protection of the structural elements from fire.

Standards for long-term care facilities are typically used to guide the provision of proper space and equipment. The most widely used manual of standards is *Guidelines for Construction and Equipment of Hospital and Medical Facilities.*[4] This document is published by the American Institute of Architects with assistance from the U.S. Department of Health and Human Services. It contains general standards as well as specific chapters on skilled nursing, rehabilitation, and outpatient facilities. However, many states develop individual standards through their departments of health.

The purpose of using standards is to give consumers, providers, and third-party payers a certain level of assurance that the facility is able to provide the services that are offered. The standards also assist architects and consultants in the development of space programs and in functional planning.

In addition to having to meet codes and standards, many long-term care facilities pursue accreditation or membership in associations that also have certain design requirements. Typically, these organizations refer to the codes and standards already discussed, but it is not uncommon for specific design issues to be addressed. One of the most commonly sought accreditations is from the Joint Commission on Accreditation of Healthcare Organizations. In the required Joint Commission reviews, members of the accreditation team may also interpret codes and standards differently than the other reviewing agencies. As a result, it is necessary to evaluate the potential impact of these accreditation facility reviews.

Because of the number and variety of codes and standards, there is a substantial amount of redundancy, especially in the area of life safety systems. However, it is the responsibility of the providers and architects to provide a safe facility design, which means having to comply with the codes. It is important to note that fire safety reports show health care facilities have proven to have excellent safety records.

Another emerging issue in long-term care design concerns new services that do not fit standard definitions. For example, subspecialty facilities like head trauma, behavioral, or Alzheimer's units may not fall into existing codes and standards categories. Standard definitions are not always applicable, and the regulatory agencies are not always flexible in their interpretations. Flexibility would allow creative approaches to providing long-term care services, but it may impact licensing requirements and therefore also reimbursement.

Reimbursement, many times, is based on specific licenses the facility holds. Third-party payers, public and private, are adamant that facilities offer standardly defined services. This creates an impediment to emerging types of facilities. However, many insurers are beginning to give recognition to creative and cost-effective forms of care.

Long-term care facilities, as well as almost every type of building, have experienced the impact of the Americans with Disabilities Act of 1990 (ADA). The ADA is designed to eliminate discrimination based on disability. It covers employment practices and calls for the elimination of architectural as well as communication and transportation barriers in public and commercial facilities. It applies to almost all types of buildings, including buildings slated for construction and those already existing. New buildings completed and ready for first occupancy after January 26, 1993, must be designed and constructed to be "readily accessible" to individuals with disabilities. A facility is also subject to the new construction requirements if a completed application for a building permit or permit extension is filed after January 26, 1993. A new building that does not meet these criteria may be considered to be an "existing facility," in which case it will be required to remove barriers in public accommodations where such removal is "readily achievable." The term "readily achievable" means "easily accomplishable and able to be carried out without much difficulty or expense."

The ADA is not enforced by state or local governing agencies, and therefore construction documents are not necessarily reviewed by these agencies (or any federal agency) for compliance with the ADA. Consequently, compliance may not be determined until proven in court. In the absence of any authoritative and binding clarification of any standards in question, it is recommended that the standards should be construed liberally (in favor of the disabled).

Even though long-term care facilities are beset with a number of codes, standards, and agency reviews, the trend is toward consistency and acceptable alternative methods and designs that demonstrate equivalent performance and quality. Coordination among federal, state, and local agencies reviews is becoming more usual as well. A thorough review of codes and standards early in the acquisition, renovation, or construction of a long-term care facility is not only appropriate but required.

SITE CONSIDERATIONS AND SELECTION

Before beginning the development of a new long-term care facility, careful attention should be given to site appropriateness, whether the organization owns an existing site or is acquiring a new site. If site acquisition is required, purchasing a site based on low cost alone can result in major problems, even to the point that the property can be developed only at extreme cost (or not at all). The following issues should be carefully considered before settling on the final site.

Location

The facility's location can have a major effect on the organization's ability to serve residents and to attract and retain qualified physicians and employees. Road accessibility and proximity to other related facilities can improve the image of the facility and its chances of success. When evaluating a location, consideration should be given to the distance between the site and related health facilities and other types of facilities, such as shops, churches, restaurants, financial institutions, recreational facilities, and the availability of public transportation.

Zoning

Checking zoning regulations is extremely important, primarily to ensure that the type of facility planned will be authorized to be constructed by the reviewing authorities. If the zoning is not appropriate, the question should be raised as to whether rezoning is possible and, if so, how long the rezoning procedure would take. Various site restrictions such as setbacks, height restrictions, and easements should be carefully evaluated. In addition, zoning regulations regarding the adjacent land should be ascertained. The site assessment should also include the types of future development permitted in the surrounding area. Obviously, adjacent and surrounding land compatibility is important to ensure the facility will have suitable neighbors.

Property Size and Usability

A mistake often made in land acquisition is the selection of too small of a site or a site configuration that is difficult to build on. In addition to space for the building itself, there must be sufficient space for access roads and parking, appropriate landscaping, and possible expansion. Available utilities should be ascertained, as should the need for any preconstruction site modifications. Factors affecting usability include drainage, subsurface conditions (e.g., the water table), topography, and existing vegetation. If part of the site is on a flood plain, it should be determined how much of the site is usable outside of the flood plain.

Intermediate care and skilled nursing facilities of 100–120 beds typically require approximately 5 acres of developable land, while the addition of housing facilities, dependent on the number of living units, can push developable land requirements into the 20-acre range. Sufficient acreage should be included for outdoor activities for residents.

Site Amenities

Although subjective, the attractiveness of a potential site is a consideration. If objectionable noise or odors or other negative factors such as heavy traffic exist, alternative sites should be evaluated. Positive factors include attractive views, interesting topography, and available trees or vegetation.

PUBLIC AND ADMINISTRATIVE SERVICES

A long-term care facility typically has an area for receiving the public and an area to house the administration of the facility. The nature of the public area will depend on the services provided and size of the facility. Public reception begins at the front door and lobby. The front door usually opens into a vestibule that provides an air trap between the exterior and the lobby. The lobby should be designed so it is sufficiently large to receive visitors and residents but also provides a control point for those entering the facility. The lobby should have access to public toilets, a drinking fountain, and a public telephone. Other possible amenities may include a newsstand and even a small convenience store or gift shop to provide essentials to residents. The reception area should be directly adjacent to the lobby and be readily accessible to those entering the facility. It may consist of a desk or counter in the lobby or an enclosed room with a window opening into the lobby. The reception function is sometimes combined with the switchboard function. If the switchboard function is at this location, it is prudent to provide a communications closet to house telephone equipment.

Administrative functions, depending on the level of care provided, include administrative office and business office functions. The administrative area usually includes space for the administrator, the chief financial officer, possibly an assistant administrator, and often a director of nursing. It also usually includes space for secretarial support as well as a coffee bar, a coat closet, a conference room, a copy room, a supply closet, and sometimes a private toilet. The business area may provide space for a number of employees involved in accounts receivable and payable and in insurance. Many facilities provide private rooms or cubicles for resident registration or account review. The business area also may include a copy room, a supply room, an auditor's office or conference room, and rooms for other support activities. Smaller facilities may combine many of these operations, both in terms of space and staffing.

Areas often accessible to the public as well as residents include dining facilities and recreation and group activity rooms. Use of these areas by family members, friends, and even other members of the community can be encouraged to good effect. For example, many long-term care facilities provide special discounts for the elderly in their dining facilities so that elderly persons living independently may be exposed to the facilities they may ultimately require. Encouraging public use of recreation and group activity rooms is also an excellent way of exposing outsiders to activities within the facility, including education courses, arts and crafts activities, games, and social events.

Guidelines for Construction and Equipment of Hospital and Medical Facilities requires that the combined area for dining and recreation in a skilled nursing facility should be based on a total of at least 30 square feet per bed or be at least 225 square feet total. The factor may be reduced to 25 square feet per bed if the facility has 100 beds or more. At least 14 square feet of this number is to be provided for dining. Additionally a minimum of 50 square feet of storage for equipment and supplies is to be provided at or near the recreational area. Sheltered workshops may also be available for residents and outpatients.

DIAGNOSTIC AND TREATMENT SERVICES

Long-term care services do not traditionally focus on diagnosis or treatment—beyond what is required to maintain maximum levels of health and independence. Individuals are typically diagnosed and treated in an acute care setting, but they may require ongoing treatment and maintenance after transferring to a long-term care facility. This treatment and maintenance function usually only requires minimal area.

Exam Room

Generally a multipurpose exam and treatment room of 100–120 square feet is sufficient for typical medical interventions, such as routine examinations or minor treatment. The room should be flexible so it can be used for a wide range of services, including routine physical examinations and gynecological, proctological, ophthalmological, and even dental examinations. Minor treatment may also occur, so adequate lighting is essential. A lavatory for handwashing should be provided within the room. A work counter, storage cabinets, and a writing surface are also essential. A nearby toilet is sometimes desirable, not only for resident use but also for specimen collection. This exam room may be located in a central area or in a resident care unit.

Physical and Occupational Therapy

If rehabilitation therapy is part of the program for long-term care, physical and occupational therapy services should be provided. Physical and occupational therapy space requirements vary according to program and equipment. Generally, the therapy departments are combined in one location unless more extensive rehabilitation services are provided. Space requirements for providing minimal physical and occupational therapy services include an administrative and clerical area, patient reception area, supplies storage, personal effects storage, clean and soiled utility rooms, a janitor's closet, access to the conference room for in-service training, and convenient access to toilets, including a toilet for handicapped persons. If outpatient services are provided, other requirements include convenient access from parking areas, covered entrances for patient drop-offs during inclement weather, and dressing rooms and shower facilities. *Guidelines for Construction and Equipment of Hospital and Medical Facilities* is a good resource for more detailed planning.

Pharmacy

Each facility must plan for the procurement, delivery, and proper distribution of pharmaceutical products. Although a pharmacy does not have to be on site, 24-hour access must be provided.

RESIDENT CARE SERVICES

Long-term care services are provided in a variety of areas within a facility. This section primarily addresses resident rooms and nursing units and discusses general design considerations. It also contains several sample floor plans that indicate new directions in resident room and nursing unit design.

Resident Rooms

The resident room in a long-term care facility is generally where the resident interacts with nursing and medical staff and his or her family or friends. Much of the resident's daily routine occurs there. Although many facilities have multibed rooms to encourage social interaction, there is a growing trend toward private rooms or at least more privacy in multibed rooms. Configurations of multibed rooms are changing to give more privacy to each resident than is provided by a cubicle curtain (see Figure 13-1).

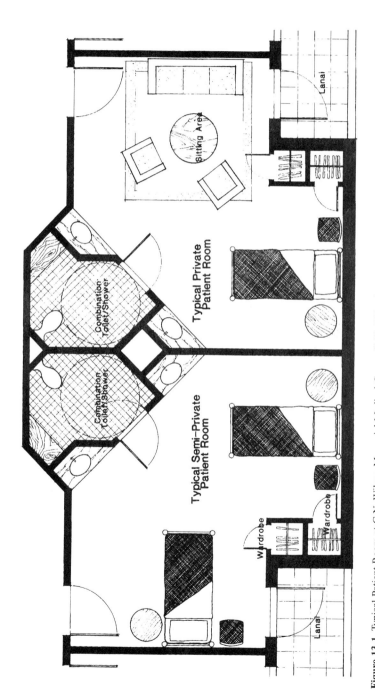

Corridor

Sitting Area

Lanai

Combination
Toilet/Shower

Combination
Toilet/Shower

Typical Private
Patient Room

Typical Semi-Private
Patient Room

Wardrobe

Wardrobe

Lanai

Figure 13-1 Typical Patient Room at G.N. Wilcox Memorial Medical Center Skilled Nursing Facility, Lihue, Hawaii. *Source:* Courtesy of HKS Architects, Dallas, Texas.

More room space is needed in a long-term care facility than in an acute care setting because of the greater length of stay. Many newer designs provide an area for sitting and a desk for writing. Wardrobe requirements also exceed those for acute care facilities, and wheelchairs must be accommodated. Resident rooms must meet minimum standards. Most codes require a minimum of 120 square feet for a private room and 100 square feet per bed for multibed rooms. These space requirements are exclusive of toilets, closets, wardrobes, alcoves, and vestibules. Multibed rooms cannot contain more than four beds, and only one bed can intervene between another bed and the window. All resident rooms must have an operable window of sufficient size for natural light and ventilation. The window may be keyed if the key is kept at the nurse's station. A sink for handwashing is not required if one is provided in the nearest toilet, but it is advisable to have a sink in multibed rooms. This allows residents to wash even if the toilet is occupied.

Toilet and Bathing Facilities

The toilet and bathing facilities in a long-term care setting often differ from acute care types of facilities. For example, it may be decided that bathing facilities should not be readily accessible to residents except when assisted by an attendant. This is an especially good policy for older residents or residents who have been brain damaged and whose equilibrium is in question. One solution is to centralize bathing facilities and provide showers and peninsular bathtubs that are equipped with hoists or devices to ensure safety. In skilled nursing facilities, a minimum of one bathtub or shower must be provided per 12 beds. In addition, residents must have access to one bathtub per nursing unit and to a handicapped shower in the centralized facilities. Bathing areas must also have associated areas for drying and dressing as well as space for attendants and wheelchairs. However, for reasons of convenience and flexibility, the long-term care facility may choose to provide bathing facilities in each room. Regardless of location, access to a nurse call in the bathing areas is important because of the possibility of falls.

The current trend is toward showers instead of tubs. Statistically fewer accidents occur in showers, probably because of the relative ease of walking directly into the washing area. One related issue is the height of the rim around the shower basin. Many propose no rim, only a sloping floor to the floor drain. The advantage of this design is that there is no tripping hazard and it is relatively easy to roll a resident into the area using a shower chair. The disadvantage is that water sometimes spreads onto the floor area. This problem can be remedied in two ways. First, a small sill of one-half inch or less could provide a small barrier to the water without being an obstacle for the resident. Second, a flush drain could be installed as the barrier between the shower and remaining area. It is important to note that this approach is more costly than installing a conventional shower basin.

Conventional shower basins are still popular and are used in most facilities. The rim of conventional basins is not a major obstacle for ambulatory residents but does act as a barrier for shower chairs. There are also seamless acrylic stalls with integral grab bars and a seat that are designed for health care use. However, any properly designed shower in a long-term care facility should have grab bars at the periphery. Also, a showerhead fixed to a flexible hose is to be preferred over a fixed head, since it allows attendants to bathe residents more thoroughly.

A handicapped-accessible toilet should be provided on each unit, and this toilet can serve as a resident training toilet. If centralized bathing facilities are provided, residents must have access to a toilet that does not require them to pass through a public area. This toilet can also serve as a training toilet.

The resident room toilet should also contain a water closet, handwashing lavatory, mirror, paper towel dispenser, and shelf for personal hygiene items. The water closet should preferably be placed at handicapped height. This sitting height is more easily attained by elderly and infirm residents. It is also advisable to have grab bars on each side of the toilet to ease access. These bars may be the swing-away type. A nurse call should be within easy reach of the toilet in case of a resident fall. Sometimes the nurse call is placed between the toilet and the shower so as to serve both areas. The handwashing lavatory must be at an appropriate height to serve sitting and standing residents. The handwashing fixture's valves should be provided with wing blades for easy operation. The mirror is best located above the lavatory, but it should have a tilting mechanism for residents in a wheelchair. The shelf for the storage of personal hygiene items should be within easy reach of the lavatory. Toilets and bathing facilities must be appropriate for the specific type of care provided. In addition, provisions for handicapped residents must meet applicable codes and standards.

The Resident Care Unit

The resident care unit comprises individual resident rooms and the support area. The support area at a minimum includes the nurses station, a staff toilet, access to the staff lounge, a medication room, a nourishment station, clean and soiled utility rooms, a peninsular tub, access to the exam room, an activity room, a janitor's closet, wheelchair and stretcher storage, storage for personal belongings, and general storage. The size of the resident care unit can vary according to the services. For example, a 60-bed unit may be appropriate for skilled nursing care (see Figure 13-2), whereas a smaller unit would be adequate for Alzheimer's care (see Figure 13-3). *Guidelines for Construction and Equipment of Hospital and Medical Facilities* recommends that at least 5 percent of the total beds be in

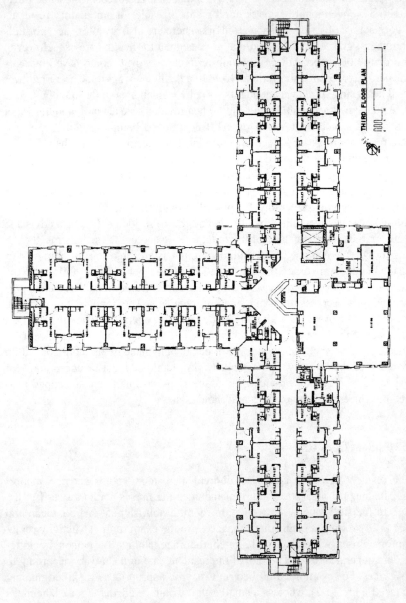

Figure 13-2 Skilled Nursing Facility Plan. *Source:* Courtesy of HKS Architects, Dallas, Texas.

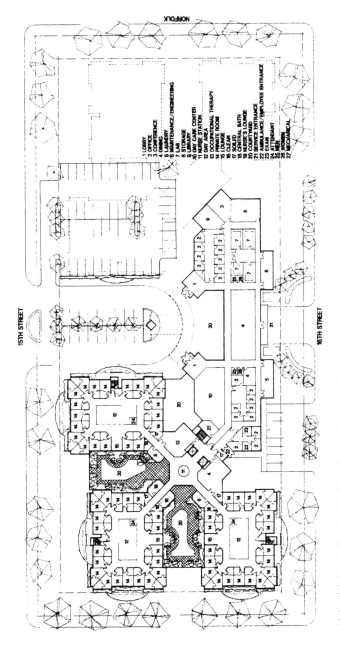

Figure 13-3 Alzheimer's Care Facility Plan. *Source:* Courtesy of HKS Architects, Dallas, Texas.

private rooms that have toilet and bathing facilities. Many of the support functions may support more than one resident care unit if conveniently located.

The nurses station should be centrally located. Ideally, it should permit viewing of all resident corridors if not the door openings into each room. The activity room should preferably be located near the nurses station for observation purposes. Also, it is common for residents to congregate around the nurses station; so if the activity room is nearby, it may reduce corridor congestion. The nurses station location should allow observation of those entering and exiting the unit. The nurses station should include areas for medical charting, administrative duties, and storage of supplies, and it should be near handwashing facilities.

Several support functions must be convenient to both the nurses station and the exam rooms. The medication preparation area should be within, or at least within sight of, the nurses station. The nourishment station may be outside of the nurses station, but it must be conveniently located. The nurses working on the unit should also have easy access to a staff toilet and lounge. Clean supplies and linen may be kept in a single clean utility room. The soiled utility room should contain a work area, a storage place for soiled linen, a waste receptacle, and a clinical service sink. Wheelchairs and stretchers should be stored in alcoves or equipment storage rooms and not in corridors.

The activity room is a popular gathering place within a long-term care facility. Some of the amenities that are desirable include natural light, views, and flexibility of layout. Since many residents may be somewhat restricted physically, the exposure to natural light and views provides an orientation to time of day and season. Access to outdoor courtyards can also be beneficial to residents, since it reduces the closed-in feeling many residents experience during their long lengths of stay. The layout may include both quiet and noisy activity areas. The areas may need a physical or acoustical separation to mitigate conflict of activities. The quiet area could be used for reading, watching television, or listening to music. The noisy area could be used for games or other social activities. Long-term care facilities are often able to attract volunteer groups that provide various kinds of entertainment, such as choir groups. It is suggested that this be considered when planning the area.

Design Considerations

Long-term care facilities must be designed specifically with residents in mind. Many of the residents suffer with mobility, hearing, seeing, and equilibrium problems. Consequently, many design issues need to be resolved. For example, it is important that corridors be equipped with handrails on both sides and have minimal protrusions so as to reduce bumping and tripping. Sharp edges, slippery floor finishes, and tripping hazards are unacceptable. Walls should be protected from wheelchair hubs and footpads to prevent unsightly damage. Changes in floor levels and communicating stairs should be avoided. Floor patterns must be as unconfusing as possible to those with eyesight problems, who may interpret darker colors as steps or level changes. Contrasting colors at the wall base assist those with seeing problems in identifying the change of planes. Contrasting colors for door frames can help in the identification of openings. Doorways should be adequate for passage by patients in wheelchairs, walkers, canes, and other orthotic or prosthetic devices. Graphics should be easily readable and easy to find. Design features that aid orientation and wayfinding are generally desirable.

BUILDING SUPPORT SERVICES

A long-term care facility needs certain support functions to provide for proper delivery of care. These functions have their own space requirements, including food preparation and distribution areas, general storage, a housekeeping area, and employee facilities.

Dietary

The dietary services area includes a receiving area, refrigerated and dry food storage, a preparation area, a serving and dining area, a clean up and washing area, a staff toilet, and a waste removal area. Distribution of food, either through a servery or tray carts, should be planned carefully.

Meals can be served in a central dining area, in the activity area of a nursing unit, or in the resident's room. They can also be delivered to nursing units using thermal trays or hot and cold carts. Dietary services are an important component of long-term care from both a clinical and an enjoyment perspective.

General Storage

General storage consists of a receiving dock, breakdown area, work area for the purchasing clerk, and general storage area. Supplies are delivered by a variety of trucks, including 18-wheelers, semi-tractors, bobtails, and vans, so it is important that the dock facilities be flexible. The breakdown area is usually adjacent to the dock and is used to unpack larger containers. A trash dumpster is usually nearby for discarding waste. The purchasing clerk typically has a view of the dock area, the general storage area, and the dispatchment of items from the stores. The general storage area includes open shelves accessible by corridor rows. Secured storage may be required for more expensive items to prevent pilfering.

Housekeeping Area

The housekeeping area is a storage area for cleaning supplies and some cleaning equipment, such as floor buffers and vacuum cleaners. The housekeeping area is augmented by janitor's closets located conveniently throughout the facility.

Employee Facilities

Employee facilities within long-term care facilities vary significantly depending on number of employees. In many cases, the facilities consist only of a lounge and toilets. However, larger facilities will also contain locker and shower areas. This area should be designed according to program need.

Engineering Services

Engineering services are responsible for operating and maintaining heating, ventilation, and air conditioning systems. General maintenance is usually also one of the responsibilities. Grounds maintenance may be contracted out or provided on site by engineering services.

MECHANICAL, ELECTRICAL, LIGHTING, AND PLUMBING DESIGN CONSIDERATIONS[*]

General Considerations

Support systems, such as the mechanical, electrical, lighting, and plumbing systems, are often overlooked in relation to the overall architecture of a long-term health care facility until they cease to function properly. In most cases, the users are the elderly, and this simple fact is neglected by many support system designers. The physical problems of the elderly, such as decreased vision, decreased hearing, and arthritis, should affect the selection of engineering systems. Yet the

---

[*]This section is contributed by Rick Rome, P.E., CCRD Partners, Dallas, Texas.

high standards and intricate design details used for hospital facilities are usually not required for long-term facilities.

Another support systems design issue sometimes overlooked concerns building codes and state standards. Several states do not have separate standards for long-term facilities. In many other states, these standards are simply modified hospital standards. In all cases, these standards prescribe what is minimally acceptable in the design of the systems. However, many designers use these standards as if they reflected the best options available. Combine this with the fact that many of the standards are based on young to middle-aged users rather than senior citizens and it is no wonder that many inferior systems are designed and installed.

Mechanical Systems

The mechanical systems comprise the heating, ventilating, and air conditioning systems and the various subsystems that support them. The majority of the basic design concepts for these systems are established by the American Society of Heating, Refrigeration and Air Conditioning Engineers, the local building codes, and state standards.

- The design temperature for the heating season should be 75°F to compensate for the increased sensitivity of older people to colder temperatures.
- Insulated and tinted glass should be used in the rooms to limit the temperature gradient at the glass and to reduce the glare experienced in the room.
- Unlike state standards for hospitals, many state standards for long-term care facilities do not specify the filtration efficiency that the supply air to the rooms should have. Eighty percent final filters should be considered for the supply air, which matches most state requirements for patient rooms.
- Many states do not specify the number of air changes of outside air that should be introduced into each room. It is recommended that a minimum of two changes of outside air with six changes of supply air per hour be provided. This should adequately ventilate the space and prevent stale air.
- Exhaust air change rates of two to four per hour should be provided to reduce the institutional odors that are often experienced.
- Heat lamps in the bathrooms provide the elderly with additional comfort after bathing.
- Air supply diffusers should be designed for low terminal velocities in the range of 25 feet per minute, thus reducing the feeling of drafts within the space.
- Thermostats with larger numbers should be utilized for ease of viewing by residents.

Electrical Systems

Electrical power and special systems in long-term care facilities are very tightly controlled by NFPA 70 (National Electric Code), with little room for variation. Additional considerations are discussed below.

- Electrical outlets should be located 24 inches above the finished floor for easier accessibility.
- Two TV outlets should be provided in each room, one 12 inches below the ceiling for a wall bracket location and the other 24 inches above the floor for mounting a TV on a stand.
- Emergency nurse call switches should be provided in two locations—one at the bed and one in the bathroom. Integration of lighting, television, and intercom controls into the call station at the bed is recommended.
- When establishing the fire alarm system for the facility, consideration should be given to the reduced hearing capacity of the elderly. Solutions include decreasing the space between speakers, providing higher wattage speakers, and locating smoke alarms in the resident's rooms.

Lighting Systems

When considering lighting for the living areas in a long-term care facility, care should be devoted to providing lighting that renders colors truly and gives character to the room. In addition, proper placement of light fixtures, either in the ceiling or on the wall, can provide an appropriate stimulus for the residents.

- Because of the illumination needs of the elderly, maximum illumination levels of 50 foot-candles should be provided in the living and bed areas, and 25–30 foot-candles in the corridors.
- Proper emergency lighting in the rooms and corridors can assist in preventing any confusion. Corridors should be designed for an emergency lighting level of 3–5 foot-candles instead of the more common 1 foot-candle level.
- Glare caused by a strong light source or windows at the end of a hallway can confuse an elderly person and obscure the definition of the space. This problem can be minimized by utilizing diffused light sources.
- Aging eyesight impacts the ability to perceive depth and discriminate details. The eye also has a difficult time adjusting to lighting changes. To aid with these problems, sudden changes in lighting level should be avoided. Moving from a dim corridor into a bright room can cause temporary blindness and

possibly even cause a trip or fall. Provision of lighted vestibules between a bright room and dimmer corridors can minimize such problems.

- Light fixtures that provide true color rendition are preferable, particularly in resident bathrooms.
- The use of illuminated light switches is recommended because of the limited night vision of many of the elderly.

Plumbing Systems

Plumbing systems are tightly controlled by the local building codes, the state health codes, and the National Fire Protection Association.

- Wrist blade faucet trim is recommended on all patient lavatories.
- Installation of a fixed or fold-down seat in the tub or shower should be considered. A detachable spray head is recommended for bathing.
- A slip-resistant finish on the floor of the tub or shower should be provided, with integral grab bars on the walls.
- The domestic hot water temperature should not be higher than 110°F, nor lower than 100°F.

CONSTRUCTION OPTIONS

There are a variety of construction approaches available in delivering the completed long-term care facility. The most common has been the conventional design-bid-construct approach. This approach follows a sequential pattern: First the architect and engineers prepare design documents; next general contractors submit bids; then a construction contract is awarded, typically to the lowest bona fide bid submitted; and finally the construction phase begins. The primary advantage of this approach is that the organization receives a firm cost before construction begins, although there is no assurance that bids will be within the established budget.

An alternative approach is to establish a design-construct team that includes the contractor. The contractor is thus involved during the design phase and has the ability to provide a negotiated construction contract with a guaranteed maximum price after the full project scope is established. In this approach, construction management techniques are often utilized. Construction management is the process of including construction expertise in the formative stages of a project in order to provide construction concept and cost-control input. The construction manager is responsible for cost estimates and budget control, design review for constructability, construction scheduling, prepurchasing of critical materials and equipment, and direction of all construction activities. When appropriate, the design-construct team approach affords the opportunity to start construction before all design documents are complete.

A third alternative is the design-build approach, where a single-source "turn-key" organization or a consortium consisting of an architect and a contractor is hired to develop a building design and to provide a fixed price. Since plans are typically in a preliminary form when the fixed price is established, a greater level of risk is placed on the builder, and there is the possibility that the quality of the construction may be reduced as unknown costs appear.

Variations or combinations of these methods are possible, depending on specific contract requirements. The advantages and disadvantages of available approaches must be weighed in light of the facility's needs before a plan of action tailored to the specific requirements can be initiated.

COST ESTIMATING

Throughout the design of a long-term care facility, estimates of probable construction and development costs should be reviewed in order to control the cost of the completed project. Costs per square foot are often quoted, but the variety of components included may differ. As a result, comparison of costs per square foot of various projects can be misleading.

It is recommended that cost control be approached by formulating a total project budget containing not only construction costs but all other developmental investments made by the long-term care facility. A common format for budgeting includes the following.

- *Building cost.* Typically the cost for the structure and all internal space and systems. This cost typically includes expenditures for all construction within five feet of the building exterior.
- *Site development cost.* Commonly includes cost of all construction work outside of the five-foot building line. This construction consists of non-building development such as extensions of existing utility services, new utility services, site lighting, grading, walks, drives, parking lots, and landscaping.
- *Fixed equipment cost.* Includes cost of all items that are installed before completion of the building and that are a part of the construction contract, such as lockers, food service equipment, laundry equipment, and any medical equipment fixed to the building.

- *Construction cost.* The sum of the building cost, site development cost, and fixed equipment cost, with appropriate provision for inflation and estimating contingencies.
- *Land cost.* All costs of land, including purchase price and cost of site preparation, not included in the construction cost.
- *Movable equipment cost.* Includes the cost of depreciable equipment that typically has five years of life or more and is not normally purchased through construction contracts. Movable equipment comprises large items of furniture and equipment that have a reasonably fixed location in the building but are capable of being moved.
- *Professional fees.* Fees for services provided by various professionals involved in the project development, including architectural and engineering services.
- *Owner's contingency.* Funds set aside to provide a buffer to absorb normal growth in schematic design and design development, variations in bidding, unforeseeable construction conditions, and change orders.
- *Administrative cost.* Includes costs for such items as soil tests, site survey, legal fees, printing costs, and related expenses that the owner must pay in connection with building construction.
- *Financing cost.* Cost of interim financing that may be required for land acquisition and construction. Estimates of this cost should be established.
- *Total project cost.* The sum of all development costs listed above.

Not only is it necessary to prepare a detailed budget initially and have all members of the design team and the owner in full agreement on it, but it is also necessary to update the estimate often to incorporate current selections of building elements and systems and to confirm current prices in the marketplace.

EMERGING DESIGN CONSIDERATIONS

Long-term care facilities are facing unprecedented change. Demographically, our population is growing older and will be requiring more long-term care than ever before. Concurrently, hospital reimbursement is encouraging shorter and shorter lengths of stay—thereby encouraging transfer to long-term care facilities. As hospitals become super acute tertiary facilities, long-term care facilities will become more like hospitals of the past. In fact, many new hospitals that have moved to new quarters are converting their old buildings into various types of long-term care facilities. Many of these facilities are offering new services, including care for individuals with Alzheimer's disease, head injuries, and cancer.

In general, the acuity of the long-term care residents' conditions is increasing. Many facilities are also providing a hybrid of various services to accommodate residents' needs. As reimbursement allows long-term care facilities to provide a setting for extended care, these facilities over time will play a larger role in the delivery of health care services.

The design of long-term care facilities provides a unique challenge, since the care needs of residents must be balanced against their ongoing desire for the highest level of independence possible. Facilities can and should provide an attractive homelike ambience rather than the more common institutional atmosphere. In addition, careful attention must be given to making provisions for the full continuum of long-term care in order to support the variation in level of independence.

The architect should be involved in new facility development early on in order to assist in addressing the myriad issues that arise throughout the planning of a project. Siting the buildings; sizing the complex; establishing the appropriate layout; choosing building materials, finishes, and mechanical and electrical systems; and establishing reasonable construction cost expectations are all part of developing long-term care facilities that will effectively serve their residents.

As the population in the United States continues to mature, the long-term care facility will continue to emerge as a major type of health care building. The expanded need for new and updated facilities will provide the opportunity to develop facility designs that recognize and support resident dignity and contribute to the improvement of care.

NOTES

1. *AIA Document B-141—Owner/Architect Agreement* (Washington, D.C.: American Institute of Architects, 1987 edition).
2. American Hospital Association, *Selection of Architects for Health Facility Projects* (Chicago: American Hospital Association, 1975).
3. J.A. Wilkes, *Encyclopedia of Architecture* (New York: Wiley, 1988).
4. American Institute of Architects, *Guidelines for Construction and Equipment of Hospital and Medical Facilities,* 1987 ed. (Washington, D.C.: American Institute of Architects Press, 1987).

Case Study 13-1

Planning a Child-Care Center

Seth B. Goldsmith

The Good Folks Nursing Center of Northampton, Massachusetts, is a 150-bed skilled nursing facility. The administration is interested in renovating the facility's empty 1,500-square-foot general storeroom into a day-care center for children of employees (and other children, if necessary). A marketing study indicates that there is a need for these child-care services and that if the home opens an attractive and well-staffed facility there should be enough demand to make the project self-supporting. However, the administrator is uncertain about regulatory impediments to such a project and is interested in receiving a memo that details likely regulatory problems. Relevant regulations appear in Exhibits 13-1-1 through 13-1-3.

* * *

Exercise

1. Prepare a memo to the administrator detailing the feasibility of the home developing a day-care center in light of the attached regulations.

Exhibit 13-1-1 Code of Massachusetts Regulations

105 CMR 151.500 Storage Areas:

(A) General Storage. A general storage room or rooms shall be provided in each facility with a total of at least 10 square feet per bed for 100 percent of the total beds authorized.

281

Exhibit 13-1-2 City of Northampton Use Regulations

Section 5.1—Applicability of Use Regulations. Except as provided in this Ordinance, no building, structure, or land shall be used except for the purposes permitted in the district as described in this article. Any use not listed shall be construed to be prohibited. Uses permitted by right, by special permit, or by a variance granted under the provisions of Section 10.9, shall be subject, in addition to the use regulations contained in the Article, to all of the other provisions of the Ordinance.

Section 5.2—Table of Use Regulations. The Table of Use Regulations [see Table 13-1-1] is hereby declared to be a part of this Ordinance. In the Table, the following designations shall apply:

"A"   shall designate uses allowed by right in the district indicated.

"SP" shall designate uses allowed in the district indicated, but only with a special permit granted by the Zoning Board of Appeals subject to the provisions of Articles X and XI.

"PC" shall designate uses allowed in the district indicated, but only with a special permit granted by the City Council subject to the provisions of Articles X and XI.

"PB" shall designate uses allowed in the district indicated, but only with a special permit from the Planning Board subject to the provisions of Articles X and XI.

"—"   shall designate uses not allowed in the district indicated.

Any use that is accessory to a principal use allowed under the Table of Use Regulations shall be allowed only in connection with the bona fide operation of a principal use allowed under the Table of Use Regulations, and subject to the provisions of Section 5.3 where applicable.

Note. See also:

Article VI for dimension and density regulations

Article VII for sign requirements

Article VIII for parking and loading regulations

Article X.11 for Site Plan Review/Approval requirements

Section 5.3—Accessory Uses. Any use that is accessory to a principal use allowed by right shall be allowed only in connection with such allowed principal use. Any use that is accessory to a principal use allowed by special permit, and that is not specifically included in the original special permit, shall be allowed only after issuance of a new special permit. Cessation of a principal use shall require cessation of any accessory use that is not otherwise allowed as a principal use. The Building Inspector shall be responsible for determining what uses are principal, and what uses are accessory.

Section 10.10—Special Permits. Certain uses, structures, or conditions are designated within the Table of Use Regulations as requiring a special permit. Such permit shall be granted only after application to a hearing by the special permit granting authority and subject to the provisions of Chapter 40A of the Massachusetts General Laws and this Ordinance. The special permit granting authority responsible for hearing a particular proposal shall be that board or other entity designated by the coding in the Table of Use Regulations. In situations where there is no specific board indicated as having the authority to issue a special permit, the special permit granting authority shall be the Board of Appeals.

continues

Exhibit 13-1-2 continued

1. Application for a special permit shall be made to the Building Inspector on forms provided for that purpose, accompanied by the required fee. Specific rules governing the application and fee shall be adopted by each special permit granting authority along with its rules of procedure and shall be applicable to those special permits that are under its jurisdiction. When the application has been received in a completed form as defined by said rules, a copy shall be forwarded to the City Clerk. The stamp of the City Clerk shall designate the date of filing. Copies shall also be delivered to the special permit granting authority, to the Planning Department, and to such other departments and boards as may be determined in the rules of the special permit granting authority.

2. Special permits shall only be issued following public hearings held within sixty-five (65) days after filing of an application. Advertising and notice of hearing shall be conducted by the Planning Department subject to the rules of procedure adopted by the special permit granting authority having responsibility for the particular proposal in question. Costs of advertising and notification shall be paid by the special permit granting authority.

3. Before granting an application for a special permit, the special permit granting authority, with regard to the nature and condition of all adjacent structures and uses, and the district within which the same is located, shall find all of the following general conditions to be fulfilled:

   (a) The use requested is listed in the Table of Use Regulations as a special permit in the district for which application is made or is so designated elsewhere in this Ordinance.

   (b) The requested use bears a positive relationship to the public convenience or welfare.

   (c) The requested use will not create undue traffic congestion or unduly impair pedestrian safety.

   (d) The requested use will not overload any public water, drainage, or sewer system or any other municipal system such an extent that the requested use or any developed use in the immediate area or in any other area of the City will be unduly subjected to hazards affecting health, safety, or the general welfare.

   (e) Any special regulations for the use as set forth in Article XI are fulfilled.

   (f) The requested use will not unduly impair the integrity of character of the district or adjoining zones, nor be detrimental to the health, morals, or general welfare. The use shall be in harmony with the general purpose and intent of the Ordinance.

4. The special permit granting authority shall also impose, in addition to any applicable conditions specified in this Ordinance, such additional conditions as it finds reasonably appropriate to safeguard the neighborhood or otherwise serve the purposes of this Ordinance, including, but not limited to, the following: front, side, or rear yards greater than the minimum required by this Ordinance; screening buffers or planting strips, fences, or walls, as specified by the special permit granting authority; modification of the exterior appearance of the structures; limitation upon the size, number of occupants, method and time of operation, time duration of permit, or extent of facilities; traffic features in accordance with the regulations of loading or other special features beyond the minimum required by this Ordinance. Such conditions shall be imposed in writing, and the applicant may be required to post bond or other security for compliance with said conditions in an amount satisfactory to the special permit granting authority.

Table 13-1-1 Table of Use Regulations

	District												
	Residential					Business				Industrial			Conser.
Principal Use	RR	SR	UR-A	UR-B	UR-C	CB	GB	HB	WB	GI	SI	BP	SC
—Medical center, including accessory medical research and associated facilities													
—Automotive repair or automobile service station													
—Pool or billiards hall, bowling alley, amusement arcade, teen center													
Home occupations	SP	SP	SP	SP	SP	A	A	SP	A	—	SP	SP	—
Tourist home/bed and breakfast	SP	SP	SP	SP	SP	—	—	—	SP	—	—	SP	—
Community Facilities													
Church or other religious use or any educational use that is religious, sectarian, denominational, or public	A	A	A	A	A	A	A	A	A	A	A	A	—
Any other private school, college, or university	SP	SP	SP	SP	SP	SP	—	—	SP	—	—	SP	SP
Private day nursery care or kindergarten (licensed or unlicensed)	SP	SP	SP	SP	SP	SP	SP	—	SP	—	—	SP	PC
Family day care (in the home)	SP	SP	SP	SP	A	A	—	A	A	—	—	SP	PC
Membership club	SP	SP	SP	SP	SP	A	A	A	A	—	A	SP	—
Outdoor commercial recreation use	A	A	A	A	—	A	A	A	A	PC	A	SP	SP
Municipal facility	A	A	A	A	A	A	A	A	A	A	A	A	PC
Heavy public use (See Section 11.6)	PC	PC	PC	PC	PC	PC	PC	PC	PC	PC	PC	PC	PC
City or nonprofit cemetery, including any crematory therein	A	A	A	A	A	—	—	—	—	—	—	A	—
Historical association or society (may include the residence of a caretaker)	A	A	A	A	A	SP	SP	SP	SP	A	A	A	SP
Hospital	SP	SP	SP	SP	SP	SP	SP	SP	SP	A	A	A	—
Facilities for essential services	A	A	A	A	A	A	A	A	A	A	A	A	SP
Power plant	—	—	—	—	—	A	—	—	—	PC	A	—	—
Municipal parking lot or structure	PC	PC	PC	PC	PC	PC	PC	PC	PC	PC	PC	—	PC
Bridge, tunnel	PC	PC	PC	PC	PC	PC	PC	PC	PC	PC	PC	—	PC
Private utility, substation, or similar facility or building	SP	SP	SP	SP	SP	SP	SP	SP	SP	SP	SP	SP	SP
Small-scale hydroelectric generation	SP	SP	SP	SP	SP	SP	SP	SP	SP	SP	SP	SP	SP

A: allowed by right; PC: allowed by special permit from the City Council; —: not allowed; SP: allowed by special permit from Zoning Board of Appeals; PB: allowed by special permit from the Planning Board.

Chapter 14

Adult Day Care

Richard S. Lamden, Concetta M. Tynan, and Janice Warnke

As advanced health care improves and increases the longevity of older persons, so do the options for care. In the forefront of the rapidly growing home and community-based services is adult day care (also referred to as adult day health or adult day health care). This often underutilized service provides a unique setting for persons who require some assistance with tasks of daily living but do not need 24-hour care. Through the provision of a structured day program in a safe, supervised setting, functionally impaired elderly and disabled adults are able to remain in the community, and caregiving families can maintain their employment. The provider notion of prevention is the mainstay of adult day care. Through early involvement in a program, a client can maintain some independence while gaining a renewed sense of self-worth. The large costs, both financial and human, when nursing home placement is premature and inappropriate force society to seek and utilize new alternatives.

Inherent in the continuum of care philosophy is the premise that services provided must meet the individuals' needs and be offered in the least restrictive environment. It is incumbent upon service providers to be aware of options available so that clients can be directed and referred to the service that can best meet their needs.

THE HISTORY OF ADULT DAY CARE

Adult day care, in the form of day hospitalization, originated in Europe and was implemented most successfully in Great Britain under the pioneering direction of Lionel Cosin. Responsible for the first developments in the United States in the 1960s, Cosin developed a therapeutic day program at Cherry Hospital in Goldsboro, North Carolina, that was intended to prepare patients for discharge by teaching and promoting independent living skills. Early expansion of centers was due, in part, to the efforts of a grass roots movement that pushed for recognition and funding. However, development of new centers was inhibited as a result of the general lack of expertise regarding the concept and implementation of adult day care.

The advent of Title XIX and XX reimbursement during the 1960s allowed low-income elderly to begin accessing the services in small numbers. The competition for limited funding with other essential services, particularly nursing homes, caused slow growth and center closures. In spite of difficult beginnings, centers expanded from a mere 15 in 1973 to over 2,100 currently. A major force shaping the future and destiny of adult day-care services was the development of national standards in 1984 by the National Institute of Adult Day Care (NIAD). This organization, a constituent unit of the National Council on the Aging (NCOA), has from its inception strived not only to increase the visibility of adult day care but also to set forth guidelines for practitioners as an impetus toward professionalism.

DEFINING THE CONCEPT

Adult day care fills the gap between loosely structured senior centers and full-time residential care. It is important to differentiate adult day care from the other two types of services. Both senior centers and adult day care offer meals, recreation, and socialization. The latter, however, has as its main framework an individual plan of care, and it serves more impaired clients. The primary distinctions between adult day care and nursing homes are the amount of time individuals use the services and the acuity level. Adult day care, as the name implies, provides care during daytime hours. The client returns to his or her residence at the end of the day.

Having been developed as a fragmented service defined according to treatment emphasis (e.g., medical, psychiatric, or social), adult day care emerged with a lack of direction and multiple types of programs. Although programs were flexible and responsive to the specific needs of clients and locales, the diverse models of care created confusion. As the representative body of the providers, NIAD established generic guidelines and standards intended to be used as a tool by practitioners for defining, planning, and implementing quality care:

> Adult day care is a community-based group program designed to meet the needs of adults with functional impairments through an individual plan of care. It is a structured, comprehensive program that provides a variety of health, social and related support services in a protective setting during any part of a day but less than 24-hour care.
>
> Individuals who participate in adult day care attend on a planned basis during specific hours. Adult day care assists its participants to

remain in the community, enabling families and other caregivers to continue caring at home for a family member with an impairment.[1]

Recognizing the program diversity necessary to adapt to the changing needs of the population served, the generic position is emerging as the dominant model. Regardless of definitions, the center and staff must be able to respond fully to the needs of the clients.

PLANNING AND DEVELOPING THE SERVICE

Adult day care serves a broad range of people. It can provide structure and mental stimulation for a person with Alzheimer's. It can provide socialization, nutrition, and health monitoring for someone who is frail and isolated. Or it can offer rehabilitation and respite for a young stroke victim and the working spouse.

Though characteristics vary, clients tend to fall into two general categories: (1) adults with emotional, mental, or physical impairments who require structured care in order to maintain independent functioning, and (2) adults with disabilities who require restorative and rehabilitative services in order to attain maximum independent functioning. It is necessary for the adult day-care center to define the target population it intends to serve so that programs and staff can meet the clients' needs.

Prior to developing an adult day-care center, it is prudent to thoroughly analyze the reasons for wanting to establish it. Existing organizations need to examine their mission statement and goals to ascertain the need for and compatibility of this service. New organizations need to carefully assess the appropriateness of developing a day-care facility. Since adult day care is not typically a high revenue producer, the rationale may be to create a continuum of care so that clients can be retained in the system. Independent centers may focus more on community needs.

Planning and developing an adult day-care center begins with a feasibility study. This is not as difficult as it sounds. One needs to locate individuals who represent the community in the area of services for the aging and set up a meeting to discuss the development of a facility. An initial brainstorming session could evolve into the creation of a formal planning committee.

The planning committee should undertake a needs and feasibility assessment to answer such questions as these:

- Is there a need? Is there a gap in the continuum of care? Is there a target group needing this service?
- What funding sources are available for maintaining the program? Are they private or public?

- Is there community support for such a program?
- What is the best location? Is it accessible to those who will be attending? If the program will be housed in an existing building, how much renovation is necessary to meet regulations?
- Is the program accessible by public transportation? Is it going to provide transportation for clients?
- Will the staff necessary for the program be hard to find?
- What, if any, is the competition?

After these questions are addressed, the committee might then turn its attention to the paper work and filings necessary to become a legal entity, including

- the preparation of a pro forma budget, including startup costs
- the identification of job categories and the development of job descriptions and personnel policies
- the creation of a plan for publicity and marketing
- the development of admission policies
- the establishment of a certification or licensing process and the development of operating policies

In planning for the development of a physical structure to house adult day care, several steps should be taken. Licensing and regulation play a vital role in the implementation process.

In many states, the department of health services (or its counterpart agency) usually is the agency responsible for the adoption, administration, and enforcement of regulations. It is the purpose of the department to supplement the efforts of conscientious providers by establishing and enforcing minimum standards of operation, including standards for facilities, equipment, and personnel.

Organizations contemplating the establishment of an adult day-care program should complete and submit an application requesting licensure to the department of health services, usually on a form prescribed by the department. Generally licenses are issued annually.

Any change of ownership, administration, or location of a licensed adult day-care program will require a new application for licensure.

Upon receipt of the application for licensure, it is customary for the licensing agency to schedule an appointment to inspect and investigate the space, the planned program activities, and the standards of care being proposed by the facility.

A well-designed facility is vital in providing and supporting adult day-care activities. In fact, the environment plays a significant role in improving the clients' social interaction and functional capacity. Of prime consideration in planning a facility is safety and security. The clients should be able to move through the center with ease.

The facility should be warm, inviting, and homelike and should allow for the performance of activities of daily living, promote social contact, and stimulate the visual, tactile, auditory, and olfactory senses.

The site should have sufficient space to accommodate the number of clients being served. It is common practice for state licensure to require a certain number of square feet per client, excluding offices, reception area, restrooms, and hallways.

The site should have adequate access for handicapped vans, which may be used to drop off clients. It should be within easy reach of public transportation and not be located on a very busy road, making ingress into the area difficult. There should be spaces identified for handicapped parking and a ramp for easy access to the building without the need to climb stairs.

The site should also have a covered area for exterior recreation where clients can enjoy gardening and other activities. The area should have outdoor furniture and benches for seating. The reception area should make visitors and clients feel welcome and be attractively decorated with soft colors. The reception area serves as a central center where clients are checked in. A phone should be placed in this area for clients to use if they need to make a call. A closet nearby for outer garments and rainwear is a nice convenience.

Since some clients may be wheelchair-bound, there should be wheelchair-turning space of at least 5' × 5' in entrance doors and restrooms, door opening widths of at least 32", thresholds level with the floor, lever-type controls on faucets and doors, grab bars at all toilets, angled mirrors at sinks, and at least 29" clearance under sinks and 27" clearance under tables.

Adjustable blinds to protect elderly persons' eyes from the glare of sunlight should also be considered, as should the use of parabolic filters in fluorescent lighting. Chairs should be vinyl laminated with high backs and round arms, and there should be a clear kick space below the front edge of the seat. Tables should be round and laminated. All furniture edges and corners should be rounded because of the possibility of falls.

An adult day-care center includes a kitchen for the preparation of meals and snacks. The kitchen may be designed for therapeutic use (e.g., helping impaired adults to relearn cooking skills).

Because the elderly need fluid frequently, a water fountain (handicap accessible) should also be provided. And, of course, a fire extinguisher should be readily available (usually in the kitchen area).

The equipment needed for day care includes most equipment that would be customary for a reception area, offices, a nurse's office, restrooms, a kitchen, a conference room, and classrooms. In purchasing equipment, it is necessary to keep in mind the new ADA rules as they relate to the handicapped.

Equipment for activities might include beach balls, adaptive sports equipment, quilting supplies, puzzles, frames, books, ceramic supplies, games, bingo prizes, seasonal decorations, paints, theatrical props, a movie projector, a television, a VCR, a stereo, a radio, a computer, a sewing machine, a kiln, and a large clock.

Minimum staffing is in most cases determined by state licensure. Because of financial constraints, the team consists of professionals (social worker, registered nurses, etc.) and nonprofessionals working together, including a director, a secretary (depending on size of the center), an activity coordinator, an activity assistant, and in some cases a certified nursing assistant. There should usually be two staff members for the first ten clients. With larger clienteles, the ratio of staff to clients should be 1:8. The number of positions will vary depending on the size and scope of the program.

At the time of the licensure inspection, it would be beneficial to have a personnel record for each employee. The record should include a verification of an annual tuberculosis skin test, an annual chest x-ray, or a physician's statement noting no symptomatic evidence of current pulmonary tuberculosis disease and current documentation of certification for CPR and first-aid training. A food handler certificate should be included for staff who are responsible for serving and supervising meals or snacks if the local health department requires it.

The facility should have adequate insurance, including the minimum property and casualty coverage applicable in the state as well as appropriate liability coverage.

Once the inspection has taken place and the license has been obtained, it must be conspicuously posted in the center. This license is not transferrable from facility to facility. Although the rule may vary slightly from state to state, a separate license is required for each location when more than one facility is operated by the same person or agency.

If a center is to achieve success, it must be attentive to the uniqueness of each new applicant entering the program. Like other needs-driven services (e.g., hospital care, nursing homes), adult day care is approached reluctantly by most consumers. Decisions for admission are generally executed by a family member, caregiver, or casemanager, and this often results in resistance. Integrating a new client requires forethought and sensitivity if maximum acceptance and adjustment are to be achieved.

During the initial inquiry, it is necessary to evaluate the appropriateness, needs, and interests of the potential client. A brief screening by the social worker can determine the functioning level of the applicant and type of intervention needed. A visit to the center is crucial for the applicant and family or caregiver so that the program can be explained and demonstrated. A home visit by a staff member can provide further insight into the applicant's need for service and can begin to establish a trusting relationship. A medical release, completed by the primary physician, indicating absence of tuberculosis should be obtained prior to or upon admission. Enrollment is completed when financial and transportation arrangements are finalized and admission documents and contracts are discussed, signed, and distributed.

Matching a staff person and a well-adjusted client with the new client for a minimum of one week can often ensure a positive transition. It is recommended that an interdisciplinary assessment (e.g., by activities, nursing, and social work staff) be completed within the first week so that a care plan can be developed. The assessment should include a health profile, a social history, a review of support systems, ADL (activities of daily living) skills, mental and emotional status, strengths, needs, activity interests, and community and financial resources. An initial discharge plan is developed that determines alternative services should the client leave the program. The plan incorporates input from each team member and provides the framework for all intervention. The selection of problems to be dealt with, goals, and approaches by each discipline allows for coordination of services and guides all staff activity. When possible, clients and families need to be involved so that full understanding and cooperation can be achieved.

IMPLEMENTING THE PROGRAM COMPONENTS

Having established how the center will serve the client, program implementation begins with a dual focus—on the goals and objectives of the program and on those of the client. With the core essential services in place (i.e., health monitoring, nutrition, personal care, social work, and therapeutic activities), the staff can concentrate on how to assist the client in complying with the plan of care in order to increase or maintain his or her functioning level.

Emphasis on wellness and health maintenance is the mainstay of the program. Although enrollment requires a physician's release and a tuberculosis test, many clients neglect routine medical care, thus hastening physical decline. Health supervision by the center's registered nurse, even only a few times per week, can help a client to maintain his or her capacity for self-care and community residence. The initial nursing assessment, which identifies the client's diagnosis, medical history, medications, diet, mobility, orientation, and bowel and bladder control, establishes the client's health status so that the nurse can observe and react to changes of condition. Monitoring of blood pressure, pulse, and weight is performed monthly. In compliance with physician's orders, medications, treatments, and supplemental feedings can be administered. Supportive nursing for colostomy or ileostomy maintenance, nail and foot care, gastrostomy tube feeding, bowel and bladder training, maintenance therapy, health monitoring, and so on, can also be made available. Acting as a liaison, the nurse communicates concerns to the primary physician and family or caregiver. If indicated, referrals are made to rehabilitation therapists and other health services in the community.

Health education is provided on an individual and group basis. The center's nurse is primarily responsible for any emergency care needed.

As a major component of health care for the elderly and disabled, good nutritional diets and habits are a necessity often neglected. The provision of a well-balanced meal or snack, even if just once a day, can ensure at the least a minimum level of nutrition. Prescribed therapeutic diets and supplements should be included in the center's menu. Clients needing feeding assistance or special adaptive equipment should be accommodated. A registered dietitian, either on staff or acting as a consultant, can provide the expertise necessary to properly monitor clients' diets. All staff, particularly direct care staff, should be present during snacks and meals to assist with and oversee food consumption. Cultural and ethnic preferences as well as seasonal and religious food celebrations need to be observed, if possible. For clients unable to prepare food at home, arrangements should be made for the provision of home-delivered meals.

Assistance with and training in activities of daily living (e.g., ambulating, bathing, dressing, grooming, and toileting) are essential if the functional capacity of clients is to be maintained or improved. Physical decline can often be delayed when independent functioning is encouraged. A functional status report completed by the registered nurse prior to admission and reviewed at care conferences is instrumental in determining the abilities and disabilities of the client. Direct care staff must be knowledgeable about safe body mechanics as they relate to transfer and ambulation. Heavy-care clients (e.g., those who need two-person transfers or who are bowel incontinent or total feeders) require special consideration.

Decline or loss of mental or physical functioning affects all aspects of a person's life, including family relationships. Increased dependence, functional losses, and role changes may cause stress and anxiety. The social worker is instrumental in helping the client and family to acknowledge and accept the need for services and to make a smooth transition into the program. Through individual and group counseling, feelings and issues can be discussed and resolved. Since many clients come to adult day care with numerous problems, referrals often need to be made to other community resources.

Diminished participation in social, recreational, and community activities promotes decline in personal growth and the ability to enjoy life. The goal of an activity program is to keep clients interested, involved, and active while at the center. Though providing fun and enjoyment is one objective, the underlying purpose is to stimulate and motivate individuals so they can reach their highest functional potential. All activities should be designed for persons with different goals and levels of ability. Selection of specific crafts, groups, games, field trips, entertainment, and so on, should be based on the individuals' needs and abilities. Staff expertise, environmental limitations, and budgetary constraints also must be considered.

Hamill and Oliver point out that "the purpose of therapeutic in contrast to diversional activities is to stimulate changes in the participants' ability from dysfunctional to functional."[2] Therefore, individualization of activities is vital. Initially and at each care conference the following objectives are focused on:

* identifying the client's current abilities
* preventing further deterioration
* improving function to the highest possible level

Appropriate activities are then identified and planned.

Transportation is an essential part of any adult day-care program. Without it, the program could not exist. In 1986, Von Behren conducted a study that uncovered a variety of transportation solutions.[3] In 56 percent of the centers, staff provided transportation, 32 percent of the centers contracted for transportation, while 10 percent relied on public transportation.

In those communities where special-needs transportation systems exist, it may be possible to engage the appropriate organizations in developing a transportation program. Some programs function more successfully by purchasing vehicles and developing their own transportation system. Many programs utilize a combination of transportation options. No method of transportation the adult day-care center chooses is without its problems, but the program that provides its own transportation tends to exercise more control over its operation.

The dynamic growth of adult day-care facilities over the past 20 years provides a clear indication that adult day care will be a vital part of the long-term care continuum. Although many models exist, this chapter has focused on the overall concept. The model used as the basis of the chapter is a large adult day-care program that serves approximately 80 people per day and is located on the same campus as a 161-bed nursing care facility. The adult day-care program has been in operation since 1967.

NOTES

1. National Council on the Aging, *National Institute on Adult Day Care, Standards and Guidelines for Adult Day Care,* 2d ed. (Washington, D.C.: National Council on the Aging, 1990), iv.

2. C.M. Hamill and R.C. Oliver, *Therapeutic Activities for the Handicapped Elderly* (Gaithersburg, Md: Aspen Publishers, Inc., 1980).

3. R. Von Behren, *Adult Day Care in America: Summary of a National Survey* (Washington, D.C.: National Council on the Aging, 1986), 19.

Day Center: Overempowerment

Janice Warnke

Recognizing the need for elderly clients to feel a sense of belonging and purpose, a new adult day care director took steps to ensure expanded opportunities for client input. The monthly resident council, whose agenda and meeting was formerly conducted by the staff, was turned over to newly elected client officers (i.e., president, secretary, and treasurer). Topics for discussion were generated by the officers, who encouraged the participants to share concerns, complaints, and ideas. At the behest of the president, committees were formed to address specific client issues (i.e., activities, finance, and food). Revenues generated from craft sales, which previously were part of the operational revenue, were maintained within the program and utilized to supplement the meager craft supply budget. A ledger was kept by the director's secretary of all account activity (sales and expenditures). At the monthly resident council meeting, the treasurer reported on all activity of the craft fund, and suggestions for future craft projects and purchases were elicited. As the year ensued, less interest was shown by the clients, and as ideas for spending the money waned, the fund continued to grow. At the end of December, the unspent $900.00 was closed out with the year's budget, thus leaving a zero balance. The status of the craft fund was explained by the director at the January resident council meeting. She encouraged clients to become more involved and cautioned them that unspent money at the end of that year would suffer the same fate. After several months had transpired, a controversy developed among some of the clients who were now wondering where "their" money went. The director held numerous meetings with the officers, finance committee members, and various clients to reiterate what had been previously explained. Confusion and anger over the money predominated the next resident council meeting. Numerous clients sent letters to the board president, executive vice president, and clergymen, with copies to the local daily newspaper. They alleged that the agency had stolen their money, and they wanted a full accounting.

* * *

Discussion Questions

1. By virtue of their mental and/or physical impairment(s), adult day care clients are unable to function independently within the community. Do these clients, who are unable to manage their own lives and require professional daytime services, have the ability to make decisions regarding craft funds?
2. If allowing client input promotes involvement and self-esteem, why were the results of the director's efforts so negative and problematic?
3. What was the basic flaw in the course of action taken by the director?
4. How could the situation have been handled differently to provide a better outcome?
5. Is the establishment of a resident council a good idea?
6. What learning benefits should directors derive from this experience?

Chapter 15

Assisted Living in Alternative Residential Environments

Anne K. Harrington

Assisted living is a "hot" concept in long-term care and aging. It's also the subject of considerable controversy. Some believe that it is an entirely new option for elders and represents the wave of the future in supportive residential living. Others think that it is merely a new phrase for housing and services that have been available for years. Without waiting for consensus, many state policy makers are working on plans to implement assisted living programs as they scramble to find alternatives to "budget buster" Medicaid accounts. This chapter sorts through some of the key issues and examines the significance of this new alternative for the nursing home industry.

WHAT IS ASSISTED LIVING? A MASSACHUSETTS CASE STUDY

Confusing Terminology

"Assisted living" is a phrase used by many (including the American Association of Homes for the Aging [AAHA]) to designate a wide variety of residence-with-supportive-services alternatives for older people. Places that offer assisted living services may be known as rest homes, board and care homes, group foster homes, continuing care retirement communities, elder housing, or congregate housing, to name just a few of the designations. Because they provide more than housing, assisted living settings can serve elders who are quite frail.

Note: The term "rest home" has been widely accepted and used for years. Some providers, however, feel that this language is outdated and somewhat misleading. These homes are no longer primarily a place of respite for people who may be discharged from a hospital prior to their return home. Although the term has been retained throughout this chapter because of its likely familiarity to readers, "assisted living facility" or "residential care facility" is more appropriate.

Source: Reprinted from *Continuum,* January/February, April, and June 1992, Association of Massachusetts Homes for the Aging, with permission of Anne Harrington, Ph.D. © 1992.

As defined by Robert Newcomer and Leslie Grant, this type of living (which they generically label "residential care") "refers to the provision by a non-relative of food, shelter, and some degree of protective oversight and/or personal care that is generally nonmedical in nature."[1]

By protective oversight and personal care, the authors mean supervising residents' medications, helping them with one or more of their functional needs such as bathing or grooming, cleaning residents' rooms, doing their laundry, and assisting with arranging transportation or other support services.

Not all would agree that assisted living should be so broadly defined, however. Advocates of a narrower definition often have specific characteristics in mind such as the arrangement of the physical space or the degree of personal choice and control that they feel is unique to assisted living.

While there is no universal agreement about its fundamental characteristics, perhaps more importantly, confusion about assisted living is due to ambiguity about the type and intensity of client needs, the quality of care, and the actual services provided in the different settings.

Using the broad definition of assisted living as applied to a traditional array of residential options for older people, for instance, are all rest homes or all board and care facilities or all continuing care retirement communities the same? Are they consistently different from each other in predictable ways—ways that consumers can readily understand? Looking at rest homes in particular, do all rest homes serve clients with similar physical and mental needs? Do they offer a menu of services that is the same from one setting to another? Do they cost the same? The answer to all of these questions is an emphatic no.

Rest Homes As Assisted Living

Massachusetts rest homes are as different from each other as the older residents who live in them. Some of them are very "upscale"; others cater to a moderate or a low-income clientele or a mixed population. Some of the buildings are small and homelike. Others are large and more impersonal. In some, the majority of the residents are the deinstitutionalized mentally ill. In others, the homes reflect the genteel tradition of a bygone era.

At the core of rest homes and other assisted living communities, however, is a mission to serve older people who are, by and large, physically healthy.

Jane Bellegarde, administrator of Merrimack River Valley House in Lowell, Massachusetts, talks about the historic mission of rest homes. In the past, the typical old age home served people who were mostly independent and able to take care of themselves but who needed general supervision, monitoring of medications, and some form of assistance with functional needs. Many seeking admission may also have been unable to continue to do housekeeping, meal preparation, and maintenance chores associated with living alone. At the time of admission, they were expected to be mentally alert, with only very mild confusion, if any, and able to walk and move around unassisted. As they got older, if some of the residents became more confused or developed a medical problem, they were moved to a nursing home. Others were able to live out their days in the home.

Although there have been many changes since then, today's rest homes and other forms of assisted living continue to see themselves as an important part of the continuum of elder care. As in the past, they believe that they offer a homelike residential experience for a largely independent population at a lower cost than a nursing home. By and large, most tend not to provide medical services, unless on a special basis or unless the home has nursing beds (and trained nursing staff).

Beyond this core of similarity, however, assisted living providers offer highly differentiated services in different kinds of settings to different populations at costs that can range from $30 a day to more than three times that amount, excluding extra supportive services (continuing care retirement communities excepted).

What Do State Regulations Say?

If the existence of state regulations is any measure, Massachusetts rest homes (or level IV resident care facilities, as they are called) *are* different from other types of assisted living. Unlike congregate housing and all the other residential alternatives, licensed level IV homes must conform to a significant amount of regulation and to preset reimbursement ceilings.

Let's start with the state's idea of what a rest home is. In Massachusetts, it is a facility that provides "a supervised supportive and protective living environment and support services incident to old age for residents having difficulty in caring for themselves and who do not require level II or III nursing care or other medically related services on a routine basis."[2] In other words, it's not a nursing home. It's a home that provides supportive services to people who do not have regular medical needs.

What about the staffing? What does the state require? One "responsible person" must be on the premises at all times. Not a nurse or a nurse aide. A responsible person. This is defined as a mature high school graduate 21 years or older who speaks English and the primary language spoken by residents. For homes with less than 20 beds, responsible persons should be available during the waking hours in a ratio of 1 person to 10 residents. For larger homes, a minimum of one responsible person should be available 24 hours a day for each unit (up to 60 beds).

What about medications? Who handles that? Can medications be self-administered? Perhaps. The regulations also allow for administration of certain medications by a person who has successfully completed one approved training course on dispensing medications. One course. Otherwise, a free-standing level IV home must have a licensed consultant nurse for 4 hours a month per unit, a consultant dietitian to review special diets every 3 months, and a cook "as needed." The nurse must review medications every 6 months and provide services to residents in the case of a "minor illness of a temporary nature." Also, social services should be provided as needed, along with 20 hours of activities "suited to the needs of residents."[3]

Although Massachusetts requirements for level IV homes cover many things, from the physical plant and equipment and supplies to how often the bed linen should be changed, rest homes are not much different from other types of assisted living environments when it comes to who is supposed to live and work there. What is offered is supposed to be based on the needs of residents who are more independent than frail. *(Note:* Community Support Facilities are a special type of licensed level IV home in Massachusetts. More than 50 percent of their residents have some mental illness diagnosis, and for that reason these facilities have many more regulations and staffing requirements than conventional level IV homes.)

Changing Needs—Increasing Frailty

Since July 1991, Massachusetts Medicaid officials have implemented a policy of making it more difficult for older people with "light care needs" to get into a nursing home. Rest homes are getting more referrals from people who have multiple needs. They are also seeing more dementia and emotional problems.

Rosalyn Piro, administrator of the Caldwell Home in Fitchburg, Massachusetts, is seeing people "with lots of dementia needs" as well as people who are incontinent. (Incontinence is a big issue for these facilities because of the demands for more staff, more laundry, more supplies, and hotter water. Traditionally, level IV facilities do not admit people who are incontinent.) In response to a hypothetical situation, she says that she might be willing to take in someone with mild dementia needs. She has a nurse consultant six hours a week and is able to provide "lots of personal care." In evaluating a person with dementia, she assesses her other residents' needs and considers how much supervision the applicant requires.

For Bellegarde in Lowell, Massachusetts, the new realities of who is seeking admission to her home cause her to "worry about the expectation level for level IVs." Applicants are more frail, sometimes confused or emotionally troubled, and some have "transfer assist" needs (i.e., they need help moving from one place to another). But in addition to more physical and cognitive needs, many requesting admission are in their 90s! Since the resident average age is already 88 years, she expects new residents will be pushing that average higher—and will require more services as well.

Valerie Emerton, administrator of the German Home in Lawrence, Massachusetts, sees the same change—people seeking admission who are in wheelchairs, others with oxygen or insulin requirements, and people who are incontinent.

Who Pays?

Funding sources have a lot to do with what kind of assisted living a person qualifies for and the services available in that setting. In HUD-financed elder housing, many residents receive monthly rent subsidies from the federal government. Until recently, however, federal assistance has not paid for supportive services, with the notable exception of HUD's Congregate Housing Services Program. (HUD has now acknowledged this need through a commitment to fund service coordinators, but matching demand to limited funds has been a vexing problem.) In Massachusetts-subsidized congregate housing, limited state home care dollars have restricted services to residents with the highest levels of frailty.

Unlike most other types of assisted living, rest homes offer a program of supportive services for *all* residents. Supplemental Security Income (SSI) and Emergency Aid to the Elderly, Disabled, and Children are two of the more common forms of public assistance that can help to defray expenses. If a person qualifies for SSI, for example, he or she must have income below approximately $720 a month and no more than $2,000 in assets. The state will supplement the difference between this income and the rate that the state allows the home to charge. Selling a home as part of "spending down" to qualify for SSI is common.

Massachusetts sets a cap on the rates that a licensed level IV home can charge its publicly subsidized residents. Unfortunately for level IV homes, the Massachusetts Rate Setting Commission uses a payment formula that reimburses facilities for costs based on what happened two years earlier. Consequently, if a home incurs increased costs, as many did in 1991 in response to tougher Medicaid nursing home eligibility requirements and frailer applicants to rest homes, these are not reflected in the state's allowable rates until two years later. There is no mechanism for appeal. Because the state maintains no historical data on resident health status, it has no information on which to base a rate adjustment due to changed needs.

State Policies for Community-Based Residential Programs

The Massachusetts example demonstrates that in many respects there is little to distinguish a rest home from a congregate home (defined as providing private or shared quarters along with some shared common space such as dining and socializing areas) or from a board and care home (an unlicensed boarding house with services). The major difference is the presence or absence of state regulation and licensure. (In licensed level IV homes, significant regulations apply as compared with other types of assisted living. Available penalties for breaking the rules include being cited by the state Department of Public Health, fines, delicensure or decertification, and, in very egregious circumstances, criminal prosecution.) The major similarity across these settings is the people whom they serve. Although there have been some changes in recent months, it is the same population of elders who are looking to get their needs met wherever they live! It is really habit and history that is causing rest homes to be viewed as down-sized nursing homes.

As Massachusetts implements two new programs—a group adult foster care program and a managed care program in publicly funded housing—important public policy questions emerge. What's going to happen in the rush to create new community-based alternatives to nursing homes? When personal care services are reimbursed through Medicaid's adult group foster care program, will more regulations be added to elderly housing to make *them* safer and more protective environments? Will they too become more medicalized and therefore more government controlled? Or will they be allowed to grow and diversify as elder housing and congregate housing and board and care homes have traditionally been allowed to do? And what about the state's policy for rest homes? What group of older people should they serve and what reimbursement is appropriate, given the level of need of their residents? Is it time for a more flexible state approach that incorporates rest homes as one type of assisted living?

WHAT'S BEHIND THE NEW BUZZWORDS: "HOSPITALITY MODEL," "CATERED LIVING," AND "RESIDENTIAL ALTERNATIVES"?

Imagine that you are a provider of services to older people and that you are in charge of a residence with supportive services. Most of your residents are in their eighties. Some are very independent. They may take public transportation, do volunteer work either in your facility or elsewhere, or drive their own cars. Many, though, are quite frail. They require some type of assistance—perhaps a reminder to take medications or assistance with meals, housekeeping, transportation, bathing, or getting dressed.

In this hypothetical scenario, is it possible to say with certainty what type of residential setting is being described? Is it a rest home? A board and care home? Congregate housing? Senior housing? A continuing care retirement community?

Without more information, it could be any of these settings. Knowledge of the needs of the residents and the services offered are typically not enough to determine which form of assisted living is being provided.

An identical floor plan could belong to a congregate housing site, a level IV facility (a rest home), or a board and care home. In these settings, each resident may have his or her own private room and shared common areas such as a dining room or a place to socialize with friends. Staffing patterns could also be similar—aides, kitchen staff, housekeeping staff, transportation staff. Nursing might be available on staff or as needed (through contracts with local home health agencies).

What if we add another piece of information? Our residence serves primarily private-pay clients. Does this help us to narrow it down? Not necessarily. All forms of assisted living may be offered on a private-pay basis. If, on the other hand, our residence serves a low or moderate income group, we have ruled out most continuing care retirement communities, which tend to serve a more affluent population.

If, after thorough investigation, we discover that this residence is regulated and licensed by the state and the facility is in Massachusetts, we are ready to solve the mystery. We have identified a rest home. Had we been told that it was an unregulated facility, we would still be in the dark. The possibilities would still include senior housing, congregate housing, board and care homes, and the non–health care areas of continuing care retirement communities.

The point is that there are many different types of assisted living settings offering services for independent, frail, and sometimes even very frail older people. Labels alone offer little help in identifying what goes on in them.

Just How New Is Assisted Living?

Housing with supportive services provided by a nonrelative (our definition of assisted living) has a long history, as we saw in the Massachusetts example. Terms like *senior housing, congregate housing,* and *rest home* were used to differentiate one form of supportive residential living from another. The fact that the physical layout and the needs of clients living in congregate housing were often very similar to those for rest homes and unlicensed homes was ignored. The variation from one rest home to another or from one congregate housing site to another was also ignored.

It was the differences between these environments that counted. After all, rest homes were state-regulated and licensed. They evolved from a more medicalized model of health care. Weren't they just a step down from nursing homes? What about much of the senior housing funded by the federal government in the 1960s? Weren't these residents really more independent? And weren't people living in congregate housing somewhere between independent living and "custodial" care—but closer to independence?

Beyond the different labels, funding sources, and government regulations or lack thereof, there was also an important reality for residents. They knew that if they developed more needs, they would have to move somewhere else. Where they went would depend on the level of assistance they required and the amount of money they had. Perhaps it would be to congregate housing or a rest home or a nursing home. But maintaining independence (or faking it) was as real as the fear of having to move someday.

To today's older consumer, the newer assisted living communities may seem entirely different. They frequently offer self-contained apartments. There may be more "amenities." Supportive services may be purchased separately or included in the monthly fees. Prices may be "upscale" and there may be an entrance fee in addition to the monthly fees. For residents, there's another crucial difference: It is okay to need assistance.

However, all assisted living environments, old or new, share a common philosophy that focuses on the independence of the resident and the residence itself as a person's home.

Shifting Priorities: Medical Model Is Out, Hospitality In

Government policy makers caught on. They knew all along that people living independently had a variety of unmet needs. However, it took a fiscal crisis of enormous proportions to begin a massive shift in outlook and funding priorities at the federal and state levels.

We are seeing evidence of that shift today. The new priorities are to create and fund nonmedicalized residential alternatives for independent and frail elders. To limit the use of nursing homes through changed Medicaid eligibility criteria and make them more like subacute hospitals. To keep the middle class from "spending down" to Medicaid and to recoup expended funds from their estate if they require publicly financed assistance. And to create "managed care" programs for older adults that hopefully prevent or postpone institutionalization. Driving it all is the government's fiscal motivation to save public dollars, limit spending, and restrict Medicaid access.

The medicalization of elder care is presumed to be the cause of budget buster state Medicaid programs. Consequently, the medical or hospital model has lost favor in the eyes of government policy makers, who now speak of its limited usefulness for the majority of older people. Studies are widely quoted that document older people's desire to live in their own homes. Nursing homes, solidly rooted in the medical model, are "out," appropriate only as a last resort. Protective, supervised environments are passé.

What's "in" is the hotel model. Maintaining independence through supportive services offered in a residential, homelike setting. Developing a contractual relationship between the individual who pays the rent or fee for housing and services and the provider.

The model has important implication for staff, who, like the hotel concierge, make arrangements for residents basically responsible for their own "evenings out." Implicitly and explicitly, the resident is the ultimate decision maker, responsible for requesting and using services and programs.

Licensure and Regulation

Assisted living requires a new set of ideas about state licensure and regulation. The medical model uses the acuity of the individual as its benchmark. Government reimbursement follows need, primarily defined in terms of health care. In Massachusetts nursing homes, the places of greatest need for chronic care, the case mix Medicaid reimbursement system uses a scoring system to identify residents as somewhere between "light" and "heavy" care and bases its reimbursement to facilities on these scores, with more money paid for heavier care residents.

Assisted living challenges all that. If a resident becomes very frail and wishes to remain at home, he or she may not have to go to a nursing home. Theoretically, that resident can live in an assisted living setting as long as he or she wishes to remain there, can pay for services, and is permitted to by the assisted living contract. A move may be unnecessary. Given the level of need that can be met in assisted living, acuity may not be the defining difference between regulated and unregulated environments. It all depends on what state regulations permit.

Consultant David Roush argues that a critical factor in future state decisions about whether a community is regulated or not should be the kind of relationship that gets structured between providers and older people. In assisted living environments, the relationship often works out as follows: "I (the consumer) am the decision maker. This is my home. I choose the services. I want you (the provider) to remind me to take my medications or help me to get dressed in the morning. I am still in charge of my life." Perhaps in these situations, there may not have to be regulation or licensure.

On the other hand, if a provider must exercise direct responsibility for care and services, similar to what happens in a hospital or a nursing home, where there is a significant degree of protective oversight and supervision, then perhaps that environment *should* be regulated and licensed.

In a situation like Massachusetts, however, where the state is still working out its position on assisted living, providers can be caught in a quandary about liability issues, licensure, and regulation. Fear of liability and state regulation drives many, often at the advice of counsel, to make distinctions between acts that require licensed health care workers (and that may, therefore, trigger facility licensure and regulation) and acts that do not.

One area where this plays out is the distinction between reminding residents to take their medications and actually dispensing medications. Medication reminders arguably can be done by anyone regardless of setting or staff qualifications, since the final decision to take the medication belongs to the resident. On the other hand, dispensing medications, unless performed by an outside vendor like a certified home health agency, may require facility regulation and licensure.

It is common to find assisted living providers instructing their nonmedical staff to set out trays with medications in individual compartments and to offer medication reminders. Many have also developed arrangements with home health agencies for nurses to make visits as needed. This avoids potential liability problems and regulatory oversight by the state, they hope.

Providers interested in avoiding regulation may also use great caution from the outset in deciding the number and type of services they will offer, whether services will be offered on site or off, and whether they will be performed by their own staff.

Government officials may have little experience with this type of supportive living. Should it be subject to regulation? If so, how much? What type? By whom? If not, what are the risks? Assisted living opens up whole new areas for federal and state decision making about where to draw the line between consumer protection and individual risk. It also raises questions about what services and programs should be funded, and for whom.

The consensus that seems to be emerging in Massachusetts and elsewhere is that the medical model of assistance is too expensive and may not be appropriate for assisted living.

Who Is Really Served in Assisted Living?

Who really needs assisted living? Why do older people make the change to assisted living in the first place? Although precise statistics are nonexistent and figures depend on how one defines "assisted living," Victor Regnier, author of *Best Practices in Assisted Living,* estimates that about 40 percent of the people coming into assisted living have some degree of confusion (probably mild) and 40 percent have trouble with incontinence.[4] There is undoubtedly some overlap in these numbers due to older people who have difficulty in both areas. In the experience of Bill Carney, an assisted living consultant who manages the John Bertram House in Salem, Massachusetts, his state's numbers are lower than the national figures. He believes that approximately 33 percent have some confusion and 33 percent have urinary incontinence. "If you eliminated [people with] incontinence and confusion," states Carney, "you'd eliminate most of the clients seeking supportive environments."

In states still debating their views on alternative environments, many assisted living providers who serve a cognitively impaired group of residents may feel that they are not free to make independent decisions about what is in the residents' best interest. The issue of medication administration is a case in point. For example, asks Carney, what happens if a resident with manic-depressive tendencies chooses not to take his or her medication? What if that resident becomes agitated and disturbs other residents? What is the responsibility of the provider in this situation? Is a hands-off policy appropriate?

Sorting Out the Questions

Assisted living raises many unresolved questions. The following list is an attempt to identify some of the critical ones:

- What's the right model for assisted living? Considering some of the people being served in assisted living environments, is "hospitality" the best model for people who may have cognitive problems or who take psychotropic medications?
- Who is at risk? What is the risk? What is the role of the provider in minimizing risk (e.g., the overnight supervision of very frail elders at risk of nursing home placement)? What is the role of the state in setting up safeguards?
- Should there be regulation? If yes, should it be based on a health model, a consumer protection model, or some hybrid?
- What amount of state regulation is desirable and what entity should do the regulating?
- Are there aspects of the current regulatory and certifying system that work well? What are they? Where are they?
- What are the parts of the system that do not work well and create obstacles to providing supportive services?
- What about licensure and certification? Should places be licensed or the people who work in them? Should licensure or certification be limited to health caregivers or should it be broad enough to include personal care assistants?
- Should there be a special category of residential care facilities that serve primarily older people with cognitive impairments who may also have other needs (e.g., incontinence)?
- If regulations establish only basic consumer protection safeguards to protect against fraud, abuse, and negligence, should the state also encourage the voluntary adoption by providers of a higher set of assisted living standards?

- What are fair admissions criteria? Can providers legally refuse admission to those who may upset the mix of healthy and infirm?
- What kind of services can appropriately be provided in assisted living settings?
- Can or should the state expect cost savings from these assisted living alternatives?
- Is nursing home placement prevented or postponed?
- If older people are being diverted into community-based settings by Medicaid policy makers, what system of checks and balances can be set up to ensure appropriate placement and care?
- What about private-pay elders? Do new state programs serve their needs? Are costs for supportive services going to be driven up for people not eligible for publicly funded programs?
- What happens to those who "spend down" in assisted living? Where do they go? How do they access services and housing? What is the provider's responsibility? What is the state's responsibility?

These and many other questions need to be publicly discussed and debated. The recognition that the current long-term care system cannot continue presents a unique opportunity for states, providers, and consumers.

STATES ARE SCRAMBLING TO FIND ALTERNATIVES TO NURSING HOMES

In states all across the country, massive experimentation is taking place. It involves the redirection of millions of dollars from nursing homes to community-based residential programs, affects thousands of older people, and promises to fundamentally reshape the way retirement housing is provided in the future. Consumers, state regulators, and the whole spectrum of elder service and housing providers are all being affected.

The driving forces behind the state-by-state experiments include consumer desire to "age in place" in home and community-based settings, state and federal governments' desperation over budget buster Medicaid programs, and a recognition that cost-effective innovation is the only way to avoid fiscal and programmatic collapse in the near future. Reliance on increasingly restrictive Medicaid benefits or other old ways of doing business just will not suffice.

This experimentation has a name. It is called assisted living. As we have seen, there is little agreement about how to define it, design it, or fund it. Whether and how to regulate it or license it. Whether to develop one basic statewide model or take a more laissez-faire approach. Whether to target it to the poor, the rich, or everyone in between. Whether it is the great new wave of the future or just another passing fad.

Regardless of the lack of consensus, this form of residential living appears to be taking hold and consumers are fueling a growing demand. In Oregon, developers cannot build assisted living communities fast enough; waiting lists in existing communities are commonplace.

What accounts for the excitement? After all, we have had various sorts of housing with supportive services in the past, such as congregate housing and rest homes. HUD has also acknowledged the need for adding services and service coordinators to public housing.

Narrowly defined, however, assisted living is new. Depending on who you talk to, it may refer to a specific kind of physical environment—a private apartment, private bath, kitchenette, and a locking door on the outside of each unit, for example. But the physical setup is meant to be just a reflection of a much broader philosophy that emphasizes privacy, expanded care choices, respect for individuality, personal decision making and control, and maximum independence—all within a homelike environment. Given the needs of residents who typically require assistance with such things as bathing, dressing, and medications and who may also be confused or incontinent, this option can meet the needs of frail older people and do it in a "consumer friendly" way.

Given a lack of policy, leadership, and funding for assisted living at the federal level, states have become de facto labs for experimental programs and new regulations. Sometimes, a state starts an assisted living program after a provider develops the initial concept and makes it work in the private sector; then the state agrees to step in and fund it for a Medicaid population. That is what happened in Oregon. In other states, it may take an out-of-control budget to get policy makers seriously interested in figuring out how to create and fund community-based alternatives for frail elders.

Regardless of how states get into it, however, two things are certain. Every state in the nation is taking a long, hard look at assisted living and assessing its viability. And secondly, with programs being created and implemented on a state-by-state basis, it is clear that each state regulating assisted living will probably do it differently.

Oregon

Oregon has a highly successful track record in providing residential alternatives like assisted living and adult foster care. Medicaid nursing home utilization by people over age 65 has shown a steady decline since 1982. According to Dick Ladd, administrator of the Senior and Disabled Services Division, nursing home costs account for a significantly smaller percentage of Oregon's total long-term care budget than in other states—about 65 percent in Oregon vs. more than 90 percent in most other states.[5]

Assisted living is defined in the regulations as "an apartment complex that provides nursing home level non-medical support in a way that allows for increments of service to be added to or taken away from a client's total care package as that client's condition changes." The assisted living unit shall consist of "single occupancy units [220 square feet] with lockable doors, private bathrooms, and kitchenettes." These are the "key structural ingredients," according to Rosalie Kane et al., *Meshing Services with Housing: Lessons from Adult Foster Care and Assisted Living in Oregon.*[6]

Although assisted living is defined very specifically in terms of the physical environment, the rules about providing services are more ambiguous. They do not stipulate a basic core of services or required staffing levels. Instead, providers must have the ability to meet the needs of residents at all times.

According to Keren Brown Wilson, developer of the first private assisted living project in the state and one of the contributors to Oregon's assisted living regulations, 24-hour 'care capability' for "providing or coordinating routine nursing care such as medication management, injections, nail and skin care, dressing changes, health monitoring, non-skilled catheter care, and other nursing tasks" and other types of required capabilities put a lot of responsibility on providers.[7] They must be proactive on the resident's behalf—identifying needs and preferences and making sure that needs are met. This applies even to ancillary services. In her words, "It is the responsibility of the provider to act as a case manager [for each resident.]"*

Generally, to meet nursing needs, assisted living providers either contract directly with a nurse or hire a nurse on staff. This nurse is responsible either for providing direct care or supervising unlicensed staff whom he or she authorizes to perform certain tasks (e.g., medication administration). There is very little use of third-party providers, Wilson explains. It's simply too expensive to contract with an outside home health agency, for instance, whose own overhead would get factored into the final bill.

Residents are typically in their mid-eighties and require assistance with multiple activities of daily living. Many have need of incontinence care, Alzheimer's assistance, or some type of routine nursing care such as dressing changes, medications, or injections. Eighty-four percent are "mobility impaired." Some require behavioral intervention and supervision. The majority need 24-hour "custodial" supervision.

At the higher end of impairment, one 87-year-old resident has had two strokes, a fractured hip, is unstable when walking unassisted, is confused, and has an in-

---

Note: Keren Brown Wilson interviewed by telephone 5/20/92.

dwelling catheter and a colostomy. This resident is being served appropriately in assisted living, despite these multiple needs.

The success of Oregon's program can be measured in several ways. One is the declining utilization of nursing homes. Another is its cost-effectiveness. Assisted living costs, on average, about 80 percent of the Medicaid nursing home rate for level III residents (according to Kane's report). In addition, assisted living seems to provide an empowering milieu for residents so they tend to do more for themselves and may even improve, especially when they move into assisted living from another more restrictive setting. Improved behavioral outcomes were reported by Kane et al. in their study. Finally, there have been no problems with liability so far. Despite some controversy about the Nurse Delegation Act, no provider has been sued.

Of the many factors that have contributed to Oregon's success in designing and implementing a workable program, a few stand out, including these:[8]

- A consolidated bureaucratic apparatus for gaining access to all elder services, both at the state and local level. Consumers and providers deal with only one entity at each level; state officials are able to make tough budgetary decisions about programs because all of the aging programs are administered by one agency.

- A comprehensive philosophy and clear vision about what assisted living is. This includes a vocabulary defining new roles, responsibilities, and relationships in this environment (e.g., "managed risk," "shared responsibility," and "bounded choice").

- A flexible, nonprescriptive regulatory approach.

- A law that permits nurses to delegate responsibility for certain routine tasks to less skilled staff acting under their supervision (known as the Nurse Delegation Act).

- A commitment by regulators, providers, and residents to work things out as problems or differences of opinion arise.

- A single assessment process that prescreens everyone interested in nursing home placement, including privately paying clients.

- A five-tiered reimbursement system that compensates providers based on the intensity of resident need.

- Care plans that are developed and agreed to by staff, residents, and families.

- A needs-driven, personalized approach to care for residents who are or may become quite frail. Services are "unbundled" and made available only when needed.

- An outcome-based system (i.e., the state evaluates providers based on resident outcomes, not on the temperature of the water or the date on the fire extinguisher).

Oregon now has 785 assisted living apartments in 18 licensed facilities and hopes to add 1,000 more units by the end of 1992, according to a preliminary report of the National Academy for State Health Policy.[9] Of the existing licensed facilities, there is an average of about 50 units per site. When these sites reach capacity, about 24 percent of the residents will be receiving Medicaid assistance.

It's important to point out that nursing homes continue to play an important role in Oregon. Although a wide range of physical and cognitive frailty and aging in place is accommodated in assisted living, residents who become totally and permanently bedfast and are unable to ask for assistance are not considered suitable for this environment. (However, an exception is possible if a facility can demonstrate that it can safely meet the needs of such a resident.)

Washington

The state of Washington is developing a new assisted living program that is similar in many ways to Oregon's. The program, sponsored by the Department of Social and Health Services, is intended "to test a variety of service models within assisted living standards proposed by the Department." According to Charles Reed,[*] Assistant Secretary, the state hopes to have contracted for 180 units of assisted living by late August 1992. (Forty-five are currently in operation and have been for a year.)

The statewide demonstration involves a low-income population who would otherwise qualify for intermediate nursing care (ICF or level III care). A flat rate of $45 a day has been set. This is higher than the $20 a day rate for state-funded congregate care but only 58 percent of the ICF-level nursing home rate. Medicaid waivers and Title XIX personal care monies are being used to fund the program.

All units must be private, 220–square foot, handicapped-accessible apartments with private bathrooms, refrigerators, and "cooking capacity" (i.e., a hot plate or microwave). Congregate meals are required, along with access to common areas. Services include personal care, behavior management, incontinence care, and specified nursing services, such as medication administration and injections. Facilities have the option of providing additional services such as therapies, sterile dressing changes, and catheter and ostomy care.

---

[*]*Note:* Charles Reed interviewed by telephone 5/18/92.

Because Washington has no nurse delegation act, implementation of the staffing aspect of the program differs from the Oregon model. Nurses are required to be on staff and available for unscheduled resident needs 24 hours a day. (In Oregon, there is no required staffing pattern and unlicensed staff can perform many care tasks.)

The state expects to contract with existing licensed boarding homes rather than build new assisted living facilities. Of the state's 12,000 licensed board and care beds, 3,000 are state-funded congregate. Assisted living is seen as an important alternative that fills in the gap between congregate and nursing home care. And with the state projecting that it will be at nursing home bed capacity by the year 2005 (its bed limit is 45 per 1,000 residents), the assisted living demonstration will provide valuable information about alternative residential living for frail elders.

Florida

Florida has a new law that allows providers to care for more impaired residents than in its regular adult congregate housing program. The regulations, now finalized, apply to a new licensure category called extended congregate care (ECC). ECC homes have to be dually licensed both as adult congregate living facilities and as extended congregate care facilities. Oregon's Keren Brown Wilson consulted with Florida state officials in the development of the program.[*]

Although the law is in place, reaching agreement on the regulations was more difficult. The state was temporarily mired in controversy with its for-profit nursing home association about the scope of proposed regulations, which would allow assisted living providers to care for some of the same type of residents as nursing homes. State officials worked out a compromise and implementation is underway.

Initial admission rules are similar for all congregate facilities. To get in, a resident must have a statement from a physician or nurse practitioner indicating that he or she does not require 24-hour nursing care, can have needs met in a nonmedical, non-nursing facility, has no apparent sign of infectious disease, is capable of self-administration of medications with assistance or supervision, and is capable of "self-preservation in an emergency"—with staff assistance. In addition, the medical report must stipulate whether the individual is independent in daily functional needs or requires supervision or one-on-one assistance.

What the state will permit as residents "age in place" in assisted living is defined in the new rules and is unique to ECC facilities. ECC residents can be bedridden for up to 14 consecutive days and can be totally dependent in up to three activities of daily living—dressing, grooming, toileting, bathing, and eat-

---

[*]Note: This section describes the Florida regulations as of September 1992.

ing. (An exception is made for quadriplegics, paraplegics, and people with muscular dystrophy or multiple sclerosis or other neuromuscular disease as long as they can communicate their needs and do not require facility assistance with complex medical problems.)

Residents become ineligible for aging in place in extended congregate care when one of the following needs or situations arises: a condition that requires 24-hour nursing supervision, more than 14 consecutive days of being bedridden, four or more functional impairments, cognitive impairment to the point where the resident cannot make simple decisions, treatment for level 3 or 4 pressure ulcers (sores), needs beyond transfer assistance, danger posed to self or others, or a medically unstable condition in a person with special health problems for whom no therapy regimen has been established.

To emphasize the importance of giving residents choices, Florida requires that providers must offer a minimum set of choices such as remaining in the same room, participating in activities sponsored by the facility, being part of the service planning, and taking part in local community activities.

Besides setting up criteria for admissions, discharge, and personal decision making, Florida's regulations highlight another important difference in its assisted living program—its adaptation to congregate housing and life style. Shared quarters and shared living space differentiate its assisted living program from those in many other states, particularly Oregon. In Florida, semiprivate rooms and apartments are permitted, along with private rooms and apartments. In shared quarters, there can be up to two residents to a room (four in other congregate facilities). The amount of square footage is also significant. It is okay to have a very small private room or even small shared quarters! In private quarters, for example, the minimum is 80 square feet of usable floor space per room. Bathrooms can be shared by as many as four residents. And because it is a congregate facility, the amount of shared living and socializing space is stipulated.

Meals may illustrate another part of the difference, although it remains to be seen how the new rules for extended congregate care get played out. Residents living in all congregate settings "shall be encouraged or assisted to eat at tables in dining areas." Given the congregate nature of extended care facilities, there is an implied expectation that meals will continue to be served in a group setting. How does this fit in with the requirement in the proposed rules that extended care facilities must give residents choices, especially about participation in activities of the community? What if some choose to eat alone in their own rooms or apartments? Which one will be encouraged—eating with others or making a personal decision?

As in all congregate facilities, unlicensed staff will be allowed to get medications, do reminders, open the bottle or container, and steady any part of the resident's body. "Self-administration" of medications means that the final act of putting medication in the mouth is done by the resident. What is defined as "administration of medication" to a resident is limited to licensed professionals.

Extended congregate care regulations contain many other requirements for licensure, including the types of staff needed, training, resident service plans, record keeping, allowable services, and the development of facility-specific mechanisms to encourage residents to make personal choices and decisions and facility-specific policies and procedures to allow residents to age in place.

New York

The New York model is least like the others described in this chapter. According to a new law effective in January 1992, assisted living is defined in terms of the providers who offer it and the types of residents who need it. It is not defined in terms of a private room or apartment or a prescribed amount of square footage. Assisted living is a hybrid that combines supportive housing with home care services. The aim is to provide housing and needed services "in the least restrictive environment possible" to people who are medically eligible for nursing home placement. Assisted living is expected to offer a more intensive level of services than is available through "adult homes" (comparable to residential care facilities) or "enriched housing" (similar to congregate housing).

Under the current proposal, the Assisted Living Program (ALP) must be doubly licensed—as an adult home or enriched housing program *and* as a home care or certified home health agency or as a long-term home health care program. In addition, projects must be located in areas of unmet need. To pay for services, the provider will get either a private rate payment or a capitated payment (50 percent of the resident's RUGS classification for nursing home care) for Medicaid-eligible residents. (Covered services include nursing, personal care, home health aides, therapies, medical supplies and equipment, personal emergency response, and adult day health.) Funding for the housing portion will be based on SSI or private payments.

Residents who are in need of continual nursing or medical care, are chronically bedfast or chairfast, or are cognitively or physically impaired to a point that compromises safety are ineligible for assisted living under the proposed regulations.

Two state agencies and various divisions expect to regulate the program. The Department of Social Services (DSS) will have general oversight. However, each of the component parts will be separately regulated. The Department of Health will regulate the home care agency. The DSS's Division of Medical Assistance will be responsible for personal care. And the DSS's Division of Adult Services will review and regulate the housing.

New York hopes to eventually have 4,200 assisted living units, which are expected to save an estimated $61.8 million in averted nursing home costs, according to the National Academy for State Health Policy report.[10]

SUMMARY

Assisted living is a form of residential living that is highly variable from one state to another. In Oregon, it is called "assisted living," in Florida "extended congregate care," in Rhode Island "sheltered care," in Pennsylvania "personal care," and in Colorado "alternative care." It not only has different names, it can actually look physically different, offer different services, and be staffed differently. It can be suitable for frail people who would otherwise be in a nursing home and may need "regular nursing care" (Oregon) or it can exclude people because they cannot walk or move about without staff assistance (current regulations in New Hampshire). It can be part of a major state initiative intended to divert people from nursing homes through expanded community-based alternatives and restricted nursing home access (Massachusetts proposal) or be just another type of residential living available to older people (Colorado). It can involve new construction (Oregon) or existing housing (Washington).

By its very nature, then, assisted living can take many different forms and serve widely different needs. Each state has tailored its assisted living policies to its own spectrum of available services, its own financing constraints, and the nature of the state itself. A program for a state that has fewer than three million residents many of whom live in rural areas (Oregon) may not work in a densely populated area that forces greater economies of scale (New York).

Perhaps the greatest strength of assisted living is its adaptability to a wide range of needs of people as they age and its strong emphasis on individuality and consumer choice. Perhaps it matters less whether resident rooms are private or shared and whether the unit is an apartment with its own kitchen and bathroom. As long as consumers get to decide, they will "vote" their preference. A critical role for states is to figure out where to draw the line between encouraging flexibility, independence, and reasonable risk and providing adequate resident safeguards.

NOTES

1. R. Newcomer and L. Grant, Residential Care Facilities: Understanding Their Role and Improving Their Effectiveness, in *Aging in Place: Supporting the Frail Elderly in Residential Environments,* ed. D. Tilson, (Glenview, Ill.: Scott, Foresman & Co., 1990).

2. Department of Public Health, *105 CMR 150.000–159.000: Long-Term Care Facilities* (Commonwealth of Massachusetts, 1990), 597.

3. Ibid.

4. V. Regnier et al., *Best Practices in Assisted Living: Innovations in Design, Management, and Financing* (Los Angeles, Calif.: University of Southern California, 1991).

5. M. Southwick, Reforming the Long-Term Care System, Oregon-Style, in *Continuum: A Report on Aging and Long-Term Care in Massachusetts,* vol. 2, no. 4, ed. A. Harrington (Boston, Mass.: Association of Massachusetts Homes for the Aging, 1991).

6. R. Kane et al., *Meshing Services with Housing: Lessons from Adult Foster Care and Assisted Living in Oregon* (Minneapolis, Minn.: University of Minnesota, 1990), 113.

7. K.B. Wilson, Assisted Living: A Model of Supportive Housing, in *Advances in Long-Term Care* (New York: Springer Publishing, in press), 1–2.

8. Ibid. Also, K.B. Wilson, Assisted Living: The Merger of Housing and Long-Term Care Services, in *Long-Term Care Advances: Topics in Research, Training, Service, and Policy.* Vol. 1. (Durham, N.C.: Duke University Center for the Study of Aging, 1990).

9. R.C. Ladd et al., *Building Assisted Living into Public Long-Term Care Policy: A Discussion Paper* (National Academy for State Health Policy, 1992).

10. Ibid.

The Johnsons

Stephen R. Roizen

Mr. and Mrs. Johnson moved into Laureldale Retirement Community in 1987 when it opened. At that time they were both physically active and mentally alert. They never got along very well, however. He was often verbally abusive and when he was, she became quite submissive. Over the six years that the Johnsons lived in the community, Mr. Johnson's health began to fail. He was hospitalized, placed in the community's nursing home for rehabilitation, and then placed in the assisted living center.

After several weeks, Mr. Johnson was recovered and strong enough to return to his apartment to live with his wife. The problem was that some days he said he wanted to return, and other days he said he wanted to stay in assisted living. The same was true for Mrs. Johnson. One day she would ask staff why Mr. Johnson had not returned, and on other days she said she was much happier now that they were not living together. After the first few weeks of Mr. Johnson's move to assisted living, Mrs. Johnson ceased coming to visit Mr. Johnson and Mr. Johnson ceased asking to be brought back to the apartment to see his wife.

The family was not much help. For example, when Mrs. Johnson had a 90th-birthday celebration, one daughter came from the other side of the country and was joined by her sister who lived near their parent's retirement community, but despite requests to meet with the community's nurse or director, they avoided staff and left immediately following the party. Mr. Johnson refused to attend his wife's party.

On another occasion, the daughter who lived across the country ordered a telephone with built-in sound amplification for the hearing impaired so Mr. Johnson would be able to talk to his grandchildren. The daughter wanted him to be able to tell her children about their family heritage and for them to have relationships with their grandfather. The day the phone company came to install the phone, he complained to staff that he did not want the "damned thing" and demanded that it be removed.

Mr. Johnson had occasional falls when he changed positions from lying down to standing up. It was easier for staff to monitor his condition with him living in assisted living. However, his wife could have observed him and called for help from staff, if needed, were they living in their apartment together.

The staff were in a quandary. The Johnsons were not adjudged to be mentally incompetent, but they were very difficult to serve. They had a 50-year history of a dysfunctional marriage. Mr. Johnson, at times, verbally abused caregivers. The administration did not want to financially exploit the couple (who were paying for both an apartment in the independent living section and a unit in the assisted living section). However, the Johnsons changed their minds from one day to the next, making it unclear what to do. The children refused to return the staff's phone calls.

* * *

Discussion Questions

1. Who should decide the disposition of Mr. Johnson?
2. How should the management handle the Johnson situation?

Mrs. Quirck

Stephen R. Roizen

When Mrs. Quirck moved to Heatherland Suites Assisted Living Center three years ago, she was 87 years old and had been living in an intermediate care facility for over four years. She was paying privately for her care from her life savings and received only $350 per month in Social Security benefits. The marketing staff estimated that she would have enough money left to pay privately in the assisted living center for about three years.

The administration decided to allow the admission after considering Mrs. Quirck's age and health status. They believed that before she used up her resources, she would age and become more frail and then be able to be admitted to a skilled nursing facility on Medicaid. After all, she would be 90 by then. She was already wheelchair dependent for ambulation due to her severe arthritis, and her heart condition was progressive.

During the course of the three years, several things happened:

1. Mrs. Quirck's condition did not deteriorate as much as anticipated. She was somewhat more frail, but had more or less plateaued. Mrs. Quirck, like so many others who moved into Heatherland Suites, seemed to thrive on the structure provided; the nutritious menu; the freedom from worry about shopping, cooking, and cleaning; and the assistance with dressing, bathing, and medication. Medication compliance, social interaction, and improved nutritional status seemed to add years to the lives of many residents who otherwise would have deteriorated living at home in isolation.

2. The state had moved to a much more restrictive definition of nursing home care and had instituted a rigid screening program to ensure that Medicaid did not pay for care that could be provided in a less costly setting, for example, adult foster care or in-home, community-based care.

3. Mrs. Quirck's daughter had died and now Mrs. Quirck was totally alone with no living relatives and nobody to assist her in relocating or in making other decisions about her future. In fact, the only close friend she had was a

Heatherland staff member who had worked at the nursing home where Mrs. Quirck had previously resided and who had been an advocate for Mrs. Quirck after joining Heatherland Suites' staff.

Mrs. Quirck might qualify for nursing home care, but it was questionable. Further, she was doing well at Heatherland, and there seemed to be no reason, other than financial, to relocate her. Staff, especially her friend and advocate, would have been very upset if Mrs. Quirck was moved to a nursing home. Her unit at Heatherland was a cozy little apartment with a kitchenette and private bath. It was furnished with her own things and decorated as she liked it. She followed her own schedule and her life was not dictated by nursing home rules, policies, and regulations. She had no roommates to interfere with her life style and she was generally very happy.

Administration did not know what to do. If they did not relocate Mrs. Quirck, they would lose over $2,500 per month—a sum they could hardly afford to absorb, especially when there was a waiting list with others who could afford to pay the full monthly service fee. There was no indication that Mrs. Quirck would fail any time soon. The financial drain could go on for several years. There was no family to help supplement the cost of care for Mrs. Quirck, and it was questionable whether she would qualify for Medicaid payment in a nursing home, although administration thought it possible since Mrs. Quirck had been receiving care for so long and had no home and no family to assist her. The care staff did not know her financial condition but would certainly advocate for her to stay where she was thriving. Finally, the administration did not want to have a reputation in the community for taking a resident's money until it was used up and then throwing the resident out on the street.

* * *

Discussion Questions

1. What are the options for treating residents who run out of money?
2. What does management do when social consciousness and ethical behavior clash with financial realities?
3. What are the consequences of Mrs. Quirck moving to another setting?

Case Study 15-3

Mrs. Childers

Stephen R. Roizen

Mrs. Childers's sister telephoned Jane, a nurse at The Maples Assisted Living Center, regarding Mrs. Childers's falling. Mrs. Childers had been falling more recently, and her sister wanted the nurse to look into the problem and then take steps to resolve it.

Jane, the RN in charge of the resident assistants at The Maples, visited Mrs. Childers and questioned her about her health. There seemed to be no change in Mrs. Childers's health status, and Jane concluded, based on her observations, that Mrs. Childers's falling seemed to be related to alcohol consumption. Mrs. Childers still had a car, but she had not driven it for several months; so there was no way she could obtain alcohol without someone acquiring it for her.

Jane questioned her staff about Mrs. Childers's falling and asked about her social patterns. She learned that her most frequent visitor was her sister. Needing to follow up with the sister and suspecting that she might be the source of the alcohol, Jane called. After the initial small talk, Jane began to probe and learned that the sister was, in fact, bringing in alcohol.

Jane explained that Mrs. Childers's falls were due to too much alcohol consumption and suggested that if her sister wanted to protect Mrs. Childers from a possible injury that might result from a fall, she should stop bringing her alcohol. Mrs. Childers's sister seemed to understand the causal relationship but did not know how she could possibly quit bringing her sister her favorite whiskey. "After all," she told Jane, "she will get mad at me." Mrs. Childers's sister was quite adamant that she wanted Jane to handle the problem and that there was no way she could possibly betray her sister by ignoring her requests for alcohol.

Jane did not know what to do. Where did her responsibility begin and end with respect to this resident? Should she make daily inspections of the apartment and remove the alcohol? Was such action a violation of Mrs. Childers's rights and privacy? Should she risk Mrs. Childers falling and fracturing her hip? If that were to happen, Mrs. Childers would need surgery, there would be a hospitalization and recovery (if she survived surgery at her age and in her condition), and she might never return to The Maples.

Jane decided to discuss the matter with Mrs. Childers's physician and learned that the doctor had advised Mrs. Childers to quit drinking years ago. (It should be noted that no mention of alcoholism appeared on Mrs. Childers's medical forms submitted to The Maples by this doctor at the time of her application for admission.) Jane then suggested that the doctor notify the state that Mrs. Childers's driver's license should be revoked due to her frailty and impaired mental judgment caused by alcoholism. Jane was afraid Mrs. Childers might try to drive under the influence of alcohol and was especially likely to if Jane was successful in convincing the sister not to bring in alcohol. Mrs. Childers might then try to obtain the alcohol herself.

Jane was dismayed by the doctor's response. Despite the fact that Mrs. Childers was in her late 80s and lived in an assisted living center where there was no need for her to drive, the doctor refused to write the letter. He understood that in this state only a doctor could write such a letter in order for the Department of Motor Vehicles to take action but believed he would be violating his doctor-patient relationship by doing so.

Jane did not know what to do and went to the administrator for advice. How was she going to protect this poor woman from injury to herself and possibly to others? She felt that her hands were tied. Mrs. Childers did not think she had "a drinking problem." She had consumed several drinks a day her whole life. She did not see any need to stop now. Her sister, her only kin, wanted the problem solved, but would not participate in the solution. And the doctor was no help at all.

* * *

Exercise

1. Develop a management policy to deal with these situations.

Discussion Questions

1. In this situation how protective of the resident should the assisted living facility be? Are there public policy rules that are likely to have an impact on what the facility can or cannot do?

Chapter 16

Strategic Planning in Long-Term Care

Mark E. Toso

INTRODUCTION

Within the health care community, the elderly population has been viewed as a market segment that requires special attention because of its large impact on resource requirements and because of the aging of American society. In 1950, 16.9 percent of the American population was over 55 years old. In 1980, 20.9 percent of the population was over 55 years old. Table 16-1 indicates that the trend toward an older population will increase dramatically from the year 2000 to 2050. In the year 2000, 22.0 percent of the population will be over 55, and in the year 2020, 30.9 percent of the population will be over 55 years old.[1] The graying of the American population is one of the most significant demographic changes of the 20th and 21st centuries.[2] Despite the difficulties facing health care organizations today, the planning process must begin to deal with the health care needs of members of this market segment, the so-called baby boomers, as they begin to march past age 65 in the year 2010.

Table 16-2 indicates that the payment amounts for Medicare and Medicaid have grown at an average annual rate of 9.7 percent, from $88 billion in 1983 to $153.1 billion in 1989. Nursing home expenditures have grown from $2.1 billion in 1965 to $43.1 billion in 1988. Medicare normally represents 35–45 percent of a hospital's revenues, and Medicaid represents in excess of 40 percent of a nursing home's revenues. The percentage of Medicare and Medicaid reimbursement by type of service is shown in Table 16-3. Medicare outpatient service payments grew at a compound growth rate of 21.8 percent from 1966 to 1984, and Medicaid outpatient service payments grew at a compound growth rate of 17.2 percent from 1973 to 1985. Medicare home health service payments grew at a compound growth rate of 22.8 percent from 1969 to 1984, and Medicaid home health service payments grew at a compound growth rate of 37.1 percent from 1973 to 1985.[3] These rates of increase cannot be sustained for an elderly population that is growing and a tax base to fund these expenditures that is shrinking.

Table 16-1 Actual and Projected Growth of the Elderly Population, 1900–2050

Year	Total Population*	55–64		65 and over		85 and over	
		Population*	Percentage	Population*	Percentage	Population*	Percentage
1900	76,303	4,009	5.3	3,084	4.0	123	0.2
1950	150,697	13,295	8.8	12,270	8.1	577	0.4
1980	226,505	21,700	9.6	25,544	11.3	2,240	1.0
1990	249,731	29,090	8.4	31,799	12.7	3,461	1.4
2000	267,990	23,779	8.9	35,036	13.1	5,136	1.9
2010	283,141	34,828	12.3	39,269	13.9	6,818	2.4
2020	296,339	40,243	13.6	51,386	17.3	7,337	2.5
2030	304,339	33,965	11.2	64,345	21.1	8,801	2.9
2040	307,952	34,664	11.3	66,643	21.6	12,946	4.2
2050	308,856	37,276	12.1	67,081	21.7	16,063	5.2

*Population is given in thousands.

Source: U.S. Senate Special Committee on Aging in Conjunction with the American Association of Retired Persons, *Aging America: Trends and Predictions,* 1984.

Table 16-2 Medicare and Medicaid Reimbursements, 1983–1989 (in billions)

Year	Total Payments	Medicare Payments	Medicaid Payments
1983	$88.0	$55.6	$32.4
1984	94.8	60.9	33.9
1985	107.1	69.6	37.5
1986	115.1	74.2	40.9
1987	125.2	77.7	47.5
1988	138.0	87.1	50.9
1989	153.1	98.4	54.7
Percent Growth Per Year	9.70%	10.00%	9.10%

Source: Health Care Financing Administration, *Health Care Financing, Program Statistics, Medicare and Medicaid Data Book, 1988,* U.S. D.H.H.S. Pub. No. 03270, 1988.

Table 16-3 Medicare and Medicaid Reimbursement by Type of Service

Service	Medicare (1984)	Medicaid (1985)
Hospital Inpatient	65.0%	28.4%
Physician	25.0	6.3
Outpatient	6.3	4.8
Home Health/Other	2.9	17.0
Nursing Home	.8	43.5

Source: Health Care Financing Administration, *Health Care Financing, Program Statistics, Medicare and Medicaid Data Book, 1988,* U.S. D.H.H.S. Pub. No. 03270, 1988.

Strategic planning has as one of its goals the allocation of scarce resources among competing objectives. In the 1980s, the planning processes undertaken emphasized improving market share. However, given the historically low operating margins of health care organizations and the desire on the part of the federal government, the state governments, and employers to hold down the rate of increase in health care expenditures, the 1990s' planning processes will place more of an emphasis on the financial viability of strategic plans. "Financially driven strategic planning is based upon the assumption that the results of the planning efforts should improve the organization's financial position."[4]

THE NURSING HOME INDUSTRY

The ability of the nursing home industry to adequately provide services to the elderly population in the future is not clear. Nursing homes today rely on Medicaid for 50–60 percent of their total revenues, according to Fitch Investor Services, Inc.[5] Fitch is one of three rating agencies that evaluate the creditworthiness of health care organizations, and it is the only rating agency that maintains a set of standards to evaluate the ability of nursing homes, continuing care retirement communities, and other housing options for the elderly to acquire debt in the capital markets. Given the growth in the elderly population, it is reasonable to assume that the demand for nursing homes and housing for the elderly will require significant capital investment, since most nursing homes are operating near capacity, as shown in Table 16-4.

The primary factors determining whether a health care organization will have the ability to obtain debt in the capital markets are the payer mix, the management, and the service area competition.[6] Although the demographic trends indicate that the demand for nursing homes and elderly housing should be strong, the

Table 16-4 Number of Nursing Homes, Beds, and Residents, 1967–1986

	1967	1976	1986
Nursing Homes	14,488	16,426	17,122
Beds (in thousands)	765	1,318	1,568
Residents (in thousands)	696	1,215	1,437
Occupancy Rates	91.0%	92.2%	91.6%
Beds per 1,000 (+65)	40.7	57.5	53.8

Source: Health Care Investment Analysts, Inc. and Arthur Anderson, *The Guide to the Nursing Home Industry,* 1990.

present reliance on Medicaid for financing long-term care is at best an inadequate solution. The financial stress placed upon state governments to fund Medicaid has resulted in significant cutbacks in Medicaid funding in most states. This is clearly demonstrated in Table 16-5, which shows that nursing home expenditures as a percentage of total health expenditures have declined since 1980. This decline was due, in part, to the passage of the Omnibus Budget Reconciliation Act of 1987 (OBRA '87), which eliminated the distinction between skilled nursing facility (SNF) beds and intermediate care facility (ICF) beds and ultimately

Table 16-5 Nursing Home Expenditures as a Percentage of National Health Care Expenditures

	Expenditures (in billions)		Nursing Home/ National Health Care
	Nursing Home	National Health Care	
1960	$0.5	$23.7	2.11%
1965	2.1	35.8	5.87
1970	4.7	65.1	7.22
1975	10.1	116.8	8.65
1980	20.6	219.4	9.39
1985	35.2	425.0	8.28
1988	43.1	539.9	7.98

Source: Health Care Investment Analysts, Inc. and Arthur Anderson, *The Guide to the Nursing Home Industry,* 1990.

required higher staffing ratios in nursing homes. Another significant reason for the slower growth in nursing home expenditures was the funding of home health services by Medicare and Medicaid and other payers. Home health will continue to grow in the 1990s, but it is expected that the significant increase in the over 75 population will reverse the decline in the relative size of nursing home expenditures shown in Table 16-5. Economic forecasters have projected that national health expenditures as a percentage of gross national product will continue to grow from 12 percent in 1990 to 13 percent in 1994.[7] As the population ages, a larger percentage of the health care expenditures will be spent for long-term care services.

Support for health care services for the elderly varies significantly by state. Table 16-6 indicates the number of beds per 1,000 persons over 65 and the net revenue per resident day in 1988. It shows that each state supports the funding of nursing home beds and the availability of nursing home beds based upon the political climate within each state. The midwestern states appear to have more beds available for persons over 65 than the rest of the country. The payment rates per resident day appear to mirror the cost of living within the geographic area. The most striking statistic is that 50 percent of the elderly are located within ten states (California, Florida, Illinois, Massachusetts, Michigan, New Jersey, New York, Ohio, Pennsylvania, and Texas).

Table 16-7 summarizes some national performance indicators for nursing homes. According to these data, the average nursing home has 100 beds, a Medicaid mix of 61.86 percent, a loss from operations of $1.08 per day, and a debt to asset ratio of 57.00 percent. In order to be successful in the nursing home industry in the 1990s and beyond, it will be necessary to develop a plan that is responsive to the critical issues in the specific environment (e.g., demographics, reimbursement, payer mix, and competition) so as to accomplish the organization's mission. Without financial viability, an organization's goals and objectives cannot be achieved, and it is clear that financing for long-term care will be particularly vulnerable when the baby boomers near retirement age.

STRATEGIC PLANNING PROCESS

Strategic planning is the process of allocating the financial and human resources of an organization to meet its goals and objectives. The planning process evaluates the products and services of the organization, the markets the organization serves, the structure and financial capability of the organization, and the mission statement and then makes an assessment of the alternative strategic choices available to the organization. Based upon an assessment of these factors and others, the health care organization develops strategies regarding its markets, products, and services that allocate its resources in the most effective manner.

Table 16-6 Nursing Home Statistics by State, 1988

State	Net Revenue per Resident Day	Beds per 1,000 Persons Aged 65 and over	Population over 65 (1980) (in thousands)	Rank (1980)
Alabama	$41.19	42.9	440	10
Alaska	na	40.0	12	51
Arizona	na	36.5	307	28
Arkansas	na	58.0	312	27
California	57.62	38.4	2,214	1
Colorado	55.30	60.0	247	33
Connecticut	74.45	65.8	365	26
Delaware	62.40	53.5	59	48
Florida	63.24	27.5	1,688	3
Georgia	39.18	58.2	517	16
Hawaii	88.69	16.8	76	45
Idaho	53.95	45.8	94	41
Illinois	42.66	86.9	1,262	6
Indiana	54.87	86.4	585	13
Iowa	38.13	84.4	388	24
Kansas	38.27	87.1	306	29
Kentucky	42.96	62.3	410	21
Louisiana	34.98	70.7	404	22
Maine	62.89	53.9	141	36
Maryland	60.94	52.8	396	23
Massachusetts	70.72	63.5	727	10
Michigan	50.49	44.7	912	8
Minnesota	53.82	84.7	480	18
Mississippi	38.60	53.9	289	31
Missouri	51.50	68.8	648	11
Montana	50.27	61.6	85	43
Nebraska	na	77.2	206	35

Table 16-6   (continued)

State	Net Revenue per Resident Day	Beds per 1,000 Persons Aged 65 and over	Population over 65 (1980) (in thousands)	Rank (1980)
Nevada	60.45	26.5	66	47
New Hampshire	71.32	62.6	103	40
New Jersey	75.12	42.7	860	9
New Mexico	61.17	45.7	116	38
New York	82.68	41.7	2,161	2
North Carolina	52.06	32.9	603	12
North Dakota	54.70	74.2	80	44
Ohio	53.50	67.3	1,169	7
Oklahoma	54.59	72.7	376	25
Oregon	54.32	38.0	303	30
Pennsylvania	65.04	48.3	1,531	4
Rhode Island	55.37	63.9	127	37
South Carolina	44.11	33.1	287	32
South Dakota	na	80.9	91	42
Tennessee	40.06	53.4	518	15
Texas	38.68	61.6	1,371	5
Utah	54.01	47.9	109	39
Vermont	63.77	57.8	58	49
Virginia	57.07	39.3	505	17
Washington	58.82	54.0	432	20
West Virginia	55.41	36.0	238	34
Wisconsin	53.20	86.7	564	14
Wyoming	51.76	60.8	37	50
United States	51.27	53.6		

Source: U.S. Senate Special Committee on Aging in Conjunction with the American Association of Retired Persons, *Aging America, Trends and Projections,* 1984, and Health Care Investment Analysts, Inc. and Arthur Anderson, *The Guide to the Nursing Home Industry,* 1990.

Table 16-7 Nursing Home Industry National Averages, 1988

Indicator	Median Value
Beds	99
Occupancy Rate	95.61%
Medicaid Percentage	61.86%
Net Revenue per Resident Day	$51.27
Expense per Resident Day	$52.35
FTEs per Average Daily Census	0.74
Total Profit Margin	1.20%
Current Ratio	1.42
Average Age of Plant (years)	7.45
Debt Service Coverage Ratio	1.21
Long-Term Debt:Total Assets (%)	57.00%

Source: Health Care Investment Analysts, Inc. and Arthur Anderson, *The Guide to the Nursing Home Industry,* 1990.

Figure 16-1 provides a schematic of the planning process that health care organizations have typically followed. In order to serve the long-term care or elderly market most successfully, it is critical to know the elderly market.

Environmental Assessment

Internal Profile

The internal profile evaluates the past utilization and financial performance of the organization. It indicates the kind of patients the organization has historically served, where the patients have historically lived, and what referral patterns exist. Based upon this information, the historical service area is defined. The internal profile also outlines the organization's human resources (i.e., managers, nurses, physicians, and other health care professionals). The human resource profile might include a description of the perceptions that employees, community members, and clinicians have of the organization based upon interviews with key individuals within the organization and from the community. Perceptions can have as much influence on an organization as facts.

One of the most critical components of the internal profile is a description of the financial capacity of the health care organization, including a list of its SWOTs (strengths, weaknesses, opportunities, and threats). This capability

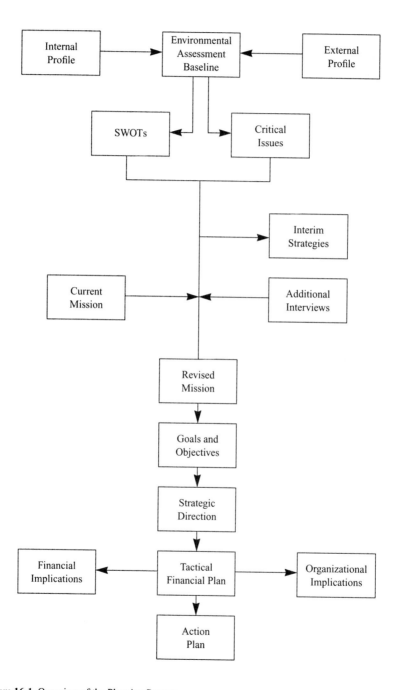

Figure 16-1 Overview of the Planning Process

defines the limits within which decision making should occur. After evaluating the internal data and preparing the internal profile, management should be able to define the strengths and weaknesses of the organization based upon its present position. See Exhibit 16-1 for a list of the most important data to include in the internal profile of a long-term care facility.

External Profile

The external profile of the elderly market should focus on the items listed in Exhibit 16-2. After evaluating the external factors affecting the health care organization's environment, the planning group should be able to make an assessment of the opportunities and threats that the health care or long-term care organization currently faces.

Exhibit 16-1 Internal Profile Data of Special Relevance for Long-Term Care Facilities

1. Patient Profile
   • Demographics
   • Patient origin
2. Elderly utilization by service
3. Elderly utilization by physician
4. Elderly utilization by DRG
5. Discharge planning experience
   • Administratively necessary days and experience
   • Policies and procedures experience
   • Placement success or failure
   • Service gaps

Exhibit 16-2 External Profile Data of Special Relevance for Long-Term Care Facilities

1. Service area demographics
   • Population by type, by age, by area; historical and projected; age groups 55–64, 65–74, 75–84, 85+
   • Sex
   • Marital status
   • Home ownership
   • Income
   • Employment
   • Race and ethnic characteristics
   • Third-party payer mix changes
2. Sociographics
   • Living situations
   • Support systems
3. Health status

continues

Exhibit 16-2 (continued)

4. Competitor profile
   - Types of competitors
     — Other hospitals (elderly utilization, elderly programs)
     — Long-term care facilities
     — Home health agencies
     — Ambulatory care facilities
     — Physicians
   - Utilization by service
   - Market share by service and by area
   - Charge structure of competitors
   - Known future plans for expansion or contraction
   - Existing referral patterns for competitors
5. Nuances of the elderly market
   - Elderly culture
   - History of programs for the elderly
   - Factors of importance to the elderly
     — Family and friends
     — Social activities
     — Financial concerns
     — Independent living
   - Preferred characteristics of particular programs
6. Evaluation of unmet health needs
   - Current
   - Projected
7. Health care human resources availability
   - Nurses
   - Technicians
   - Managers
   - Physicians
8. Regulatory changes
   - Certificate of need laws
   - Reimbursement changes
     — Medicaid
     — Medicare
     — Long-term care insurance
     — Home health
     — Managed care programs
     — Other payers
   - Third-party payer mix changes
9. Technology changes
10. Political environment
    - State government's future plans
    - Federal government's future plans
    - Insurance companies' future plans
    - Managed care companies' future plans
    - Organization support within political structure
    - Licensing requirements

The Elderly Market

The elderly market is heterogeneous and has many levels of segmentation. It includes the following dualities: independent living versus assisted living; living alone versus family or group living; fully functional versus functionally limited; good health versus chronic medical problems; full faculties versus mental impairment; affluent versus economically disadvantaged; and employed versus retired.

People in this multisegmented market are seeking a wide range of services, and therefore many opportunities exist for long-term care providers. Among the desired services are daily living support services provided in the home, social services for the independent healthy, care for chronic conditions in an outpatient setting, complete care in a residential setting, intensive inpatient care for the acutely ill, and caring support for the dying.

Services currently provided to the elderly are often not designed for the elderly. In order to provide appropriate services, health care organizations serving the elderly must be sensitive to the characteristics, needs, and preferences of those being served. Accessibility problems, including transportation, scheduling, and spatial configuration problems, should be addressed. Many services needed by the elderly are currently not provided, primarily because of lack of funding or because of the high cost of providing the service.

Additionally, the provision of services to the elderly usually occurs in the absence of coordinated care planning and management. This is unfortunate, since many providers may be involved, such as a hospital, physician, nursing home, home health agency, or day-care program. In addition, appropriate providers of acceptable quality may not be available, and reimbursement is not consistent across providers (and is even nonexistent for many). The lack of coordinated care planning and management leads to suboptimal care for some elderly patients and a discharge crisis for many hospitals. Physicians can play a key role in the successful provision of services to elderly patients, a role based upon the faith elderly patients have in their physicians.

The range of services required by the elderly is associated with a range of sources of payment: Medicare, Medicaid, supplemental (Medigap) insurance, long-term care insurance, and private payment. In order to maintain financial viability, health care organizations serving the elderly must be knowledgeable about reimbursement, have the ability to market to the private-pay market segment, and manage efficiently within narrow constraints. The provision of services to the elderly is strongly influenced by regulation. As the baby boomers age, this voting block, along with organizations like the American Association of Retired Persons (AARP), will impact regulation that affects funding for services to the elderly population.

What services and products can health care organizations provide to the elderly market? Table 16-8 presents a matrix consisting of care sites versus elderly patient care status and identifies some of the services that have been offered. Table 16-9 presents a matrix showing the typical payers for the services listed in Table 16-8. Providing services to the elderly community requires that the reimbursement for cost-efficient services be improved. Recently, long-term care insurance added home health care as a benefit, which allows the elderly to plan financially for care in the home. Health care planning for the elderly must anticipate the changing reimbursement and insurance climate in order to be in a position to provide the services that will be necessary.

Critical Issues and Planning Assumptions

If there are immediate threats to the health care or long-term care organization providing services to the elderly, interim strategies should be developed. In the absence of immediate problems, the focus should be on the future. Using an analysis of the strengths, weaknesses, opportunities, and threats, the organization should identify the critical issues confronting the organization and develop the planning assumptions that will be used to develop alternative strategies. The planning assumptions also define the criteria for the analysis of alternative strategies (Exhibit 16-3).

The Organization's Mission, Goals, and Objectives

A mission statement defines the purpose of the organization. A mission statement can be very simple and short or it can be very specific. For example, it might include a lengthy description of the organization's goals, functions, and services, the community it serves, and its relationship to other providers. In order for the mission statement to have any significance, it must be understandable to the employees of the organization and the market it serves. The mission statement should provide the foundation for future growth consistent with the values and beliefs of the people who run the organization. Two sample mission statements follow:

> The organization will provide a full range of primary and secondary health services to the service area population, along with selected tertiary programs.

> The organization will provide a continuum of services to the senior residents of the area, coordinating services as needed to ensure optimal care. This continuum may include acute care, long-term care, and supportive home and community services.

Table 16-8 The Elderly Market Service Matrix

Care Site	Care Status					
	Independent Good Health	Chronic Condition	Acute Illness	Rehabilitation Recovery Assistance	Permanent Living Assistance	Terminal Illness
Specialized Facility				Rehabilitation hospital	Alzheimer's psychiatric hospital	Hospice
Residential	CCRC Retirement community	CCRC Congregate living Assisted living		Skilled nursing facility	Skilled nursing facility Rest home Respite	Skilled nursing facility
Inpatient Facility	Membership programs	Membership programs	Diagnosis Treatment	Transition unit	Swing beds	End-stage care
Outpatient Facility	Routine maintenance Education	Diagnosis and treatment of disease Information	Follow-up	Outpatient rehabilitation		
Community	Social activities Health screening	Social activities Day care Monitoring			Family counseling	Family counseling
Home	Services Transportation	ADL assistance Home health Durable medical equipment				

Table 16-9 The Elderly Market Payment Matrix

Care Site	Care Status					
	Independent Good Health	Chronic Condition	Acute Illness	Rehabilitation Recovery Assistance	Permanent Living Assistance	Terminal Illness
Specialized Facility				Medicare Medicaid Commercial insurance	Medicaid Private pay Grants	Medicare Private pay
Residential	Private pay	Private pay		Medicare Medicaid LTC insurance Commercial insurance	Private pay Medicaid LTC insurance Commercial insurance	
Inpatient Facility	Private pay	Private pay	Medicare Medicaid Commercial insurance Private pay	Private pay	Medicare	
Outpatient Facility	Medicare Commercial insurance Private pay	Medicare Commercial insurance Private pay	Medicare Commercial insurance Private pay	Medicare Medicaid		
Community	Private pay	Private pay Medicaid			Private pay	Private pay
Home	Private pay	Medicare Private pay LTC insurance	Medicare Private pay		Medicare Private pay	

Note: The payment sources are continually changing; however, the above payers have historically been the primary payers.

Exhibit 16-3 Criteria for the Analysis of Strategies

- Consistency with mission and values
- Fulfillment of goals and objectives
- Market demand or unmet need
- Impact on market reputation
- Impact on market share
- Impact on competition
- Barriers to entry
- Partnership potential
- Impact on health care professionals
  — Physicians
  — Nurses
  — Technicians
- Need for new health care professionals
  — Physicians
  — Nurses
  — Technicians
- Fit within product portfolio
- Resources required (capital, human, other)
- Management expertise
- Capacity issues
- Financial impact
  — Reimbursement changes
  — Insurance changes
  — Profitability potential
  — Cash flow requirements
  — Financing requirements
- Control
- Degree of risk
- Responsibility and timing

The strategic planning process will generally not change the purpose of the organization. The goals and objectives set by the organization to accomplish the mission will change as the environment changes. This can easily be seen in today's increasingly competitive health care environment. As the environment changes, it will become necessary to determine whether the organization can accomplish its original mission. For example, many health care organizations were established to provide a full range of health care services. Because of the greater competition, some can no longer provide the full range of services and remain financially viable.

A detailed set of goals are established that determine what must be done in order to accomplish the mission of the organization. The objectives of the organization include measures of performance that allow management to determine whether the goals have been achieved. The goals and objectives follow from the mission and further define the direction of the organization. Three sample objectives follow:

To capture ___ percent of the long-term care market as defined by skilled nursing beds.

To serve at least ___ percent of the elderly acute care market.

To reduce the annual number of administratively necessary days by ___ percent.

Strategic Direction and Action Plans

The long-term care organization must evaluate the alternative strategies using the criteria for analysis established previously. The selection of a set of strategies to follow will be based upon both subjective and objective criteria. If individual strategies meet the requirements for the criteria for analysis but the sum of several strategies is not within the ability of the organization, then the organization must develop a method to rank the strategies and ration the organization's capital and human resources in the most efficient way possible.

The strategic planning process must identify short-term, intermediate-term, and long-term strategies. For those strategies that can be implemented immediately, action plans (or business plans) need to be prepared. Appendix 16-A contains an outline of elements that might be included in an action plan.

STRATEGIC IMPERATIVES IN LONG-TERM CARE

At the beginning of this chapter, it was noted that the elderly population will require more health care services because of two factors: the increase in the absolute numbers of the elderly population, and the increase in longevity of the elderly population. Additionally, the federal government, the state governments, employers, HMOs, and other payers will pressure the health care system to control the rate of increase in health care expenditures. These trends are in conflict with each other and will bankrupt the system if reasonable alternatives are not developed.[8]

The role of strategic planning in a health care or long-term care organization is to deal with the realities of the present and anticipate which changes will occur in the future. However, without changes in the financing system for health care services for the elderly, reasonable access cannot be ensured by health care or long-term care organizations as they exist today. The financial vulnerability of the long-term care industry will require planners to focus on the financial viability of the services being offered if the organizations are to accomplish their mission.

NOTES

1. U.S. Senate Special Committee on Aging and the American Association of Retired Persons, *Aging America, Trends and Projections* (Washington, D.C.: Government Printing Office, 1984).

2. Ibid.

3. U.S. Department of Health and Human Services, Health Care Financing Administration, *Health Care Financing, Program Statistics, Medicare and Medicaid Data Book, 1988,* HCFA pub. no. 03270 (Baltimore: HCFA, 1988), 7,10–11.

4. M.C. Jennings, What Is Financially Driven Strategic Planning? *Topics in Health Care Financing* (Gaithersburg, Md.: Aspen Publishers, 1988), 1–8.

5. Fitch Investor Services, *Not-for-Profit Nursing Home Rating Guidelines* (New York: Fitch Investors Services, 1991).

6. Ibid.

7. Bernstein Research, *The Future of Healthcare Delivery in America* (New York: Sanford C. Bernstein and Co., April 1990).

8. J. Tedesco, *Financing Quality Care for the Elderly* (Chicago: The Hospital Research and Educational Trust, 1985), 20–21.

Appendix 16-A

Long-Term Care Action Plan Elements

I. Definition of strategy
   A. What type of service will be provided by the organization?
   B. What needs will be met by the service?
   C. Who will operate the business? What provider?
   D. What services or products will be offered?
      1. To which segments?
      2. When?
      3. Where?
      4. At what price?
   E. Are there any special constraints or limitations?
   F. What results are expected?
   G. What guidelines exist to monitor performance?
II. Primary market research
   A. Techniques
      1. Surveys
      2. Focus groups
      3. Interviews
   B. Populations
      1. Physicians
      2. Consumers
      3. Patients
      4. Referral sources
      5. Discharge placements

III. Secondary data sources

    A. Census data

    B. Home health agencies

    C. Senior centers

    D. State agencies

    E. Trade associations

    F. Churches and synagogues

IV. Internal data sources (health care system or long-term care provider)

    A. Patient origin

    B. Age profile (segmented by sex, area, 5-year increments)

    C. Payers

    D. Physicians serving the elderly

    E. Referral sources

    F. Admissions/days/ALOS

    G. Outpatient visits

    H. DRGs

V. Market analysis or plan

    A. Product or service definition

        1. Place description

    B. Target market segments

        1. Description

        2. Size

        3. Future trends

    C. Competitor profile

        1. Current and anticipated

        2. Performance and image

        3. Future plans

        4. Potential threats

    D. Regulatory climate

        1. Favorable or unfavorable

        2. Future changes

    E. Price determination

F. Promotional plan
1. Media selection
a. Print
b. TV
c. Radio
2. Direct mail
a. Timing
b. Target audiences
c. Budget

Development of Demand Projections

VI. Organizational structure
A. Long-term care facility (system)
B. Hospital cost center
C. Separate corporation, hospital owned and operated
D. Joint venture
1. Physicians
2. Another hospital
3. Developer
4. Long-term care provider
5. Other
E. Management contract
1. By hospital
2. For hospital
F. Lease arrangement
VII. Legal and regulatory requirements
A. Contractual arrangements
1. Partners
2. Management firms
3. Vendors
B. Licensing requirements
C. Certificate of need

VIII. Resource requirements

    A. Personnel

       1. Development

       2. Operations (clinical, management, and marketing)

    B. Facility

       1. Space

       2. Construction

       3. Utilities

    C. Equipment

    D. Supplies

    E. Marketing

       1. Upfront

       2. Ongoing

    F. Outside professional services

       1. Legal

       2. Accounting

       3. Architectural

IX. Projected financial performance

    A. Costs

       1. Project costs

       2. Operating expenses

    B. Revenues

       1. Demand projections

       2. Reimbursement assumptions

       3. Private-pay assumptions

    C. Financing needs

       1. Project financing

       2. Working capital

    D. Financing sources

       1. Mortgage

       2. Bond issue

       3. Sponsor equity

       4. Grants

     5. Philanthropy

X. Incremental financial forecasts (five years)

    A. Income statements

    B. Cash flow statements

    C. Balance sheets

Assessment of Financial Feasibility of Action Plan

The Webster Home
for the Aged: Next Steps

Seth B. Goldsmith

The Webster Home for the Aged (WHA) is a nonprofit community nursing home now in its 50th year. During its existence, the WHA has had three sites, the latest of which is a 160-bed facility located on a 32-acre site in Timber Creek. The home, which is entirely certified by Medicare, maintains close to a full occupancy.

Presently, the WHA operates with a staff of 176 full-time-equivalent persons, of whom 67 percent are in nursing, 10 percent in food services, 9 percent in housekeeping, and 5 percent in laundry.

Over the past few years, the resident population has changed from a younger and less physically debilitated group to one that now has an average age of 86 and an average length of stay of just under three years. Approximately 79 percent of the residents are paid for by Medicaid, 6 percent are paid for by the State Commission for the Blind or the Veterans Administration, and the remaining 15 percent pay privately for their care. Data from a recent resident survey indicate that 83 percent of the residents are from the Webster-Timber Creek area.

The home is under the general direction of a 45-member self-perpetuating board of trustees that meets semiannually. Each year this board elects a 7-person executive committee that meets twice monthly, provides direction to the home's management, authorizes the expenditures of funds, and approves critical personnel decisions. This executive committee group is composed of people who have a long history of active involvement in the affairs of the home, including a number of former presidents as well as presidents of related groups such as the women's auxiliary.

FINANCES

As noted earlier, the primary source of revenue for the WHA is Medicaid payments. These payments are further subdivided into current revenues that are provided on a regular basis and an adjustment payment that is paid as many as two years after costs have been incurred. This latter payment, amounting to several hundred thousand dollars, reduces a deficit that may have been incurred in a given year.

A second source of revenue is the private payments from residents. The rate is presently set at $137.00 per day. Additional income comes from nonresident sources, primarily donations through ongoing fund-raising activities and the income from the home's $4,000,000 endowment.

As with all service institutions in the health field, the largest single expense category is salaries (and related payroll expenses). Data from the most recent budget indicate that at the WHA this expense category accounts for 73 percent of all expenses. Almost 50 percent of these expenses are for nursing services, 13 percent for dietary salaries, and 9.3 percent for the salaries and related payroll expenses of the housekeeping staff. Other areas of major expenditures were 10 percent for food and dietary supplies, 6.5 percent for building insurance and mortgage interest, and 6 percent for plant supplies and utilities.

LOCAL TRENDS LIKELY TO AFFECT THE HOME

There are approximately 38,000 nursing home beds in the state and an occupancy rate of between 97 percent and 98 percent for those beds. Recent reports from the state government indicate that approximately 4,000 more beds will be authorized in the near future. It is unclear how these beds will be distributed throughout the state, but, based on population figures, between 500 and 1,000 new beds can be anticipated for the Webster-Timber Creek area.

A second trend likely to have an impact on the home is the general perception that nursing homes in the Webster-Timber Creek area are becoming more competitive. A recent example is the level of advertising and promotion associated with the opening of the Home2000 in East Webster. As the number of beds increases, it can be anticipated that more competition (clinical or financial) will be experienced for the most desirable residents.

Finally, the Webster-Timber Creek area has seen a significant population increase of newcomers who generally have no long-term connection to the region. For example, a decade ago the younger members of the community were most frequently children of long-time residents of the area; that is no longer the case. Typically, the newcomer has no familial connections to the Webster-Timber Creek metroplex but rather is a refugee from large neighboring cities and is looking for a particular life style that the Webster-Timber Creek area offers. As many long-time friends of the home have said, the newcomers do not know of the home's existence, reputation, or needs.

ORGANIZATIONAL STRENGTHS AND WEAKNESSES

Strengths

A particular strength of the WHA is that its accommodations are among the best in the region. Despite its age, the home's physical plant appears to be in excellent condition and the grounds continue to be beautifully maintained. The space available for activities is, in general, adequate.

Second, the location of the home is excellent and has long-run viability. The home is located in an affluent suburb and proximate to other community-sponsored facilities and agencies.

The home enjoys an excellent reputation in the area. It is considered a "5 star" institution in terms of facilities and quality of services offered by staff.

The home also continues to enjoy the strong support of the community as manifested by the success of fund-raising activities and the active volunteer program.

Another strength is that there is a stable and high-quality clinical staff. The medical director and the consultant physician are respected members of the medical community. The home's commitment to medical care as manifested by its half-time medical director distinguishes it from almost every other nursing home in the region and is a particular strength.

The endowment funds represent an important strength of the home. These funds allow the home to provide those additional services and programs that distinguish it from other facilities in the region.

In terms of policy direction, the executive committee members provide an impressive number of hours of volunteer activity to the home. Particularly noteworthy is the commitment of the board president, who provides both the time and perspective that is required by this organization.

A final strength is that the management team at the home is both professionally trained and experienced and dedicated to the provision of quality services to elderly. The team has the skills and commitment to provide the management and leadership necessary to implement the board's present and future programs.

Weaknesses

One weakness of the WHA is that it lacks a clear mission. Although the by-laws provide the basic framework of a mission statement, goals and objectives are not provided in this statement. Such goals and objectives could provide the standards against which the organization would chart and evaluate its progress.

Related to this is the observation that the current functioning of the home is not in accord with the roles and responsibilities of the various organizational components as delineated in the home's by-laws. This suggests the need to either rewrite the by-laws or require the board and the committee to act within the scope of their authority and responsibility.

A second weakness is the local orientation of the home. The organization still behaves as if its mission is to serve only the Webster-Timber Creek area. There is a clear lack of knowledge and understanding of the broader community in the region. The home has, until recently, not marketed itself in an effective manner outside of a very narrow community.

A third problem is that of loss of support. Although the home continues to raise funds in impressive amounts, such funds appear to represent, when corrected for inflation, a steady decline; that is, fund raising has not kept pace with inflation. Equally important is that funds continue to be raised from the same sources. The ability of the home's activities to engage new area residents is limited. Even in the Webster-Timber Creek community, energy that might once have been directed toward home activities has now shifted to other organizations, including the new YMCA and several new and revitalized social service agencies.

The home may also be a victim of some community myths. While the home enjoys an excellent reputation in terms of quality, there is an undercurrent of animosity toward it in the community. This hostility is related to unclear admission standards that are thought to relate to the willingness and ability of a family to provide donations to the home.

Another weakness is that there has been no organized or effective program of board education. There is now an attempt by the administration to remedy this lack of knowledge, but much work still needs to be done.

Finally, there appears to be some ambiguity about the roles and responsibilities of the board and administration. As part of the planning process, these roles should be clarified. Specifically, there needs to be a clear delineation of responsibility and authority for policy and organizational administration.

* * *

Exercises

1. Develop a presentation to the board that summarizes the case study.
2. Develop a management action plan to address the issues raised by the case study and Chapter 16.

Index